Traditional Chinese Medicine

CLINICAL CASE STUDIES

Edited by
Professor Chen Keji, M.D.

FOREIGN LANGUAGES PRESS · NEW WORLD PRESS   BEIJING

First Edition 1994

ISBN 7-119-01661-X

© Foreign Languages Press and New World Press, Beijing, 1994
Published by Foreign Languages Press and New World Press
24 Baiwanzhuang Road, Beijing 100037, China

Printed by Beijing Foreign Languages Printing House
19 Chegongzhuang Xilu, Beijing 100044, China

Distributed by China International Book Trading Corporation
35 Chegongzhuang Xilu, Beijing 100044, China
P.O. Box 399, Beijing, China

Printed in the People's Republic of China

PREFACE

Traditional Chinese Medicine: Clinical Case Studies, which crystallizes the clinical experience of many of China's outstanding medical specialists of integrated Chinese and Western medicine, will soon be published in English and Chinese separately by the Foreign Languages Press and the New World Press. Among the authors are Kuang Ankun, pioneer of integrated Chinese and Western medicine and professor of the Shanghai Second Medical University, and Jiang Chunhua, famous TCM specialist and professor of the Shanghai Medical University. Each of the 140 clinical cases under review contains a TCM diagnosis, a modern medicine diagnosis, the course of treatment, and an appraisal of the clinical effects. These will not only prove instrumental in inheriting and promoting traditional Chinese medicine and giving play to the advantages of integrated Chinese and Western medicine; but they will also help clinicians to draw on the experience involved and to explore the ways and means of enhancing therapeutic effects and promoting traditional Chinese medicine.

It is widely agreed in this country that in promoting traditional Chinese medicine, the principle should be "to inherit without getting stuck in the old rut and to develop without departing from the original source." According to Professor Chen Keji, a famous medical scientist at the Academy of Traditional Chinese Medicine in Taiwan had written these words on a sheet of paper and placed it at his desk as a reminder, and a professor at the Chinese Medicine Research Centre of the Hong Kong Chinese University also made a point of expounding the meaning of these words. From these two instances it can be seen that many of our colleagues outside of the China mainland see eye to eye with us on this point.

I hope the publication of this book compiled by Professor Chen Keji will go a long way towards promoting the integration of Chinese and Western medicine in clinical practice and popularizing traditional Chinese medicine throughout the world.

June 1993
Chen Minzhang

CONTENTS

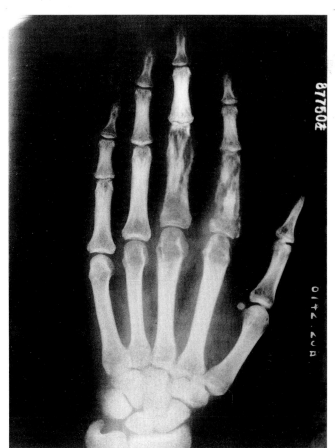

The second and third distal phalanges of the left hand have different bony density, the cortex is penetrated, with irregular blurring shape, and the sequestrum is visible.

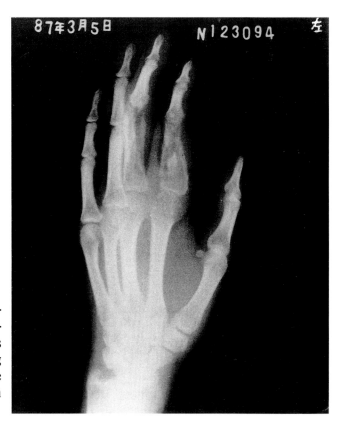

The second and third distal phalanges of the left hand have different bony density, and the cortex is penetrated, with irregular blurring shape. The sequestrum is visible and the soft tissue is fusiform with swelling.

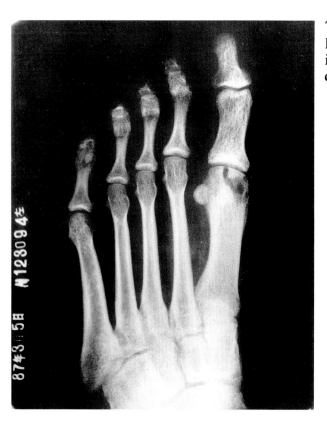

The distal part of the first metatarsal of the left foot has regional bony lesions, penetrating the metatarsophalangeal joint and medial cortex.

Remarkable repair of bony lesions, especially on the distal phalanges of the left hand, with a thin, regular-shaped cortex. The sequestrum and soft tissue swelling have both disappeared.

Remarkable repair of bony lesions, especially on the distal phalanges of the left hand, with a thin, regular-shaped cortex. The sequestrum has disappeared.

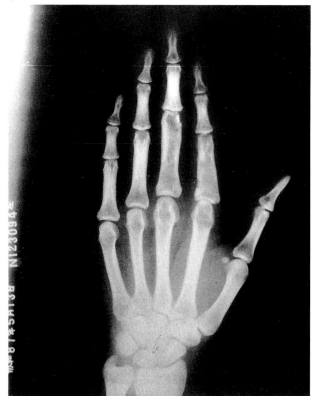

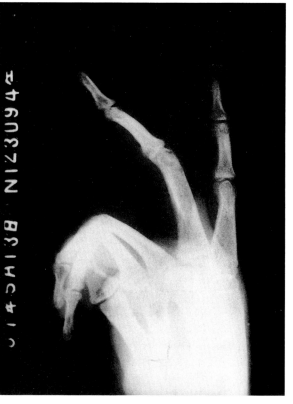

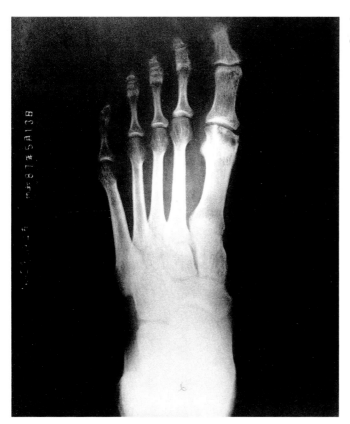

The bony lesions on the first metatarsal of the left foot have become smaller.

Remarkable repair of the bony lesions on the first metatarsal cortex of the left foot.

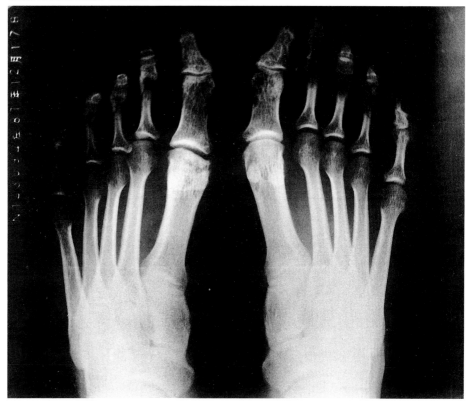

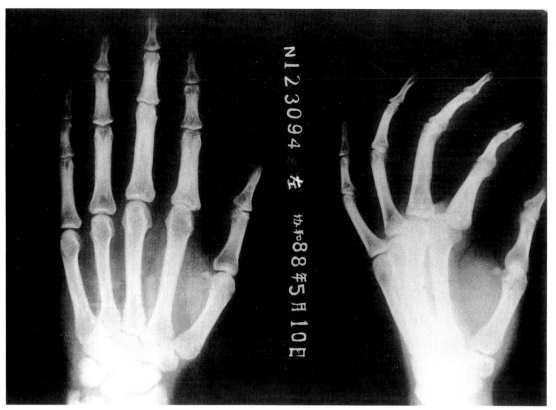

There are complete cortex, increased and identical bony density and reconstruction of the trabeculae, but the blurred line on the margin of the medulla and cortex remains.

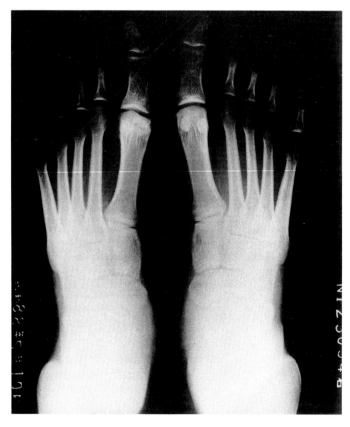

Almost complete repair of the bony lesions and reconstruction of the cortex on the first metatarsal of the left foot.

FOREWORD

Four years ago, on my lecture tour in Los Angeles and Santa Barbara, U.S.A., I was touched by the intense interest and curiosity of American scholars and American Chinese towards traditional Chinese medicine (TCM). Such interest and curiosity was more evidently displayed in the weekly clinical traditional medicine lecture and demonstration I gave in Santa Barbara's College of Oriental Medicine. Given such a strong following, it is regretful to see that there are not enough basic reading and reference materials on the subject available to those who are interested. In the bookstores, particularly those in the Chinatowns, Ii is fair to say that there is quite a number of books concerning TCM, but most of them just touch on the theoretical side. Some authors are not even clinicians, yet they can publish such enormous volumes on the subject. I felt responsible and compelled to produce a book, or a collection of clinical cases, to serve as a guide to clinical traditional medicine treatments for those who had been so enthusiastic. Dr. Jean Yu, a teacher of TCM in Minnesota and Santa Barbara for many years, agreed readily with me. Our original concept was to edit the book together, but since I had to return to China to oversee a postgraduate students' programme, the task of compiling this book was left for me to tackle alone.

This book contains my clinical experiences as well as those of Dr. Jean Yu and some renowned TCM clinicians and specialists in China. The editing took over three years of slow but continuous effort to complete. I only hope that it can be of help to practitioners of TCM. Some of the English translations of traditional medicine terminology have not been standardized. Since different authors have their own interpretations, it's not my intention here to standardize them forcefully. I rather leave them as they are so as to retain the original style and to serve a reference purpose. TCM terminology, particularly those referring to human anatomy, has different denotations as compared with those of modern medical science. These terms are capitalized throughout the text to make the distinction.

I would like to thank Mr. Chen Minzhang, Minister of Public Health of China and Professor of Medicine, PUMC, for writing the preface to this book; Dr. Nelson Y. S. Tan of the University of Hong Kong for taking time from his busy schedule to copy-edit the manuscript; Dr. Chen Kai and my graduate students Ma Xiaochang, Xia Renhui and Liao Xin, for sorting out the terminology of all the medicinal herbs. Naturally, my gratitude also goes to the Foreign Languages Press whose enthusiasm and support from the very start was essential to the publication of this book.

Chen Keji, M.D., Professor
Beijing
June 1991

ABOUT THE EDITOR

Professor Chen Keji, M.D., 59, has over 35 years of clinical experience in Chinese medicine and integrated traditional and Western medicine. He also has a distinguished clinical research background in cardiology, geriatrics, Qing Royal Medicine and anti-ageing herbal medicines. He has received several national/Ministry of Public Health academic awards in China including Coronary Heart II Project, aromatic formula for treating coronary heart disease, tetramethylpyrazine for treating acute cerebral thrombosis and hygenamine for treating sick sinus syndrome, etc. He is the author of more than one hundred scientific papers and was awarded the "Albert Einstein" World Award of Science by the World Cultural Council in 1989.

Dr. Chen is professor of clinical cardiology and geriatrics at Beijing's affiliated Xiyuan Hospital of the China Academy of Traditional Chinese Medicine. He is also a supervisor of doctoral degree students in medical research.

Dr. Chen is an academician of the Chinese Academy of Sciences, a member of the Chinese Academic Degree Council (Medicine) and a standing member of the Committee of the Chinese Association for Science and Technology. He is Vice-President of the Chinese Association for the Integration of Traditional and Western Medicine and Vice-President of the Geriatrics Society of the Chinese Medical Association. Dr. Chen has been a WHO consultant on TCM since 1979 and is an honorary advisor to three associations of Chinese medicine and acupuncture in California and New York, U.S.A., as well as to the *Journal of Phytotherapy Research* (U.K.) and the *Journal of Abstracts of Chinese Medicine* (Hong Kong). He has lectured and participated in numerous international conferences in the U.S.A., France, Japan, India, Geneva, the Philippines and Hong Kong. At the same time, he is the Deputy Editor-in-Chief of the *Chinese Journal of Cardiology* and Editor-in-Chief of the *Chinese Journal of Integrated Traditional and Western Medicine* and an editorial board member of both the *Journal of Traditional Chinese Medicine* (Chinese and English editions) and the *Chinese Medical Journal* (English edition). He is also an advisor to the *Chinese Journal of Gerontology* and concurrently serves as visiting professor of the Fujian College of Traditional Chinese Medicine and the Liaoning Academy of Traditional Chinese Medicine.

Dr. Chen graduated from Fujian Medical University in 1954. He completed advanced studies at the Institute of Cardiovascular Diseases of the Chinese Academy of Medical Sciences (1954, 1964). He studied traditional Chinese medicine under famous doctors since 1956 and is the recipient of numerous awards given by the Chinese Government. Born in Fuzhou City, Dr. Chen resides now in Beijing, China.

WORKS BY PROFESSOR CHEN KEJI

1. Clinical Experiences of Qing Royal Medicine (1990)
2. Geriatrics in China (1989)
3. Chinese Rehabilitation Medicine (1989)
4. Anti-Ageing Herbology (1989)
5. Research on Heart Diseases and Cerebrovascular Diseases (1988)
6. Research on Blood Stasis Symptom-Complex, Activation of Blood Circulation and Removal of Blood Stasis (1988)
7. Comments on "Keeping the Health of the Aged" (1988)
8. The Cream of Chinese Traditional Geriatrics (1987)
9. Comments on the Prescriptions of Empress Dowager Ci Xi and Emperor Guang Xu (1981)

1. CARDIOVASCULAR DISEASES

1.1 PRINZMETAL ANGINA PECTORIS
(SUDDEN HEART PAIN)

Chen Keji

Xiyuan Hospital, China Academy of Traditional Chinese Medicine, Beijing

Shi, 43, male, Han nationality, married, labourer. Admitted on the morning of November 8, 1977. Medical record number: 15495.

CHIEF COMPLAINT: Precordial area lacerating pain for seven hours.

HISTORY OF PRESENT ILLNESS: The patient has been having intermittent precordial area pain for the past two years. On the morning of admission at around 4 a.m., he was awakened by a sudden chest pain which was relieved gradually by taking nitroglycerine. He subsequently experienced nine more episodes of the same attack, with different degrees of severity, radiating to the left shoulder and left arm and accompanied by cold, damp perspiration, chest heaviness and shortness of breath. After occurrence of the symptoms, the patient experienced general malaise, lack of speech, shortness of breath and an inclination to seek warmth. Known hypertensive for 20 years with usual blood pressure reading at 180/100 mmHg.

PERTINENT PHYSICAL EXAMINATION & LABORATORY FINDINGS: Temperature, 36.6°C; pulse rate, 72/min; blood pressure, 200/100 mmHg. Ambulant, general condition fair. Head and EENT: Grade II retinal arteriosclerosis with chronic central retinitis; neck, negative; pulmonary auscultation negative; cardiac area percussion: heart border at left mid-clavicular line on the 5th intercostal space; cardiac rhythm, normal; heart rate, 72/min, slight diminution of the first heart sound; grade II systolic blowing murmur heard on the apex. Abdomen soft, no hepato- nor splenomegaly, no edema of the extremities. CM-2 ECG monitoring during occurrence of the angina showed ST segment elevated by 0.7-1 mv, assuming a unidirectional curve. Remitting period ECG revealed sinoatrial heart rhythm and left ventricular hypertrophy. T waves in leads I, II, aVL, aVF, V_5-V_6 low or flat. Urine protein trace. SGOT, 106 units; SLDH, 130 units. Sedimentation rate, 2 mm/hr. ß-globulin ratio, 403.2 mg%; triglyceride, 82.2 mg%. Whole blood viscosity ratio, 5:26; plasma viscosity ratio, 1:16; erythrocyte electrophoresis 22'95".

INSPECTION OF TONGUE: Dark tongue substance with pale tongue fur.

PULSE CONDITION: Taut.

MODERN MEDICINE DIAGNOSIS: 1) Coronary Heart Disease; Prinzmetal Angina Pectoris; 2) Hypertensive Disease, Grade III.

TRADITIONAL CHINESE MEDICINE DIAGNOSIS: Sudden Heart Pain; Deficiency and Cold of Yang-Qi with Blood Stasis.

THERAPEUTIC PRINCIPLES: Replenish the Qi and invigorate the Blood; warm-up the Transport Channel and alleviate the Pain.

FOLLOW-UP/COURSE OF TREATMENT: Upon admission, the patient was given IV infusion of parenteral Qi-replenishing and Blood-invigorating Compound Prescription (composed of Radix salviae miltiorrhizae, Radix paeoniae rubra, Radix codonopsis pilosulae, Radix astragali and Rhizoma polygonati) as well as aromatic and warm Kuanxiong Pill (composed of Fructus piperis longi, Herba asari, Lignum santali, Borneolum, Rhizoma corydalis and Rhizoma zingiberis recens) at the dosage of one pill three times a day. He usually complained about pain on the precordial region at about five o'clock in the morning or in the middle of sleep at night. ECG monitoring showed that at the onset of this particular pain, there was a sharp lift of the T wave followed immediately by elevation of the ST segment. When the pain was remitting, T wave was lowered and ST segment also shifted to a level lower than its initial configuration. There existed a direct relationship between the extent of T wave shift and ST segment elevation and the degree of pain experienced. Onset of the pain was also frequently accompanied by cardiac dysrhythmias. On the first day of hospitalization, there was one episode of extreme chest pain which was accompanied by frequent ventricular presystolic bigeming as well as ventricular tachycardia. The patient was stuporous, pale and perspiring profusely. There was also a severe drop in blood pressure to the extent of being undetectable. He was successfully resuscitated and succeeding course of treatment using Persantin, nitroglycerine and propranolol combined with traditional herbal medications resulted in a certain degree of remission of the angina, though it still occurred regularly even when the patient was fully rested. Both hypertension and hypotension were noted during this period. A traditional medical diagnosis of "Yang-Qi Deficiency" was given in view of the signs and symptoms of general malaise, warmth seeking, easily induced shortness of breath, unstable manifestations of tongue substance from pale to dark and the fact that the angina occurred mostly at night time. Yang-Qi Deficiency necessarily means sluggishness in the transport of the Blood-Pulse which would result in Blood stasis. Numbness and de-regulation of flow secondary to this obstructive phenomenon would be manifested as pain. To rectify specifically this pathological process, the treatment employed a large dose of a Channel-warming prescription in order to warm up the Yang and to replenish the Qi as well as to revitalize the Blood and to remove the sluggishness of its transport. Also administered were Sini Decoction and modified Danggui Sini Decoction at the dosage of once a day. The prescription was composed of Radix aconiti praeparatae, 12 gm; Rhizoma zingiberis, 6 gm; Cortex cinnamomi, 3 gm (prepared in tea form); Radix glycyrrhizae, 6 gm; Radix astragali, 24 gm; Radix angelicae sinensis, 18 gm; Herba asari, 3 gm; Bulbus allii macrostemi, 12 gm; Fructus piperis longi, 12 gm; Resina olibani, 6 gm; Resina myrrhae, 6 gm; and Radix paeoniae rubra, 6 gm. The patient was also given Kuanxiong Pill, three pills t.i.d., the last intake of which being adjusted to just before bedtime instead of right after supper. On the second day of this therapeutic regimen, the patient did not experience angina. During the next 20 days, there was only occasional slight chest pain and left shoulder or left upper limb discomfort, occurring occasionally at night. Most of these pains remitted spontaneously though some of them required symptomatic relief. The extreme chest pain which the patient experienced previously was definitely under control now and he was able to ambulate around the premises. The patient was subsequently discharged when clinical symptoms were relieved. One month's follow-up after discharge showed that the angina was essentially under control and the patient was able to go to the outpatient department for consultations regularly. Blood pressure was about 150/100 mmHg, heart sounds strong, resting ECG still showed left ventricular hypertrophy but T wave in leads I, II, and aVL, aVF and V_5-V_6 tracings were low, flat or flat to upright. The patient was admitted once more thereafter because of unprovoked sudden onset of chest pain which also occurred at night. He was treated by a combination of conventional and traditional medications such as Liver-soothing and Blood-revitalizing prescriptions together with Channel-warming ones which were able to bring the symptoms under control effectively.

DISCUSSION:

1) Prinzmetal angina pectoris is one of the relatively rare forms of angina pectoris. It usually occurs when the patient is at rest or at sleep, thus it is also known as "supine angina." ECG taken during anginal episodes usually demonstrates a progressive elevation of T wave and ST segment of corresponding leads are relatively low. In 1959, Prinzmetal systematically described the characteristics of this kind of angina which consequently assumed his namesake. Later-day investigative efforts into this disease entity showed that proximal coronary artery spasm could be one of the mechanism of actions for the onset of this kind of angina. A combination of large doses of medications effective in warming-up Blood transport channels with conventional medications has achieved a quite satisfactory outcome in controlling this type of angina.

2) Sini Decoction and Danggui Sini Decoction were first recorded in *Shang Han Lun (Treatise on Febrile Diseases)* by the famous herbal medicine practitioner Zhang Zhongjing in the early third century. Sini Decoction is used to treat patients with Yang-Deficiency of Three Yin Meridians (Foot Taiyin, Foot Shaoyin and Foot Jueyin) as well as to treat those with "preponderance of Yin-Coldness manifested as general coldness of the extremities." Danggui Sini Decoction is also a well-known prescription employed in treating ailments of the same nature; it possesses properties of warming the Jin and removing the Coldness in addition to those of invigorating and regenerating the Blood. Its application is particularly apt in patients with Qi-Yang Deficiency and Blood-Pulse obstruction. In our particular case, the angina generally occurred during the early mornings, the severe episodes of which brought about profuse perspiration, pallor, weak and thready as well as irregular and intermittent types of pulse which are all indications for the use of these particular prescriptions. To arrest the regular occurrence of angina, the patient was given Kuanxiong Pill at the dosage of nine pills a day. This unusually large dosage appeared to have an unequivocal contributing effect in regulating the flow of Qi-Pulse, alleviating the pain and removing spasms. It has

been shown previously in our experimental studies that Kuanxiong Ointment is effective in alleviating posterior pituitary hormone-induced myocardial ischemia in rabbits. It is also effective as an anti-spasmodic in smooth muscles. Application of a large dosage in this particular case had a definitive and beneficial role in controlling the course of pathology.

1.2 VARIANT ANGINA OF CORONARY HEART DISEASE (CHEST BI-SYNDROME)

He Xiyan
Jiangsu Institute of Traditional Chinese Medicine, Nanjing

Yu Youliang, 47, male, Han nationality, married, worker. Medical record number: 16174. Admitted on September 11, 1985.

CHIEF COMPLAINT: Substernal pain of three weeks duration.

HISTORY OF PRESENT ILLNESS: In the past three months, the patient experienced frequent episodes of substernal pain occurring at an interval of seven to ten days and lasting from five to 55 minutes. Radiating to the back, the pain was accompanied by fullness and a pressing sensation in the chest. Pallor, coldness of the extremities and marked cold sweating occurred when the attacks were serious, which necessitated the administration of nitroglycerine sublingually. Episodes of attack usually occurred on the way to work at about five o'clock in the morning or at times during rest. The patient had dry mouth with craving for drinks accompanied by yellowish discolouration of urine. Before admission, he took medications such as Dan Shen Composite Tablets, fast-acting, heart-saving pills and others but to no avail.

PAST HISTORY: Non-contributory.

INSPECTION OF TONGUE: The tongue proper was purplish red. Tongue coating yellowish, thin and sticky.

PULSE CONDITION: Thready and slow.

PERTINENT PHYSICAL EXAMINATION & LABORATORY FINDINGS: Blood pressure, 110/68 mmHg. General condition, fair. Cardiac border on percussion, normal. Heart rate, 64/min. Regular rhythm. Cardiac sounds, normal. Abdomen, extremities and neurological examination showed no abnormalities. Routine hematological examinations including fasting sugar, cholesterol and triglyceride normal except for serum HDL-D which was 35.9 mg/dl. Chest fluoroscopy revealed normal heart size. Electrocardiographic (ECG) recordings showed sinus rhythm, almost symmetrical T waves inversions, 0.25 to 0.5 mv, in leads V_2 through V_4. Augmentation double exercise test in the morning showed T waves in leads V_2 to V_4 becoming upright immediately and returning to inverted configurations two minutes later. No significant finding was detected in echocardiogram. A late systolic plane ventricular wave and PEP/LVET ratio of 0.4 was manifested in mechanocardiogram. Various parameters in impedance cardiogram were all within normal limits.

MODERN MEDICINE DIAGNOSIS: Variant Angina of Coronary Heart Disease.

TRADITIONAL CHINESE MEDICINE DIAGNOSIS: Chest Bi-Syndrome (Yin-Biao Deficiency Syndrome: Phlegm-Heat Accumulation, Blood Stasis and Obstruction of Qi due to Cold Condensation).

THERAPEUTIC PRINCIPLES: Nourish the Yin, eliminate Phlegm and clear away the Heat, remove Blood stasis and disperse Coldness by warming and dredging the Meridian.

PRESCRIPTION: Mai Dong Radix ophiopogonis, Fructus trichosanthis, Rhizoma coptidis, Rhizoma pinelliae, Rhizoma polygonati, Fructus ligustri lucidi, Herba asari, Flos syzygii aromatici, Fructus piperis longi, Radix salviae.

FOLLOW-UP/COURSE OF TREATMENT: Based on the signs and symptoms, e.g. fullness of chest, dry mouth with a desire for drinks, yellowish urine, purplish red tongue substance with yellowish, thin and sticky coating, thready and slow pulse, the syndrome was differentiated as Yin-deficient in nature with chest obstruction by Phlegm-Heat and Blood stasis. In addition, Excessive Biao-syndrome of Qi obstruction secondary to Cold condensation should also be considered in view of the presence of severe pain accompanied by pallor, cold extremities and cold sweating during attacks. On September 16, the patient was given prescriptions in accordance with therapeutic principles of nourishing the Yin, eliminating Phlegm and clearing away Heat, removing Blood stasis, and dispersing Coldness by warming and dredging the Meridian. This was achieved by simultaneously treating the Ben and Biao (primary and secondary syndromes) through application of both warming and cooling herbs. The prescription, taken once daily, was composed of Radix ophiopogonis, 30 gm; Fructus trichosanthis, 30 gm; Rhizoma coptidis, 4 gm; Rhizoma pinelliae, 10 gm; Rhizoma polygonati, 10 gm; Fructus ligustri lucidi, 15 gm; Herba asari, 4 gm; Flos syzygii aromatici, 6 gm; Fructus piperis longi, 6 gm; and Radix salviae, 12 gm. At about 2 a.m., September 24, the patient was awakened from sound sleep by a sudden attack of pain lasting for about 20 minutes. This pain was followed by perspiration and was relieved two minutes later after administration of one tablet of nitroglycerine. Examination on September 29 revealed thin and white tongue coating and tip of tongue proper reddish in colour. The original prescription, with Rhizoma coptidis and Rhizoma pinelliae replaced by Rhizoma polygonati odorati, 10 gm and Radix paeoniae rubra, 10 gm, was again given. On the early morning of October 5 at about eight o'clock, an attack of relatively mild chest pain with a sensation of chest fullness was induced by general physical activities which subsided spontaneously after a duration of about five minutes. ECG recorded at the time showed ST segment in lead V_2 being elevated by 0.1 mv and T waves inverted initially in leads V_2 to V_4 which later became upright and symmetrically peaked as well as U waves in the same leads being slightly inverted. Based on these clinical findings, a diagnosis of variant angina of coronary heart disease (coronary spasm) was established. On October 16, the sensation of chest fullness and dryness of mouth were relieved and the degree of chest pain during attack was lessened though not completely removed. At this point, 6 gm of Radix aconiti preparatae (prepared daughter root of common monkshood) were added to the original prescription for the purpose of warming and therefore dredging the Channels so as to relieve coronary spasms. After taking this prescription continuously for one and a half months (the doses of Radix aconiti preparatae reduced to 4 gm 35 days later), the angina attacks and all other symptoms disappeared completely even during exercise or jogging in the early mornings. Symptoms of Yin injury and flaring-up of Evil Fire manifesting as dryness of mouth and others were also absent and the patient's blood pressure was within normal range. Resting ECG recorded on October 31 showed upright T waves in leads V_2 to V_4. The patient was discharged on December 1, 1985, apparently symptomless. In the two-week follow-up period after discharge, no angina nor ECG abnormalities were observed.

DISCUSSION: This is a case of a middle-aged patient suffering from periodic episodes of substernal pain, most of which occurred during general activities in the early mornings or during rest. The pain could be severe and its duration as long as 55 minutes. ECG recordings during attack were characterized by ST segment elevation, upright T waves reversed from inversions (the so-called "false normalization") with symmetric spike shapes and slight inversions of U waves in the same precordial leads. Moreover, resting ECG revealed coronary T waves and slightly abnormal PEP/LVET's. Hematological examination revealed lowering of serum HDL-C level. Based on these findings and clinical observations, a diagnosis of variant angina of coronary heart disease was established.

By traditional Chinese medicine classification, this patient suffered from what is referred to as "Chest Bi-Syndrome." The predominant symptom of this disease entity is chest pain characterized as radiating to the back accompanied by a sensation of chest fullness. In accordance with the principle of symptom-complex differentiation, Deficiency of Yin in Ben should be considered in view of the presence of manifestations such as dryness of mouth, preference for drinks, yellowish discolouration of urine, red tongue substance and thready pulse. Blood stasis, one of the manifestations of Biao-Syndrome, was evident because of the presence of fixed location chest pain with purplish discolouration of tongue substance. In addition, signs and symptoms such as fullness of chest and thin, yellowish and sticky tongue coating indicate Biao-Syndrome of Phlegm-Heat. Moreover, the major symptom of the case, i.e. severe chest pain awakening the patient from sleep accompanied by pallor, cold extremities and cold sweating, points to the presence of Qi obstruction by Cold condensation, another important component of Excessive Biao-Syndrome. Some investigators believed that there are only three types of Biao-syndromes of angina pectoris, namely, stagnation of Qi, Blood stasis and accumulation of Phlegm-Heat, but we hold that the onset of angina of coronary heart disease, especially variant angina, is often significantly related to Evil-Cold (etiology) and Cold condensation (pathology). It is pointed out clearly in *The Classics of Sphymology* that "Jue Xin pain is caused by Coldness enveloping the Heart." *Prescriptions Worth a Thousand Gold for Emergencies* also indicates that "Coldness involving the Wu Zang (Five Solid Organs) and Liu Fu (Six Hollow Organs) results suddenly in Chest Bi." Conventional medicine also holds that occurrence of coronary spasm may be induced by coldness resulting in release of catecholamines. Lately, we have observed the rate of occurrence of manifestations of Cold condensation syndrome to be 50 percent in 20 cases of variant and spontaneous angina.

Based on principles of symptom-complex differentiation, we used Radix ophiopogonis, Fructus ligustri lucidi, Rhizoma polygonati and Rhizoma polygonati odorati to nourish the Yin and to sustain the body energy; Fructus trichosanthis, Rhizoma coptidis and Rhizoma pinelliae to eliminate the Phlegm and to clear away the Heat; Radix salviae and Radix paeoniae rubra to remove Blood stasis; and Herba asari, Flos syzygii aromatici and Fructus piperis longi to disperse Coldness by warming and dredging the Meridian. Such a recipe is in effect a simultaneous application of both warming and cooling herbs. After administration of 13 doses, Phlegm-Heat was gradually eliminated as evidenced by transformation of the sticky and yellowish tongue coating to normal. After 20 doses, signs of Cold condensation with obstruction of the Channels were also eliminated resulting in effective remission of the attacks. Once the diagnosis of variant angina was established, Radix aconiti preparatae, a potent warming herb, was added to the original prescription. The patient was consequently relieved from the symptoms with the angina placed fully under control and ECG returned to normal. No significant side effects were observed.

It is our belief that if the pain of angina is characterized as severe, colicky and sudden accompanied by pallor, cold extremities and cold sweating, or an attack due to the invasion of coldness with presence of thin, white tongue coating, slow or stringy and tense (wiry) pulse, a clinical diagnosis of Excessive Biao-Syndrome of Cold condensation could be ascertained. In such cases, greatest therapeutic effects can be achieved by using herbs possessing cold-dispersing properties.

The significant therapeutic effectiveness achieved in this case is attributed to pharmacological properties of the medicinal herbs employed. Radix salviae and Radix paeoniae rubra are coronary artery dilators which also inhibit platelet aggregation and release of TXA_2 from platelets. Rhizoma polygonati, Radix ophiopogonis, Fructus ligustri lucidi and Fructus trichosanthis have coronary vasodilation actions and are also effective in enhancing tolerance to anoxia. Herbs in these prescriptions which disperse the Evil-Cold by warming and dredging the Blood and Qi also play an important role. Herba asari, Flos syzygii aromatici and Fructus longi all contain a relatively more volatile oil which can directly or indirectly affect the coronary arteries resulting in vasodilation, thus facilitating a better coronary flow. Radix aconiti preparata, Herba asari and Flos syzygii aromatici, especially the former two, contain Higenamine which stimulate ß-adrenergic receptors in an isoproterenol-like manner thereby contributing to relaxation of coronary spasm (He Xiyan, *Chinese Journal of Integrated Traditional and Western Medicine*, 1985, 5 [11]:702). The mechanism of action for normalization of T waves seen inverted initially in resting ECG is suggested by the hypothesis of Ricci and coworkers. This ingredient acting similar to isoproterenol may improve the dysequilibrium of sympathomimetic activities of bilateral stellate ganglions leading to recovery of "neurogenic T wave inversions" (Ricci, D.R., et al., *American Journal of Cardiology*, 1979, 43:1073).

1.3 ANGINA PECTORIS
(CHEST BI-SYNDROME CAUSED BY DYSPEPSY)

Zhao Qingli

Zhang Zhongjing University of Traditional Chinese Medicine, Nanyang

Gao, 56, male, Han nationality, married, cadre. Date of first consultation and treatment: April 24, 1982.

CHIEF COMPLAINT: Frequent chest pain for three years.

HISTORY OF PRESENT ILLNESS: Two years prior to consultation, on February 6, 1980, the patient suddenly felt an oppressive sensation in the chest accompanied by profuse sweating. ECG examination showed ST segment 1.5 mm lower; it returned to normal after disappearance of pain. A diagnosis of coronary arteriosclerotic heart disease and angina pectoris was given at the time. The condition could be controlled by nitroglycerine but could not be totally removed. The patient was put under traditional Chinese medicine treatment based on principles of activating the Blood circulation to dissipate Blood stasis, soothing Chest disorder to regulate Vital Energy, warming the Yang to dredge stagnation in the Chest and eliminating Phlegm to disperse its accumulation, etc. All the measures had no clear effect on the patient's condition.

At the time of first consultation, the patient reported an oppressive, uncomfortable sensation in the chest as well as occurrence of severe paroxysmal chest pain which lasted three to five minutes each time. There were over ten episodes of such pains in a day and they often occurred after meals accompanied by profuse sweating. Suspecting the meals to be the cause of pain, the patient avoided taking too much food and his diet each day was only two to three *liang* (Chinese weight measurement, one *liang*=50 grams—*Ed.*). Easy fatigability and lassitude were also apparent.

INSPECTION OF TONGUE: Thick and greasy fur.

PULSE CONDITION: Wiry and smooth.

MODERN MEDICINE DIAGNOSIS: Coronary Arteriosclerotic Heart Disease; Angina Pectoris.

TRADITIONAL CHINESE MEDICINE DIAGNOSIS: Chest Bi-Syndrome caused by Dyspepsy.

THERAPEUTIC PRINCIPLES: Relieve Dyspepsia, regulate and activate Vital Energy.

PRESCRIPTION: Modified Pill for Promoting Digestion. Fructus crataegi, 30 gm; Rhizoma pinelliae, 9 gm; Poria, 12 gm; Pericarpium citri reticulatas, 9 gm; Fructus forsythiae, 9 gm; Massa fermentata medicinalis, 12 gm; stir-fried Semen raphani, 12 gm; stir-fried Fructus hordei germinatus, 15 gm; Rhizoma atractylodis macrocephalae, 12 gm; Radix codonopsis pilosulae, 9 gm; Fructus aurantii, 12 gm; and Honey stir-fried Radix glycyrrhizae, 6 gm; decoct in water, one dose a day.

FOLLOW-UP/COURSE OF TREATMENT:

Second consultation and treatment on April 24, 1982: After three doses of this recipe, there was only minimal chest pain and the patient had distinctively enhanced appetite; tongue coatings thin and greasy. Six more doses of the recipe were prescribed.

Third consultation and treatment on May 1, 1982: The patient reported that the pain had disappeared since last consultation and there had not been any attack. When last seen on December 15, 1983, he was in apparent good health.

DISCUSSION: Chest Bi-Syndrome as a clinical entity is quite common. Etiological factors contributing to it are diet, emotion, fatigue and Cold-Heat. Clinically, it subsumes several types such as stagnation of Heart-Blood and deficiency of Chest-Yang. Generally speaking, principles of treatment such as activating Blood circulation to dissipate Blood stasis, warming Yang with herbs of acrid taste and warm nature or clearing away Phlegm and removing evil Heat are appropriate to apply in the treatment of this disease entity. In fact, patients with coronary arteriosclerotic heart disease and angina pectoris caused by Stomach-Yang deficiency and immoderate diet are quite common. There is an account about this disease in *Plain Questions: Treatises on Viscus-Energy Going by Four Seasons* describing it as "Heart feels pain in the chest, fullness and pain over hypochondrium." In *The Golden Chamber: Pulse Symptoms and Signs of Chest Bi-Syndrome with Cardialgia and Shortness of Breath and Its Treatment*, the description of Chest Bi-Syndrome is similar to that of angina pectoris. Yue Meizhong, a famous contemporary physician of traditional medicine, points out even more clearly that "the underlying pathogenesis of this disease is insufficiency of Chest-Yang with Turbid-Yin attacking the areas circulated by the Lucid-Yang . . ." and "insufficiency of Chest-Yang leads to inability of the body fluid to flow smoothly thus forming Phlegm; in Yin-Deficiency patients, Stomach-Energy is unable to descend and Turbid-Yin fails to fall, both of them stagnant in the chest causing Chest Bi-Syndrome." In this particular case, the symptoms manifested themselves after each meal and the patient apparently suffered from retention of indigested food in the stomach and ascension of Turbid-Yin. The patient was consequently treated with Pills for Promoting Digestion which are effective in relieving dyspepsia and invigorating functions of the Spleen and Stomach, thus enhancing resistance of the body and eliminating the pathogens. After putting the Vital Energy and Heart Energy in order, the oppressive feeling in the chest was naturally relieved.

1.4 CORONARY ARTERY DISEASE
(SEVERE PRECORDIAL PAIN)

Chang Xiaoxing
Hubei College of Traditional Chinese Medicine Hospital, Wuhan

Wang, 54, male, Han nationality, married, cadre. Special heart clinic number: 150.
Date of first consultation: February 10, 1987.
CHIEF COMPLAINT: Recurrent attacks of chest pain, exacerbating over the past three months.

HISTORY OF PRESENT ILLNESS: On May 1, 1984, the patient felt severe pain on the left chest and retro-sternal region accompanied by nausea, pallor and profuse sweating. He sought medical advice immediately and was diagnosed by ECG to have "acute myocardial infarction" and subsequently admitted. Having been treated in hospital for 40 days he was discharged with home medications of isosorbide dinitrate and Huo-Xin-Dan. In the following period, "angina pectoris" described as a sense of oppression or cold pain behind the sternum attacked three to four times every week, each lasting three to four minutes. This symptom could be induced by emotional excitement, overeating or tiredness. The frequency of attack increased to several times a day in November. During cold weather last year, slight exertion could induce a sensation of oppression in the chest and shortness of breath. Usual accompanying symptoms were easy sweating as well as lassitude, anxiety and vexation. He had been out of work for two years. Food intake, bowel movement and sleep were essentially normal though frequency of urination was two to three times each night.

PAST HISTORY: Healthy in the past without history of hypertension. "Bronchitis" diagnosed about four years ago because of cough which persisted for several months. Since then, the patient had colds and cough easily in the winter. A drinker and smoker, he drank about two *liang* of wine and smoked 20 to 30 cigarettes every day.

INSPECTION OF TONGUE: Tongue proper slightly red and blue with three to four ecchymotic spots at its edge. Tongue fur was white and thin with clear body fluid.

PULSE CONDITION: Slow pulse rate, 68/min. Weak when pressed hard.

PERTINENT PHYSICAL EXAMINATION & LABORATORY FINDINGS: Medium build, lethargic with dull facies. Slight puffiness on infra-orbital regions. No enlargement of thyroid glands. Blood pressure, 110/80 mmHg. Cardiac boundaries, normal; heart rate, 68/min, regular rhythm. Breath sounds decreased on both lungs with mild emphysema signs. Abdomen soft and flat. Both liver and spleen not palpable and no edema on lower extremities. No pathologic reflex elicited. Cholesterol, 225 mg%; triglyceride, 100 mg%; lipoprotein, 626 mg%; fasting blood glucose, 102 mg%; hemoglobin, 12.0 gm%. Routine urinalysis negative. ECG: sinus rhythm; Q-T: 0.33 sec; QR-type QRS's in leads III and avF; QR-type QRS's in lead II; coronary T wave-type T's in leads II, III and avF; T in V_5 level. ECG diagnosis: Old inferior wall infarction. ECG examination: Aorta widened to 38 mm; double wave lower; ventricles and atria normal in size; valvular functions normal; left ventricle posterior wall activity reduced. Impression: coronary heart disease and aorta arteriosclerosis. X-ray examination: heart size normal, slight protrusion of aortic arch, coarse markings on right lower lung.

MODERN MEDICINE DIAGNOSIS: Coronary Artery Disease; Myocardial Infarction; Labouring Angina Pectoris.

TRADITIONAL CHINESE MEDICINE DIAGNOSIS: Debility of Heart-Qi in the Heart Channel, Blood Stasis with Severe Precordial Pain.

THERAPEUTIC PRINCIPLES: Invigorate the Qi, warm the Yang and remove Blood stasis.

PRESCRIPTION: Shu-Xin Peroral Mixture, a medication prepared based on research results in our hospital, composed of Radix codonopsis pilosulae, Radix astragali, Chuanxiong rhizome, Radix angelicae sinensis, Flos carthami, Rhizoma spargonii, Pollen typhae and Fructus piperis,

FOLLOW-UP/COURSE OF TREATMENT:

Second consultation on February 14, 1987: Shu-Xin Peroral Mixture had been administered for two weeks. Sensation of oppression in chest and chest pain remitting. Angina pectoris still occurred one to three times a day. Dosage of isosorbide dinitrate reduced from four times to two times a day. The patient's symptom-complex took a favourable turn. Continued Shu-Xin Peroral Mixture.

Third consultation on March 10, 1987: Having taken Shu-Xin Peroral Mixture for a month, symptom of chest pain improved markedly and frequency of angina pectoris attacks reduced to zero to two times a day. Lassitude and asthenia remitting, too. Blood pressure normal and heart rate 80/min. Thin, white coating on the tongue was observed and there were still ecchymotic spots at its edges. No change in pulse condition. These signs indicated that Heart-Qi insufficiency had recovered slightly and stagnation of Heart-Blood alleviated as well. Continued Shu-Xin Peroral Mixture. The patient was asked to perform some suitable, light physical exercises.

Fourth consultation on April 8, 1987: The patient had been taking this prescription of invigorating Qi, warming Yang and removing Blood stasis for two months. His condition had improved significantly. Pallor, dull facies and low spirit had been eliminated. Symptoms of lassitude and shortness of breath alleviated, too. No discomfort felt on the chest. Episode of angina attack still occurred when the patient was excited or after going up three flights of stairs, but the degree of chest pain was much milder than before. Principle of treatment at this juncture was to reinforce the Heart-Yang and Heart-Qi.

Fifth consultation on May 4, 1987: Following the doctor's instructions, the patient had been taking Shu-Xin Peroral Mixture for three months now. Frequency of angina attack had been reduced from three to four times a day to one or two times a week. General condition and health status were good. On the tongue edge there were several spots, light purple in colour. Pulse condition remained the same. Blood pressure normal. ECG re-examination: Q wave on QRS, II, III and avF were the same as those before the treatment. Degree of inversion of T wave on III and avF reduced. Lipoprotein level, liver function test and routine urinalysis normal. The patient asked to pursue the same treatment. He was checked after another three months. Condition stable. He was able to work half days with administration of the prescription continued.

DISCUSSION: This patient had acute myocardial infarction (Jue-Xin-Teng) two years ago. Although he was successively resuscitated, the Heart-Yang had been damaged with indwelling Blood stasis. As such, the patient suffered heart pain which radiated to the back. These attacks occurred intermittently and with various degrees of severity. Recently, overworking and exposure to cold weather rendered the patient vulnerable to invasion by the Evil-Cold. Channels of the body were in a static state resulting in frequent occurrence of precordial pain with appearance of pallor and profuse sweating. The pathologic Evil-Cold caused Blood stasis leading to hindrance of Blood circulation. When this Blood stasis was exacerbated, pain would be detected on one specific local area. Tongue was noted to have ecchymotic spots caused by "the great Evil-Cold violating the chief Heart component." Accumulation of Evil-Cold in the body rendered the Yang-Qi insufficient. Inability of Yang-Qi to nourish the Heart was manifested by symptoms of shortness of breath and lassitude. By analyzing the history carefully as well as pulse condition of the patient, we came to the following conclusions. The cause or origin (Ben) of this case was debility of Heart-Yang while the manifestations (Biao) were results of Blood stasis secondary to Yin Evil-Cold. This is a case where manifestations of Excess and Deficiency coexisted, namely, the overt symptoms combined with an originally weakened body resistance. It is a very complex syndrome indeed. Based on traditional symptom-complex differentiation and our analysis, a therapeutic principle was established and Shu-Xin Peroral Mixture was administered continuously. After three months of treatment, the Heart-Qi disturbance and Heart-Yang imbalance were rectified and Blood stasis removed. In obtaining this satisfactory therapeutic outcome, it illustrates that our analysis of the clinical manifestations had been correct and the ensuing therapeutic regimen was suitable for this case.

1.5 CORONARY HEART DISEASE
(CHEST BI-SYNDROME)

Liao Jiazhen
Dongzhimen Hospital, Beijing College of Traditional Chinese Medicine, Beijing

A 60-year-old woman had a three-year history of hypertension and chronic persistent angina occurring two to three times every week for two years which could be controlled by angina-relieving and anti-hypertensive Chinese medicinal pills. On April 4, 1988, at nine o'clock in the evening, while watching television, she was suddenly seized by a heavy pressure sensation in the substernal area and left chest associated with shortness of breath. It became severe following urination. She took Chinese medicinal pills for rapid relief of angina three times but the heavy pressure sensation persisted. Hence, the patient went to the emergency room of Dongzhimen Hospital at 4:30 a.m. the next day. ECG showed sinus rhythm with ischemic ST-T changes. She was admitted to CCU. Her pulse rate was 80/min; respiratory rate, 16/min; blood pressure, 117/90 mmHg. Physical examinations of heart and lungs essentially normal. Liver palpable 1 cm below the right costal margin. Spleen not palpable. Results of SGOT, ESR and echocardiogram examinations were normal. The patient had anorexia, shortness of breath, weakness, spontaneous sweating, purplish discolouration of the tongue with tooth prints at its border, white and greasy coating and thready pulse. She was diagnosed as having angina pectoris secondary to coronary heart disease (CHD), and traditional symptom-complex differentiation indicated this case as "Xiong-Bi" belonging to the type of Heart-Qi deficiency and Blood stasis with accumulation of Phlegm-Wetness. On the first day of hospitalization, the patient was treated with nifedipine, 10 mg, three times daily, and oxygen administration, but she continued to have episodes of severe angina attacks. Consequently, the therapy was changed to IV infusion of tetramethylpyrazine, 120 mg in 250 ml of 10% dextrose daily. Two days later, the angina was completely relieved. Continued administration of tetramethylpyrazine for another two weeks. Re-examination by ECG revealed marked improvement. However, the patient still had signs and symptoms of fatigue, shortness of breath, purple discolouration of the tongue with thin, white fur and thready pulse. According to the theory of traditional Chinese medicine, these symptoms and signs are manifestations of Qi deficiency and Blood stasis. Tetramethylpyrazine was discontinued and the patient was treated with the TCM therapeutic principle of replenishing the Qi and promoting Blood circulation. A compound medicinal recipe consisting of Radix ginseng, Radix astragali and Radix angelicae was administered orally at the dosage of 20 ml, three times a day for six weeks. Upon completion of this course of treatment, the patient's general condition improved significantly and she was discharged from hospital on June 3, 1988.

DISCUSSION: According to TCM theories, the basic pathology of CHD is deficiency within and excess without. The majority of CHD patients manifest Qi deficiency and Blood stasis and such is the case in our patient with additional manifestation of Phlegm-Wetness accumulation. Ordinarily, she should be treated by the principles of replenishing Qi, invigorating Blood flow and eliminating Phlegm. But since the patient was suffering from severe angina attacks, tetramethylpyrazine was administered first for rapid relief of angina. In so doing, we followed the teaching that "in emergency cases, treat the acute symptoms first." Tetramethylpyrazine is a herbal drug for invigorating Blood circulation and eliminating Blood stasis. Since it can be administered intravenously, it is usually indicated in cases with frequent and severe angina episodes and in cases of acute myocardial infarction. The pain and other symptoms of angina can usually be relieved within two to four days of its administration. As soon as the angina is relieved, the recipe capable of replenishing Qi and invigorating Blood flow was used instead of tetramethylpyrazine for the treatment of Qi deficiency and Blood stasis. Such mode of treatment ensures a beneficial therapy.

1.6 PAROXYSMAL ATRIAL TACHYCARDIA (PALPITATION)

Chen Keji
Xiyuan Hospital, China Academy of Traditional Chinese Medicine, Beijing

Huang, 51, male, Han nationality, married, technician. Medical record number: 16001. Admitted on April 20, 1978.

CHIEF COMPLAINT: Palpitation, shortness of breath and chest heaviness occurring on and off for the past three months; exacerbated for the past three days.

HISTORY OF PRESENT ILLNESS: About 12 years prior to admission, the patient noticed he had "irregularity of pulse" but no specific treatment was sought. On

July 16, 1977, he was admitted twice to two different hospitals in this city because of palpitation, shortness of breath and chest heaviness brought about by physical exhaustion. Blood pressure taken then showed a reading of 160/100 mmHg and ECG recording revealed "sinoatrial conduction delay with frequent premature atrial contractions" (reading verified). He was treated with propranolol, glycoside, nitroglycerine, Persantin, Radix Puerariae Tablet and other medications but without significant alleviation of the symptoms which were accompanied by frequent occurrence of paroxysmal atrial tachycardia with the tachycardiac rate reaching a high of 170-180/min. For three days prior to admission, the patient complained of exacerbation of the same symptoms, especially after mental agitation or physical activities, which rendered the patient in a state of high anxiety. He was subsequently admitted on April 20, 1978.

PERTINENT PHYSICAL EXAMINATION & LABORATORY FINDINGS: Temperature, 36.5°C; pulse rate, 78/min, irregular; blood pressure, 120/80 mmHg to 150/100 mmHg; irregular cardiac rhythm, heart rate 86/min; normal cardiac borders and heart sounds. $A_2 > P_2$; lungs negative; liver and spleen not palpable. ECG: sinoatrial heart rate, multiple premature atrial contractions, transient and frequent atrial tachycardia, tachycardiac rate at around 150/min. Chest X-ray: bilaterally increased pulmonary markings on the lower lungs, TB calcifications at left apex and accentuation of the aortic arch. Blood chemistry: ß-globulin ratio, 330 mg%; triglyceride, 139 mg%. Hemodynamics: thrombose formation at 12 mm; dry weight, 5 mg; whole blood viscosity ratio, 6.76; plasma viscosity ratio, 1.72; erythrocyte electrophoresis, 17'40". Normal hepatic functions. Negative ultrasonography.

INSPECTION OF TONGUE: Dark tongue substance with thin and pale tongue fur.

PULSE CONDITION: Irregular, alternating between running, intermittent, slow and uneven and taut types.

MODERN MEDICINE DIAGNOSIS: Hypertensive Atherosclerotic Heart Disease; Paroxysmal Atrial Tachyarrhythmia and Sinoatrial Node Dysfunction (in consideration of past medical history of sinoatrial conduction defect symptoms).

TRADITIONAL CHINESE MEDICINE DIAGNOSIS: Palpitation; Deficiency of Qi and Yin with Blood Stasis.

THERAPEUTIC PRINCIPLES: Replenish the Qi, nurture the Yin, revitalize the Blood and soothe the Nerves (tranquilize the Mind).

FOLLOW-UP/COURSE OF TREATMENT: Upon admission and in accordance with therapeutic principles of replenishing the Qi, nurturing the Yin, revitalizing the Blood and soothing the Nerves, the patient was given propranolol at a dosage of 90 mg/day. However, there was no significant remission of the symptoms with this regimen and transient episodes of atriotachycardia still occurring frequently. Even complete bed rest could not relieve the patient from the symptoms. Hemodynamic re-examination showed thrombose formation at 11 mm; dry weight, 6 mg; whole blood viscosity ratio, 6.53; plasma viscosity ratio, 19.0 and erythrocyte electrophoresis, 29'25". The patient was given, first on May 5 and then on May 22, Coronary Heart II (composed of Radix salviae miltiorrhizae, Radix paeoniae rubra, Rhizoma ligustici

Chuanxiong, Lignum dalbergiae odoriferae and Flos carthami), 10 gm in 250 ml of 5% glucose solution by IV drip for a twenty-day treatment course which was terminated on June 2, 1978. There was only slight alleviation of the symptoms after this IV infusion while cardiac dysrhythmia persisted as well as other symptoms such as palpitation (espeically at night), chest heaviness and chest pain. Physical examination showed pale and thin tongue fur with dark tongue substance and also an irregular, alternating pulse picture from intermittent, uneven, running, slow, to taut. Further analysis of the case concluded that it fell under the syndrome of "incompetence and dysfunction of Liver in smoothing and regulating the flow of Qi and Blood" manifested as sluggishness of the flow of Qi and Blood which in turn could not properly nourish the Heart resulting in dysequilibrium of the Heart and Mind. To combat such syndrome, it would be appropriate to follow the therapeutic principle of "coordinating the Liver function and regulating the flow of Qi," as well as that of "invigorating the Blood and soothing the Mind." Prescription thus given was composed of Cortex albiziae, 12 gm; Semen biotae, 9 gm; Concha margaritifera usta, 24 gm; Caulis polygoni multiflori, 30 gm; and Rhizoma seu radix notopterygii, 12 gm. Decocted in water and taken twice a day. After taking two doses, it was noted that cardiac dysrhythmia had disappeared. On June 8, the dosage of propranolol was reduced to 45 mg/day. Thereafter, except for one occasion of premature atrial contraction (15/10 min) on June 10, daily chest auscultation and ECG examination all revealed normal cardiac rhythm. The decoction was given continuously for the next 40 days and cardiac rhythm was observed to be normal as well as blood pressure. Neither premature atrial contractions nor paroxysmal atrial tachycardia was observed thereafter. Since the patient still complained about chest heaviness, Bulbus allii macrostemi, 18 gm, Cortex cinnamomi, 6 gm, and Fructus trichosanthis, 18 gm, were added to the original prescription in conformance with the principle of "loosening the Chest and channeling the flow of Yang." Sensation of chest heaviness disappeared after addition of these herbs. Two-hour continuous ECG monitoring on June 24 did not detect any abnormality. Propanolol was discontinued on June 26. Subsequent ECG monitorings all revealed normal cardiac profiles. The patient was discharged on July 18, 1978. Laboratory examinations on discharge showed ß-globulin ratio to be 490 mg% and triglyceride, 182.5 mg%. Hemodynamic examination: thrombose formation, 9 mm; dry weight, 3 mg; whole blood viscosity ratio, 6.22; plasma viscosity ratio, 1.86 and erythrocyte electrophoresis, 24'2".

DISCUSSION: This is a case admitted to hospital because of frequent occurrence of atrial tachycardia which did not abate even with complete bed rest. It was considered to be a serious case. Before admission the patient had taken a combination of several conventional and traditional medications including propranolol at 135 mg/day, but still the atrial tachycardia occurred daily. Applying traditional symptom-complex differentiation in prescribing an appropriate prescription, the case had an extremely satisfactory outcome. Cardiac arrhythmia had disappeared and ECG reverted to normal. Symptoms have not recurred since discharge from the hospital. The main therapeutic characteristic of this case was the application of the principle of "revitalizing the Blood circulation to eliminate Blood stasis." Traditional medicine believes that "Pulse is the bodily manifestation of the Heart" and that "Heart controls the Blood circulation and the Pulse." Most cases of cardiac dysrhythmias and irregular pulse rates can be differentiated accordingly and recognized as contributing elements to Blood Stasis syndrome. To a certain extent, our case manifested a definite degree of this syndrome and it was thus appropriate for the application of Blood-revitalizing medications. The decoction used for treatment was quite strong in this aspect. This specific pharmacological property has long been recognized in the saying that "Xuancao clears away depression while Hehua removes discontent."

This case involved frequent occurrence of transient atrial tachycardia, but there was no sign of atrial flutter or atrial fibrillation. It can therefore be deduced that this kind of atrial tachycardia was not a transitional atrial dysrhythmia, which could progress further into either atrial flutter or atrial fibrillation. Though premature atrial contractions were quite frequent, they were not of the multifocal type and thus portend a more favourable prognosis.

Cardiac dysrhythmias pose a greater difficulty in management. They can be tackled by either applying traditional medicine's therapeutic principles or purely from the standpoint of pharmacological mechanisms of action of the herbs. Medications with the property of "subduing hyperfunction of the Liver and the endogenous Wind" and those with the property of "dispelling the endogenous Wind" are worthy ones for further investigation. Another approach is to look into the electrophysiological characteristics of the heart. An interesting observation is that the effect of a large dose of Radix angelicae sinensis on cardiac muscles electrophysiology is quite similar to that of quinidine. Traditional medications containing glycoside and those with antihypertensive effects appear to have certain efficacy in controlling cardiac dysrhythmias. Every single clinical case should be studied and analyzed individually to accumulate more experience in order to uncover in the myriad of clinical manifestations a common pattern of pathology and an effective mode of treatment.

1.7 PAROXYSMAL ATRIAL TACHYCARDIA (PALPITATION)

Zhou Ciqing
Shandong College of Traditional Chinese Medicine, Jinan

He, 59, male, Han nationality, married, engineer. Medical record number: 74865.
Date of first consultation: October 4, 1986.
CHIEF COMPLAINT: Palpitation, chest stuffiness, shortness of breath of one-year duration.

HISTORY OF PRESENT ILLNESS: In August 1985, these symptoms first occurred when the patient got excited. ECG examination then showed paroxysmal atrial tachycardia (4:1 atrioventricular block). The arrhythmia was put under control after injecting cedilanid. Similar episodes recurred later and he took digoxin for relief. For the next six months, the medications could not control the attacks any more. He thus consulted a TCM doctor. The patient had severe symptoms of palpitation, shortness of breath, dizziness, irritability, fatigue, nausea, insomnia, dreamfulness, sweat and anorexia. He passed soft stool two to three times a day. Tongue inspection showed red tongue tip with white, slippery tongue coating. Pulse was slippery and soft. Symptoms occurred frequently during the three months prior to admission and continued for five days before consultation.

PAST HISTORY: Positive history of insomnia, amnesia and impotence. Denied history of cardiovascular disease.

PERTINENT PHYSICAL EXAMINATION & LABORATORY FINDINGS: Heart rate, 96/min; blood pressure, 140/85 mmHg; no pathological murmur. Normal blood chemistry. Chest X-ray findings negative. ECG: paroxysmal atrial tachycardia (4:1 atrioventricular block).

INSPECTION OF TONGUE: Dark tongue substance with thin and pale coating.

PULSE CONDITION: Irregular, alternating between running, intermittent, slow and uneven and taut types.

MODERN MEDICINE DIAGNOSIS: Arrhythmia; Coronary Heart Disease(?).

TRADITIONAL CHINESE MEDICINE DIAGNOSIS: Palpitation (Phlegm-Fire Infringing the Heart)

THERAPEUTIC PRINCIPLES: Clear the Heart and dissolve the Phlegm.

PRESCRIPTION: Modified Wendan Tang. Rhizoma pinelliae, 9 gm; Poria, 12 gm; Exocarpium citri grandis, 6 gm; Fructus aurantii immaturus, 6 gm; Caulis bambusae in Taenis, 6 gm; Radix glycyrrhizae, 6 gm; Radix polygalae, 6 gm; and Rhizoma acori graminei and Semen ziziphi, 15 gm each. Decoct in water for oral ingestion, twice a day.

FOLLOW-UP/COURSE OF TREATMENT:

Second consultation: After taking six doses of the prescription, frequency and duration of tachycardiac episodes were reduced markedly. The patient had fewer complaints and was able to sleep better. Tongue with red tip and white coating. Pulse wiry, rapid and weak. Heart rate was 86/min. He still complained of palpitation, shortness of breath, fatigue and spontaneous perspiration. Continued the same prescription adding Radix codonopsis pilosulae, 18 gm; Radix salviae, 15 gm; and Radix angelicae, 9 gm. Six doses.

Third consultation: Symptoms of palpitation, chest stuffiness, vexation, dizziness and nausea had disappeared but fatigue, insomnia and dreamful sleep persisted. Tongue coating normal and pulse deep. Heart rate, 82/min and blood pressure, 130/80 mmHg. ECG: rising slope of QRS in leads II, III and avF, sluggish and dull; presence of atrial premature beat. Adopt the therapeutic principle of nourishing the Blood, invigorating the Qi and relieving mental stress. Prescription: Radix codonopsis pilosulae, 30 gm; Radix astragali, 18 gm; Radix salviae, 30 gm; Radix angelicae sinensis, 12 gm; Radix paeoniae alba, 9 gm; Poria, 12 gm; Semen biotae, 12 gm; Fluoritum, 30 gm; Semen ziziphi, 15 gm; and Radix polygalae, 6 gm.

Fourth consultation: After taking 30 doses of the modified prescription, the patient felt much better without experiencing palpitation. ECG findings essentially normal.

During six months of follow-up, a total of 95 ECG examinations were performed and results were all normal. The patient did not complain of earlier symptoms.

DISCUSSION: In TCM teachings, the cause of paroxysmal palpitation could be (1) "anxiety resulting in palpitation is of the deficiency type; paroxysmal palpitation results from Blood deficiency"; and (2) "paroxysmal palpitation results from a Heart disturbed by Phlegm-Fire." This case pertains to both of these aspects with Qi deficiency and Blood stagnation. *Report of Differentiation of Symptoms and Signs* states that "anxiety leads to Fire, Fire to Phlegm, Phlegm to stagnation in the Heart and superficial venules resulting in inadequate supply of nutrients to the Heart and the symptom of palpitation." Phlegm-Fire disturbing the Heart makes the patient dysphoric with a smothery sensation and irritability. Deficiency is the culprit behind symptoms of shortness of breath, fatigue and insomnia. Therapeutic principles for such a case would be to clear away the Heart-Fire and Phlegm and to promote Blood circulation. In addition to Wendan Tang, Rhizoma acorus was added to eliminate Phlegm and for resuscitation; Rhizoma coptidis to purge the intense Heat; and Radix polygalae and Semen ziziphi to nourish the Heart. After the second consultation, the prescription was modified by replacing Fructus aurantii with Radix angelicae, Radix salviae and Radix codonopsis to remove obstruction and to tonify the Heart. In the latter part of the course of treatment, Yirong Tang was administered to replenish the Qi and Blood and to strengthen body resistance.

Paroxysmal atrial tachycardia is usually an organic heart disease. In our case, a 59-year-old man with palpitation, without history of rheumatic heart disease, hypertension and pathologic murmur, the etiology may be due to coronary heart disease (as evidenced by elevated, sluggish and dull QRS segments in leads II, III and avF). Paroxysmal atrial tachycardia accompanied by 4:1 atrioventricular conduction also indicates the possibility of coronary heart disease. The mode of treatment employed in this case, which was based on TCM symptom-complex differentiation, is also effective in treating coronary heart disease.

1.8 SICK SINUS SYNDROME
(PECTORAL PAIN WITH STUFFINESS)

Chen Wenbin and Zhang Taihuai
First Affiliated Hospital of the West China University of Medical Sciences,
Chengdu

Mao Bixian, 51, female, Han nationality, married, cadre. Medical record number: 342949. Date of admission: December 3, 1983.
CHIEF COMPLAINT: Bradycardia with syncope for 13 years.
HISTORY OF PRESENT ILLNESS: 13 years prior to admission, the patient had an episode of syncope (bradycardia confirmed by ECG) lasting for about two minutes. She had been well apparently until four years prior to admission when she experienced

sudden sharp precordial chest pain and developed cardiopulmonary arrest soon after. With 18 minutes of emergency management, she was successively resuscitated and her heart rate, pulse and blood pressure returned to normal. ECG showed junctional rhythm, ventricular premature beats and acute myocardial infarction. Her tongue substance was pale and pulse feeble indicating exhaustion of Shao-Yin Vital Energy. The treatment was based on the principle of replenishing the Vital Energy and reinforcing the vital function. The patient was given Ginseng aconite decoction once a day and her symptoms were relieved after five months of treatment.

Three years prior to admission, Adams-Stokes syndrome recurred and a pacemaker was installed. Two years prior to admission, the patient was admitted again because of pacemaker failure. Atropine and isoprenaline were given to restore normal heart rate. One month prior to admission, an attempt to put in a new pacemaker failed. Her syncopic attacks were more severe and she was subsequently admitted to be treated by traditional Chinese medicine.

PAST HISTORY: Non-contributory.

PERTINENT PHYSICAL EXAMINATION & LABORATORY FINDINGS: Pulse rate, 42/min; blood pressure, 100/70 mmHg. Heart appeared slightly enlarged towards the left by percussion. There was no murmur appreciated and rhythm was regular. Both lungs clear. Liver and spleen not palpable. Serum cholesterol and triglyceride levels were within normal limits. Chest X-ray revealed left heart border enlarged beyond the left midclavicular line. Junctional rhythm, ventricular premature beats and extensive myocardial ischemic pattern found on ECG examination.

INSPECTION OF TONGUE: Tongue substance pale and thickly covered with white coat.

MODERN MEDICINE DIAGNOSIS: Ischemic Heart Disease; Sick Sinus Syndrome.

TRADITIONAL CHINESE MEDICINE DIAGNOSIS: Deficiency of Heart Vital Function; Stagnation of Qi and Stasis of Blood.

THERAPEUTIC PRINCIPLES: Replenish the Qi, reinforce Vital Function to promote Blood circulation and to remove Blood stasis.

PRESCRIPTION:

1. Main recipe: Radix codonopsis pilosulae, 30 gm; Radix aconiti praeparatae, 15 gm (wrap and decoct first); Radix astragali, 30 gm; Ramulus cinamomi, 12 gm; Rhizoma ligustici Chuanxiong, 12 gm; Radix notoginseng, 9 gm (taken after pouring liquid on powder); Radix salviae miltiorrhizae, 15 gm; Radix paeoniae rubra, 15 gm; and Caulis akebiae, 12 gm.

2. Modified prescription for symptomatic treatment:

a. Irritation and insomnia: Poria, 12 gm; Semen jujubae, 12 gm; and Radix polygalae, 12 gm.

b. Productive cough, nausea and vomiting: Pericarpium citri reticulatae, 12 gm; Rhizoma pinelliae, 12 gm; Poria, 12 gm; and Caulis bambusae in taenian, 12 gm.

c. Abdominal distention and loss of appetite: Cortex magnoliae officinalis, 20 gm; Charred triplet, 30 gm; Rhizoma atractylodis, 14 gm; Fructus amomi, 6 gm; Semen cardamomi, 6 gm; and Rhizoma zingiberis recens, 12 gm.

d. A-V block: Ginseng, Ophiopogon Root and Schisandra Fruit Preparation, 2 ml, IM, twice a day. Isoprenaline, 10 gm, sublingual one to three times a day until the heart rate was maintained at 60-70/min.

FOLLOW-UP/COURSE OF TREATMENT: Two weeks after treatment, the patient's palpitation subsided and no syncope occurred. Heart rate was in the range of 65-68/min and ECG showed junctional rhythm with myocardial ischemia. Three months after treatment, the patient was asymptomatic and ambulant. ECG examination indicated disappearance of myocardial ischemia. Since then, the patient has used traditional Chinese medicine for treatment continuously and was checked in our clinic periodically. She has remained healthy all along.

DISCUSSION: Four years prior to admission, when this patient was still suffering from Adams-Stokes attacks secondary to sick sinus syndrome, the diagnosis then by TCM symptom-complex differentiation was exhaustion of Shao-Yin Vital Energy. The therapeutic principle adopted at that time was to remove the obstruction in the flow of Vital Energy and to reinforce its functions. Modified decoction of Ginseng typhonii was administered for treatment. The patient responded to this management quickly and favourably. After removal of the pacemaker (in December, 1983) and during the course of treatment by traditional Chinese medicine, we adhered strictly to the Four Methods of Diagnosis (inspection, auscultation, questioning and pulse feeling) and principles of traditional symptom-complex differentiation. As a result, it was discovered that the patient had a symptom-complex of Vital Energy stagnation and Blood stasis induced by deficiency of vital function of the Heart. Since then, in addition to the principles of removal of obstruction in the flow of Vital Energy and reinforcing the vital function, emphasis was also placed on promoting Blood circulation and removing Blood stasis. In so doing, the patient's vital function was restored and Heart-Pulse tonified. Blood flow was vigorous throughout the whole body. It is evident that adhering strictly to symptom-complex differentiation in determining the mode of treatment was the key to successful outcome in this case.

In this case treatment centred around one main recipe while emphasis was also placed on symptomatic management. In so doing, the major underlying pathology could be tackled without interfering with the effects of the main recipe, which was modified as dictated by the presence of accompanying symptoms and signs. This method of treatment reflects mutual supplementation of therapeutic principles based on symptom-complex differentiation in traditional Chinese medicine.

Because of the serious nature of the disease, whenever the patient's condition seemed to fluctuate during the course of TCM treatment a small dosage of isoprenaline for a short period of time as an adjuvant treatment was administered. As soon as the pulse rate became stable again, the patient was put on traditional Chinese medicine alone. In this way, the Western medicine neither distracted from the progressive improvement of the condition nor interfered with the curative effects of traditional Chinese medicine. This mode of treatment illustrates fully the advantage of a therapeutic approach combining both traditional Chinese and modern medicine.

1.9 ARRHYTHMIA
(PALPITATION)

Chang Xiaoxing
Hubei College of Traditional Chinese Medicine Hospital, Wuhan

Li, 64, male, Han nationality, married, publishing firm compiler. Date of first consultation: July 4, 1987.

CHIEF COMPLAINT: Palpitation of six months duration.

HISTORY OF PRESENT ILLNESS: Palpitation was first experienced by the patient in mid-January 1987. The symptom persisted day and night and was aggravated when he was in a bad mood or tired from work. Sensation of fullness and heaviness in chest was frequently experienced but there was never any chest pain. Accompanying symptoms were vertigo, fatigue, lassitude, irritability, insomnia, restlessness and dreamful sleep. Although experiencing thirst and vexation, he didn't like to drink much water. Intake of food was reduced and he often felt fullness in the epigastrium. He also had constipation with occasional diarrhea. The urine was normal.

The patient was hospitalized for a total of four months on two occasions in one of the city hospitals. Initially, he was given isoptin, 120 mg daily, and later mexieletine, 400 mg per day, up to the time when he came to our clinic. Palpitation improved slightly but the patient still complained of sensation of fullness and oppression in his chest. Symptoms of thirst, vexation, insomnia and dreamfulness persisted.

PAST HISTORY: Having worked in the compiling section of a publishing house for more than 30 years, the patient suffered from insomnia because of his night-shift working hours. He had non-icteric hepatitis 24 years prior to consultation. Eight years ago, he was diagnosed as having gastroptosis by barium meal examination when he had progressive loss of weight, anorexia and fullness in the epigastric region. Symptoms were recurrent during the past ten years.

PERTINENT PHYSICAL EXAMINATION & LABORATORY FINDINGS: Thin, tired, anxious, a flushed face and dry and red lips. Thyroid glands not enlarged. Lungs clear and cardiac dullness within normal limits. Heart rate, 68/min; no heart murmurs appreciated. Blood pressure normal. Abdomen soft and non-tender. Liver palpable 1 cm below right hypochondrium, soft in consistency. Spleen not palpable. No hand tremors, no pathologic reflexes elicited. Cholesterol, 180 mg%; glyceryl triacetate, 123 mg%; lipoprotein, 510 mg%; fasting blood glucose, 102 mg%; T3, T4 and TSH normal; ECG: multiple supraventricular extrasystole and occasional ventricular extrasystole, otherwise normal. ECG submaximal exercise test (-). The patient was put under 24-hour Holster ECG monitoring on March 24, 1987. Results: supraventricular extrasystole; paroxysm; supranodal tachycardia; ventricular extrasystole; and a short paroxysmal ventricular tachycardia. U.C.G.: aorta widens slightly to 36 mm, double wave low and flat, others normal.

INSPECTION OF TONGUE: Slight purplish colour with red tip. On the anterior half of the tongue, the fur was broken away and fissured. On the remaining part, the fur was thick and light yellowish in colour.

PULSE CONDITION: String-like and irregular, 68/min.

MODERN MEDICINE DIAGNOSIS: Arrhythmia; Multiple Auricular Extrasystole and Ventricular Extrasystole.

TRADITIONAL CHINESE MEDICINE DIAGNOSIS: Palpitation (Xinji).

Symptom-complex differentiation: The patient has worked in the publishing business for a long time. Mental strain has been intense leading to damage of Heart Energy. In this process, Yin, the essence of life, was being consumed resulting in inadequate nourishment of the Heart and mental activities. Such a pathology manifests itself as palpitation, irritability, insomnia and dreamfulness. Deficiency of Yin leads to flaring up of asthenic Fire which stirs in the interior of the body randomly and is manifested on the exterior as flushed complexion, dry lips, thirst and irritability. In particular, the red tongue tip and a bare, uncoated tongue are significant evidence of hyperactivity of Fire due to Yin deficiency. If this deficiency of Yin persists long enough, Heart Energy will be consumed subsequently. Inadequate Vital Energy fails to pump the Blood into circulation and the sluggish flow of Blood leads to stasis. In short, this is a case of deficiency of both the Energy and Yin. Stasis in the Channel results in malnutrition of Heart which consequently affects the patient's mental and emotional states.

THERAPEUTIC PRINCIPLES: Invigorate the Yin, replenish the Vital Energy, activate Blood circulation to dissipate Blood stasis, and stabilize the Heart and mental state.

PRESCRIPTION: Zuo Gui-Jin with Sheng-Mai-San. Radix rehmanniae, Radix rehmanniae praeparatae, Fructus lycii, Fructus corni, Poria, Radix ophiopogonis, Fructus schisandrae, Radix salviae, Semen ziziphi, Semen arborvitae, and Radix polygalae.

FOLLOW-UP/COURSE OF TREATMENT:

Second consultation on July 15, 1987: Having taken the prescription continuously for 10 days, symptoms of irritability, thirst, dry lips, etc., were alleviated slightly. To some extent, hyperactivity of Heart-Fire was put under control. There was evidence of improvement in the patient's condition. Continued administration of the prescription. Fructus schisandrae was replaced by Fructus mori to nourish the Yin and increase secretion. The aim was to moisturize the dryness and to resolve the constipation.

Third consultation on August 10, 1987: The patient had taken a total of 20 doses of the prescription. Symptoms of palpitation, fatigue and constipation were alleviated markedly but he complained of insomnia, dizziness and tinnitus. Blood pressure was normal. He still had arrhythmia with occasional premature beats at a frequency of 0-5/min. ECG examination indicated occasional supraventricular extrasystole. The patient's face was still flushed though red colour at tongue tip was reduced slightly. A thin white fur appeared on the anterior part of the tongue replacing the uncoated and smooth appearance before, but the fur on the base of the tongue was thick and yellow. Tongue proper was slightly purplish in colour. His pulse was string-like. This clinical picture suggested that the nourishment relationship between the Heart and Kidney was still not well regulated although Vital Energy and Yin had shown signs of gradual recovery. The flaring up of Fire in his state of deficiency resulted in dizziness and tinnitus. Ding Xin Tang and Zuo Gui Yin were chosen as the prescriptions to treat this case in order to nourish the Yin and to tonify the Kidney as well as to relieve mental stress. Components: Radix rehmanniae, Radix rehmanniae praeparatae, Radix scrophulariae, Fructus lycii, Fructus corni, Poria, Semen ziziphi, Semen biotae, Dens draconis, Concha ostreae, Arillus longan, Radix salviae and Rhizoma ligustici Chuanxiong. Dosage of mexieletine reduced from 400 mg/day to 150 mg/day.

Fourth consultation on September 4, 1987: Having taken this modified prescription, the patient did not experience palpitation, vexation or thirst any more. Even though he was still experiencing insomnia, the patient felt much better. He complained of epigastric fullness and loss of appetite. The tip of the tongue was red; anterior part of the tongue had a sheet of white fur, while at its root the yellow fur had changed to a white and greasy one. Colour of tongue proper still purplish. Pulse string-like and thready. Analysis of the case at this point showed that since the patient had a long history of gastropathy, and in addition, he had been taking Yin-nourishing medications for the past two months, the function of the Spleen could be disturbed leading to dysfunction of Stomach-Qi. A prescription was prepared to strengthen the Spleen and Stomach and to relieve the mental stress. Components: Radix pseudostellariae, Rhizoma atractylodis macrocephalae, Poria, Radix glycyrrhizae, Pericarpium citri reticulatae, Fructus amomi, Rhizoma polygalae, Semen ziziphi, Rhizoma ligustici and Dens draconis. Ten doses of this prescription were taken by the patient with significant relief of epigastric fullness. He was able to ingest 300 gm more of food each day than before. Bowel movement was normal and his general condition better. Occasionally, the patient experienced palpitation when he took a walk or exercised shadow boxing. Symptoms of dizziness and tinnitus were alleviated markedly though he still had insomnia and dreamful sleep. Dosage of mexieletine was reduced further to 100 mg/day. Cardiac rate was regular at 70/min. Signs of reddened tongue tip, slight purplish discolouration of the tongue and string-like pulse were not eliminated completely. Twenty-four-hour Holter ECG monitoring showed 108 beats of supraventricular extrasystole.

After months of treatment, symptoms of Heart-Yin deficiency recovered gradually, but in view of the chronic nature of the disease, it is impossible to obtain a complete effect of the treatment rapidly. Based on the observation that the patient had responded favourably to the first prescription, the herbs in that prescription were made into 1-gram pills with honey to be taken by the patient for long-term treatment. He was asked to take the pills continuously to consolidate the therapeutic effect. For his insomnia, Nao Xin Shu was prescribed and it was suggested that he continue his Qigong breathing exercises.

The patient was last checked on November 20, 1987. Mexieletine had been discontinued altogether and palpitation occurred only occasionally. His condition was stable and his health satisfactory.

1.10 AORTIC REGURGITATION AND ATRIOVENTRICULAR BLOCK (DEFICIENCY OF HEART-YANG WITH BLOOD STASIS)

Liao Jiazhen

Dongzhimen Hospital, Beijing College of Traditional Chinese Medicine, Beijing

A 60-year-old woman with dizziness and weakness had three episodes of syncope within a period of three months. She was admitted to a special hospital for cardiovascular diseases in Beijing for examination and treatment. Diagnosis given was aortic regurgitation due to rheumatic heart disease associated with RBBB and Grade II atrioventricular block. She was treated with various conventional medications, such as atropine, isoprenaline, prednisone, etc., but without any effect. Pacemaker placement was suggested but the patient refused. She was discharged and transferred to Dongzhimen Hospital on June 4, 1987, because she wanted to be treated by traditional Chinese medicine. When seen at first consultation, she had dizziness, weakness, intolerance to cold and a slow pulse of 43/min, purplish colour of the tongue with thin white fur. Physical examination showed blood pressure to be 200/80 mmHg; heart normal in size with apical impulse downward and 3 cm to the left of mid-clavicular line in the fifth intercostal space; and a decrescendo diastolic murmur best heard at left sternal border of third interspace. Breath sounds clear. Capillary pulsations evident in the blanched nail beds. ECG showed enlarged left ventricle with Grade II atrioventricular block, and the ventricular rate was 43/min. Liver not palpable and there was no edema of the lower extremities. The remainder of physical examination showed the patient to be essentially normal. Results of laboratory examination all within normal limits.

Modern medicine diagnosis of this case was aortic regurgitation secondary to rheumatic heart disease associated with RBBB and Grade II atrioventricular block. TCM symptom-complex differentiation indicated deficiency of Heart-Yang and Blood stasis. The therapeutic principle was to warm and to replenish the Heart-Yang, and to invigorate the Blood flow. Prescription was composed of Herba ephedrae, 10 gm; Herba asari, 3 gm; Radix aconiti praeparatae, 10 gm; Fructus psoraleae, 10 gm; Radix ophiopogonis, 15 gm; Radix salviae, 15 gm; and Radix paeoniae, 15 gm. One dose daily for two weeks. In this recipe, the first four herbs are adjuvant ingredients for invigorating Blood circulation to eliminate Blood stasis, while Ophiopogon root is an auxiliary ingredient for preventing the side effects of herbs which are warm in property.

Two weeks after treatment, at the second consultation, the patient's clinical condition did not change much. In order to strengthen the effects of warming the Yang-Energy and promote the Blood flow, the second prescription was modified as follows: Herba ephedrae, 10 gm; Radix aconiti praeparatae, 10 gm; Fructus psoraleae, 10 gm; Fructus lycii, 10 gm; Semen persicae, 10 gm; Flos carthamis, 10 gm; Radix salviae, 15 gm; and Rhizoma spargani, 10 gm. In this recipe, the first four herbs warm and replenish the Heart-Yang, while the others promote Blood flow. One dose daily for one month. At the end of this treatment course, the patient's heart rate was significantly increased to 90/min. ECG revealed elimination of Grade II atrioventricular block and restoration of sinus rhythm with RBBB. Meanwhile, the clinical symptoms were almost all relieved. In order to keep up the therapeutic efficacy, the patient continued to take the same prescription.

At follow-up visit six months later, the patient was in good health and sinus rhythm maintained.

DISCUSSION: When treated with traditional Chinese medicine, slow types of cardiac arrhythmia such as atrioventricular block, sinoatrial block, sick sinus syndrome and others often obtain a favourable clinical outcome. The most common clinical manifestations of AV block are dizziness, fatigue, shortness of breath, intolerance to cold and a slow heart rate. These clinical features are considered by traditional Chinese medicine as "Coldness of insufficiency syndrome" or "deficiency of Yang-Energy syndrome." On the other hand, a majority of these cases also appear with precordial pain or sensation of chest oppression associated with purple discolouration of tongue indicating Blood stasis. In accordance with the TCM symptom-complex differentiation, the following therapeutic principles and herbs are often applied:

1) Warming up and replenishing Yang-energy;

2) Replenishing Qi (commonly used medicinal herbs are Ginseng, Radix codonopsis and Radix astragali);

3) Invigorating Blood flow to eliminate Blood stasis; and

4) Removing Phlegm and Evil-Dampness. (Obstruction of the natural flow of Yang by accumulation of Phlegm and Dampness is usually manifested as anorexia, abdominal distention, lassitude, thick and sticky coating of the tongue; Agastache eupatorium, Rhizoma zingiberis, Radix notopterygium and Rhizoma pinelliae may be used according to the patient's condition.)

1.11 COMPLETE ATRIOVENTRICULAR BLOCK (SUDDEN PROSTRATION OF HEART YANG)

Dong Quanzhen

Xiyuan Hospital, China Academy of Traditional Chinese Medicine, Beijing

Yao Yifeng, 85, female, Han nationality, married, farmer. Admitted on November 30, 1986. Medical record number: 30784.

CHIEF COMPLAINT: Stuffy sensation in the chest, vertigo and palpitation exacerbated over the past two days.

HISTORY OF PRESENT ILLNESS: Twenty years prior to admission, the patient began to have high blood pressure, 230-180/120-110 mmHg, sometimes with symptoms of palpitation and stuffiness in the chest after over-straining herself. Symptoms seemed to go away by themselves and she did not take any medication. Since 1980, occurrence of the same symptoms became more frequent; she suffered from angina pectoris regularly and her ECG showed slight changes in ST-T segment. Diagnosis made at the local hospital was "coronary heart disease, stable angina and essential hypertension, stage II." For this problem, she was treated with isosorbide dinitrate, Dansheng Tablets and other drugs. Twenty days prior to admission, she had two episodes of angina pectoris accompanied by stuffiness in the chest with burning sensation, palpitation, nausea, cold sweating and vertigo. It was only by holding on to something that she did not fall down. Six tablets of nitroglycerine were taken sublingually without satisfactory effect. The patient was subsequently admitted to this hospital on November 10, 1986.

PAST HISTORY: Chronic cough with dyspnea for more than 10 years.

PERTINENT PHYSICAL EXAMINATION & LABORATORY FINDINGS: Conscious and restless; temperature, 36.4°C; pulse rate, 46/min; blood pressure, 130/70 mmHg; respiratory rate, 26/min. Head and EENT: slight cyanosis of lips. Bilateral neck veins slightly engorged. Barrel-shaped chest; cardiac border shifts to left; heart rate 46/min with a fairly regular rhythm; heart sounds very weak; no murmurs appreciated; A2>P2. Occasional dry rales on bases of bilateral lungs. Abdomen soft; liver palpable just below the costal margin and soft in consistency; spleen not palpable. Slight pitting edema on both legs. CBC: hemoglobin, 13.7 gm%; WBC count, 7,800/mm^3; BUN, 16.7 mg%; SGOT, SGPT, TTT and TFT normal; fasting blood sugar, 92.9 mg%; serum cholesterol, 153.3 mg%; serum K$^+$, 4.75 mEq/l; Na$^+$, 140.5 mEq/l; Cl$^-$, 96 mEq/l; ESR, 40 mm/h. Routine urinalysis normal.

INSPECTION OF TONGUE: Tongue substance dark in colour with thin, yellow coating.

PULSE CONDITION: Deep and slow.

MODERN MEDICINE DIAGNOSIS:

1) Essential Hypertension, Stage II;

2) Coronary Heart Disease, Stable Angina Pectoris, Complete A-V Block, Heart Failure Degree II; and

3) Obstructive Pneumonectasis.

TRADITIONAL CHINESE MEDICINE DIAGNOSIS: Obstruction of Chest; Palpitation; Deficiency of Heart-Yang.

THERAPEUTIC PRINCIPLES: Replenish Vital Energy and invigorate the Blood, nourish the Heart and relieve mental strain.

PRESCRIPTION: Radix codonopsis pilosulae, 15 gm; Radix astragali, 15 gm; Rhizoma atractylodis macrocephalae, 12 gm; Poria, 12 gm; Radix angelicae, 12 gm; Arillus longan, 12 gm; Radix auklandiae, 15 gm; Radix salviae, 30 gm; Semen ziziphi spinosae, 15 gm; Radix ophiopogonis, 12 gm; Fructus schisandrae, 10 gm; and Fructus trichosanthis, 15 gm.

In addition to Chinese medications, the patient was also treated with IV infusion of dexamethasone, isoprenaline, ATP and Coenzyme-A. During IV infusion of isoprenaline, her ECG showed reversion of AV block III to AV block II, or sinus rhythm, but the ST-T segment depression got worse. When dosage of isoprenaline was reduced, her heart rate became slow and ECG showed AV block III again. She felt chest stuffiness, vertigo and tired as usual.

FOLLOW-UP/COURSE OF TREATMENT: On November 16, 1986, the patient was noted to be pale with cyanotic lips, restless, incoherent and with cold extremities. Her lips were markedly cyanotic. Skin wet with sweat. Pulse rate was 28/min, deep and very slow. ECG showed complete AV block with conjunctive escape beat. Pacemaker insertion was suggested but the patient's family refused to give consent and proceeded to make funeral arrangements instead.

Symptom-complex differentiation: Deficiency of Heart-Energy, prostration of Heart-Yang.

Therapeutic principles: Restore Yang from collapse, tonify Heart-Qi.

Prescription: Formula of Shengfu Decoction. Radix ginseng, 10 gm, and Radix aconiti praeparatae, 10 gm. In addition, she was given isoprenaline, 0.5 mg, and dexamethasone, 5 mg, dissolved in 5% glucose solution by intravenous transfusion.

The patient's mental state improved markedly the next day. Normal colour returned gradually and extremities became warmer and sweating reduced. She reported alleviation of chest stuffiness. Pulse was more regular and in the range of 70-80/min; ECG showed stable sinus rhythm. Her general condition was stable. The dosage of isoprenaline was reduced.

Second consultation: The patient's condition was getting better; symptoms of asthma, chest stuffiness and vertigo were relieved; her health condition remained relatively stable and free of symptoms such as palpitation of the heart and excessive sweating; ECG showed sinus rhythm without AV block; blood pressure, 120/80 mmHg; pulse rate, 80/min; respiratory rate, 18/min. Tongue proper was red and dry covered by thin, white coating. Therapeutic principle to be applied at this stage was to nourish the Yin and tonify the Qi. Prescription based on Renshen Guipi Tang. Radix ginseng, 10 gm; Rhizoma atractylodis macrocephalae, 12 gm; Radix astragali, 15 gm; Radix angelica, 12 gm; Radix glycyrrhizae, 10 gm; Semen ziziphi spinosae, 10 gm; Radix aucklandiae, 10 gm; Aurillus longan, 10 gm; and Radix polygalae, 10 gm.

The patient was discharged on December 5, 1986, and advised to have follow-up at regular intervals.

On January 17, 1987, she came to the OPD for follow-up. Her condition had remained relatively stable. Pulse rate, 80/min and blood pressure, 150/80 mmHg. The cardiac rhythm was regular. Heart rate, 80/min. There was no murmur appreciated and lungs showed no abnormal findings. Liver palpable. There was no edema on the lower extremities. Pulse was wiry and rolling. Tongue proper normal with thin, white coating. She was given Shengmai Decoction, which nourishes the Qi and tonifies the Yin, in order to consolidate the therapeutic effect. The patient was also advised to avoid over-fatigue and exposure to cold, to take the medications as directed by the physician in charge and have regular follow-ups.

DISCUSSION: This patient had suffered from hypertension and chronic coronary heart disease for many years with ECG changes; her A-V block III might have been caused by coronary atherosclerosis. In modern medicine, the routine treatment of this kind of case is administration of isoprenaline, which is a ß-receptor simulator, to increase cardiac contractility and promote atrioventricular conduction and heart rate.

But such a procedure also increases cardiac oxygen consumption significantly. Therefore, although her heart rate increased and A-V conduction improved temporarily after treatment with isoprenaline, myocardial ischemia was made worse as evidenced by deterioration of the degree of S-T depression in response to treatment. The therapeutic effect of isoprenaline in treating this case was not stable. Her ECG showed complete A-V block repeatedly when IV isoprenaline was discontinued.

Shengfu Formula consists of two medicinal herbs, namely Ginseng and Radix aconiti, which replenish Qi and restore Yang from collapse. It is indicated for the treatment of Yang prostration as manifested by pallor, vertigo, cold sweating, cold extremities and thready pulse. Modern pharmacology studies have shown that Aconiti contains higenamine which has cardiotonic actions. The results of experiments carried out on isolated rat hearts indicated that higenamine increases pulsation and improves cardiac conduction. Higenamine's pharmacological action is similar to isoprenaline, but it appears to be able to protect cardiac tissues from myocardial ischemia. Ginseng is effective in improving myocardial metabolism and cardiac tolerance to anoxemia as well as cardiac performance. The rationale for choosing both Aconiti and Ginseng to treat complete A-V block is based on theories of traditional Chinese medicine as well as on results of modern pharmacology studies.

1.12 ACUTE MYOCARDIAL INFARCTION (TRUE HEART PAIN)

Chen Keji

Xiyuan Hospital, China Academy of Traditional Chinese Medicine, Beijing

Y. L. Yi, 72, female, Han nationality, married, housewife. Admitted to the emergency room on November 27, 1972. Medical record number: 182111.

CHIEF COMPLAINT: Severe pain on precordial and post-sternal areas, numbness of the left hand fingers; chest heaviness and shortness of breath of 10 days duration.

HISTORY OF PRESENT ILLNESS: For the past five years the patient has been experiencing precordial as well as post-sternal area pain described as crushing or constricting, occurring once or twice a day lasting for about 10 minutes each episode. ECG taken on March 12, 1969, confirmed the finding of acute anterior wall myocardial infarction. She was admitted and subsequently discharged cured. Two more acute episodes were recorded in May of the same year and February of 1972; both were diagnosed by ECG as acute anterior wall infarction. The last was the fourth time that she was admitted to hospital for treatment of the same complaint.

PAST HISTORY: Positive history of cough for 15 years; pain on the right elbow, wrist, palm and finger joints for 10 years. Known hypertensive for seven years (highest reading at 190/100 mmHg).

PERTINENT PHYSICAL EXAMINATION & LABORATORY FINDINGS: Pulse rate, 90/min; blood pressure, 130/70 mmHg. Conscious, of moderate health condition and normal development. Acute sickness facies, in pain. Bilateral lung auscultation normal; cardiac border shifted leftward on percussion; regular cardiac rhythm, heart rate 96/min. Grade II-III systolic blowing murmur appreciated on apical area. Liver and spleen unpalpable. No edema on the lower extremities. Evident enlargement of proximal phalangeal joints of the right hand; proximal phalangeal joint of left little finger flexed and unable to extend. ECG showed sinoatrial rhythm; cardiac vertex significantly deviated leftward (-70°); acute generalized anterior wall myocardial infarction (QRS, V_2 and V_3 assuming a QS shape, V_4 as QR shape, QV_4 depth reaching 1.0 mv, ST in V_1-V_5 elevated, V_2-V_5 assuming an unidirectional curve, T in aVL, V_6 inverted). Chest X-ray: infiltrative TB of the right upper lobe (mostly calcified), no abnormality on cardiac shadow except slight enlargement of the right ventricle. Echocardiogram: split systolic phase of the left ventricle, the rest negative. X-ray of both hands: general osteoporotic changes of bones, significant narrowing of interphalangeal spaces of the proximal and middle joint of left fourth finger; interphalangeal surface dense with edematous changes of the surrounding soft tissues; proximal end of second metatarsal showed porous absorptive changes of the bone, in agreement with rheumatic arthritic-like changes. Blood chemistry: sedimentation rate, 50 mm/hr.; SGOT, normal; WBC, 142,000/mm³; neutrophiles, 87%; lymphocytes, 13%. Routine urinalysis: protein trace; WBC, 1-2/hpf.

INSPECTION OF TONGUE: Tongue substance dark and tongue fur pale.

PULSE CONDITION: Taut.

MODERN MEDICINE DIAGNOSIS: Coronary Artery Disease: Acute Generalized Anterior Wall Myocardial Infarction; Hypertensive Disease; Rheumatic Arthritic-like Disease; Chronic Bronchiectasis; Right Upper Lobe TB.

TRADITIONAL CHINESE MEDICINE DIAGNOSIS: True Heart Pain; Deficiencies of Qi-Yang.

THERAPEUTIC PRINCIPLES: Replenish the Qi, revitalize the Blood, warm-up and regulate the flow of Qi.

FOLLOW-UP/COURSE OF TREATMENT: Treatment employed Decoction to Promote Healing composed of Radix astragali, 45 gm; Radix angelicae sinensis, 30 gm; Radix salviae miltiorrhizae, 30 gm; Ramulus cinnamomi, 12 gm; and Pericarpium citri reticulatae, 10 gm. One to two doses per day. Parenteral Shengmaisan, 2 ml, intramuscularly, b.i.d., accompanied by digitoxin, 0.1 gm/day, and energy supplementing regimen composed of the likes of ATP, Coenzyme-A and Cytochrome-C. In view of the frequent occurrence of angina which sometimes lasted several hours, Suhexiang Pills and Kuanxiong Aerosol were added which rendered different degrees of relief. At the end of the two-month treatment course using this regimen, there was significant remission of the symptoms and the patient's condition was stabilized. She was able to sit up and do some limited activities in bed though she was afraid to ambulate around because of her strong reservation about the soundness of her condition. On March 7, 1973, at around 10:40 p.m., the patient suddenly experienced extreme pain on the right upper extremity, from the shoulders to the fingertips, which occurred intermittently. Such sensation was also felt on the inner aspect of the left thigh. She complained of precordial area discomfort, anxiety, and nausea followed by vomiting. Minimal rales appreciated on the right lung; occasional premature contraction; heart rate, 90/min and blood pressure, 120/80 mmHg; ECG taken revealed elevation of ST in V_4-V_6 as compared with previous reading; no other changes of ECG picture. She was treated with electrical acupunture shocks to the Neiguan Point going through the points of Waiguan, Laogong, Hegu and Quchi; oral intake of Zhoushi Huisheng Pill, inhalation of Amylnitrate and intramuscular injection of Demerol. Symptoms apparently subsided after this regimen. Sedimentation rate was found to be 60 mm/hr; SGOT level normal. Pulse presented as deep, thready and weak; tongue fur thin and the substance dark. Considerations ruled in as the cause of these manifestations were arterial thrombosis and acute coronary arterial ischemia. Traditional therapeutic principles of replenishing the Qi, regenerating the Pulse flow and regulating the vital function of the Stomach were applied in the form of a prescription composed of Radix astragali, 60 gm; Radix angelicae sinensis, 30 gm; Radix salviae miltiorrhizae, 30 gm; Ramulus cinnamomi, 12 gm; Pericarpium citri reticulatae, 10 gm; Fructus amomi, 5 gm; Rhizoma pinelliae, 6 gm; Fructus citri sarcodactylis, 6 gm; and Rhizoma corydalis, 10 gm. In addition, IV infusion of dextroglycan and GIK solution (glucose, insulin and potassium) were administered as well as an anti-coagulant regimen (IV heparin and oral coumarin), prothrombin activity was maintained between 20% and 30%. Angina disappeared and condition stabilized. Anti-coagulants and other Western medications were discontinued after 10 days, and the main thrust of treatment now was based on the traditional medicine principle of "replenishing the Qi and removing the Blood stasis." Prescription used was composed of Radix astragali, 45 gm; Radix salviae miltiorrhizae, 30 gm; Radix angelicae sinensis, 30 gm; Rhizoma sparganii, 18 gm; Rhizoma zedoariae, 18 gm; Hirudo, 15 gm; and Semen persicae, 10 gm; decocted in 300 ml of water and administered at the dosage of one prescription a day in four equally divided doses. Oral intake of Hirudo Powder in capsule form was also instituted three times a day. Though the patient still complained occasionally of slight chest discomfort, relief could be afforded instantaneously with the intake of Roumo Tablets (made up of Rouxiang and Moyao). Overall ECG picture was converted to one comparable with that taken before the acute attack. Since the middle of March 1973, the patient has been able to ambulate and to do certain light household chores. General condition stable.

DISCUSSION:

1) Characteristics of this case are a 72-year-old patient, of weak general constitution, a long course of illness, recurrent episodes of acute myocardial infarction which rendered the treatment more difficult since the mortality rate of recurrent myocardial infarction is two times that of the primary attack. Clinical signs indicated clearly the syndrome of Qi deficiency and Blood stasis. In addition, being long bedridden, there was dysfunction of Yang which in turn aggravated the generation of the flow of Qi and Blood. Henceforth, the most appropriate therapeutic approaches in this case were those of replenishing the Qi, invigorating the Blood and removing the Blood stasis.

2) This case also presented signs of systemic arterial thrombosis. Application of a heavy dosage of Qi-replenishing, Blood-invigorating and Stasis-eradicating herbs was beneficial in improving coronary microcirculation, recovering muscle cellular activity

and in increasing the thrombolytic activity of the body. The occurrence of this particular complication reminds us of the teaching in *Su Wen: Theories of Five Qi of Xuanming* which points out that "prolonged bedriddenness debilitates the Qi." Deficiency of Qi leads to its Stasis which in turn aggravates Blood stasis, a vicious cycle of events to be reckoned with.

1.13 HIGH BLOOD PRESSURE, DIVERTICULI (BLOOD STASIS)

Jean Yu

Santa Barbara College of Oriental Medicine, California, USA

Parenti, 76, female, white, married, musician. Medical record number: 891. Date of first consultation: October 12, 1987.

CHIEF COMPLAINT: Chronic high blood pressure, decreased appetite and intestinal gas.

HISTORY OF PRESENT ILLNESS: The patient has had elevated blood pressure for many years. She is presently on a prescription of Hydrochlorothiazide and Capoten. Her blood pressure at the time of consultation was 170/90 mmHg. She also indicated that a recent GI endoscopic examination revealed three diverticuli in her colon. She had very low appetite and considerable intestinal gas. As of late, she has been constipated and uses laxatives to help move her bowels. She did not complain of abdominal pain. She said she had chronic neck stiffness and low back pain. Her energy was high and seemed very energetic for her age. She reported that she tended to be cold and preferred warm drinks and was usually not thirsty except in the early morning. She had no spontaneous sweats. She reported her urine as normal but frequent. She arose normally once a night to urinate. She slept well but had frightening dreams which caused her to awaken in a frightened state. She had raised brown moles on her face and considerable "liver spot" discolouration. She took Estrogen (Provera) three times per week.

PAST HISTORY: The patient has had gallstones for twenty years. There are three about 3 cm in diameter. She has had no colic for years but did when they were first diagnosed. She has recently been diagnosed with diverticuli.

INSPECTION OF TONGUE: Dark body with considerable dark purple spots on the sides with a thin white coat.

PULSE CONDITION: Overall wiry and slightly slippery and very rapid (100/min).

MODERN MEDICINE DIAGNOSIS: Essential Hypertension; Diverticuli; Gallstones.

TRADITIONAL CHINESE MEDICINE DIAGNOSIS: Yin Deficiency of the Liver; Qi Deficiency of the Gallbladder; Stasis of Qi in the Spleen and Stomach; Blood Stasis.

THERAPEUTIC PRINCIPLES: Benefit digestion, improve appetite, and move Qi in the Spleen and Stomach.

PRESCRIPTION: Three doses. Fructus tritici levis, 12 gm; Fructus hordei germinatus, 9 gm; Massa fermintata medicinalis, 9 gm; Fructus crataegi, 9 gm; Fructus ziziphi spinosae, 12 gm; Pericarpium arecae, 12 gm; Radix peurariae, 12 gm; and Radix glycyrrhizae, 9 gm.

FOLLOW-UP/COURSE OF TREATMENT:

Second consultation on October 19, 1987 (one week): The patient's blood pressure was 180/95 mmHg. She reported only slight improvement of her condition. Her appetite was still not good but with some improvement in intestinal gas. Her body felt a little warmer and she had slight thirst; her stools were normal but was still using laxatives. She reported that her neck stiffness had improved but her low back pain had not. She had not had any frightful dreams. The coating on her tongue was slightly thinner. The formula was modified to move the Blood and to lower blood pressure.

Modification: Three doses. Massa fermentata medicinalis, 9 gm; Fructus crataegi, 6 gm; Fructus ziziphi spinosae, 12 gm; Pericarpium arecae, 6 gm; Radix salviae miltiorrhizae, 9 gm; Cortex moutan radicis, 6 gm; Rhizoma alismatis, 12 gm; Fructus gardeniae, 6 gm; and Radix glycyrrhizae, 6 gm. Patent medicine—Jiang Yan Tablet.

Fourth consultation on November 5, 1987 (four weeks): The patient's blood pressure was 180/90 mmHg. She reported that her appetite had improved and she had less intestinal gas and some abdominal distention. She was slightly constipated. Her neck stiffness was gone but she still had some lower back rheumatic pain. Her pulse was wiry and her tongue had lost its overall darkness, although she still had dark purple spots on the sides. The prescription was changed to tonify the Qi and Yin, to move the Blood, especially in the lower back, and to cool the Liver.

Prescriptions: Three doses. Radix pseudostellariae, 9 gm; Fructus schisandrae, 6 gm; Radix ophiopogonis, 9 gm; Caulis milletti, 12 gm; Radix achyranthes bidentatae, 9 gm; Ramulus loranthi, 9 gm; Semen cassiae, 9 gm; Flos chrysanthemi, 9 gm; Poria cocos, 9 gm; and Radix glycyrrhizae, 6 gm.

Sixth consultation on November 30, 1987 (seven weeks): The patient's blood pressure was 140/90 mmHg. She presented no major complaints. Upon questioning it was learned that her neck and lower back were both without pain or stiffness. Her appetite had improved and her digestion was generally good with some slight gas. Her stools were regular and she had discontinued laxatives. She was not arising at night to urinate and her sleep continued to be undisturbed by frightful dreams. Her pulse had slowed to 60/min and was wiry and intermittent. Further modification added Radix scrophulariae and Radix paeoniae alba.

DISCUSSION: This case presented several levels of symptoms, both constitutional and acute. Treatment of all manifestations at once, in this case, was considered unwise. The patient was treated first for the digestive and sleep problems to remove manifestations of the imbalance that weakens the body. The herbs Fructus hordei germinatus, Massa fermintata medicinalis and Fructus crataegi all improve appetite and help digestion. Pericarpium arecae is effective in moving stagnant Qi, food, water and Dampness from the Spleen and Stomach. Fructus ziziphi spinosae is specifically used for frightful dreams because it tonifies the Gallbladder Qi as well as sedates. Once the acute manifestations were substantially improved it was important to tonify the Qi and Yin of the body, move the Blood and reduce blood pressure. Caulis milletti, Ramulus loranthi and Radix achyranthes bidentatae are all herbs that benefit the lower back. Semen cassiae and Flos chrysanthemi are two excellent herbs for hypertension. (Collator: Brock Haines)

1.14 ARTERIOSCLEROSIS, HYPERTENSION AND RENAL FAILURE (DEFICIENCIES OF THE SPLEEN AND KIDNEY)

Kang Ziqi

Department of Medicine, Peking Union Medical College Hospital, Beijing

Li, 74, male, cadre. Medical record number: 389668.

CHIEF COMPLAINT: Dizziness and weakness for three months, vomiting for a month.

HISTORY OF PRESENT ILLNESS: The patient has been suffering from systemic hypertension for 20 years. Blood pressure used to be 160/110 mmHg. He was treated by Qigong for about a year which rendered the blood pressure normal. For the last three months, the patient had been in a bad mood and suffered from dizziness, headache and insomnia. No special treatment was given. During the past month, he experienced itchiness and had nausea and frequent vomiting. He had not had any food for a few days accompanied by thirst, constipation and oliguria. Urine was yellow in colour and frequency of nocturia increased.

PAST HISTORY: Non-contributory.

PERTINENT PHYSICAL EXAMINATION & LABORATORY FINDINGS: The patient had a dull facies. Lips appeared cyanotic. Skin rough and elasticity poor. He had a uremic breath. BUN level, 80 mg%; creatinine, 6 mg%; CO_2C_p, 25 vol%; hemoglobin, 5.2 gm%. Urinalysis: protein, (++); WBC, 0-2/hpf, RBC, 0-1/hpf.

INSPECTION OF TONGUE: Pale tongue proper with blood stagnation *ban* (subcutaneous hemorrhages coalesce to form reddish purplish patches), tooth marks on the borders with thin and yellow coating.

PULSE CONDITION: Deep thready with mild, rapid pulse.

MODERN MEDICINE DIAGNOSIS: Arteriosclerosis Secondary to Systemic Hypertension; Renal Failure.

TRADITIONAL CHINESE MEDICINE DIAGNOSIS: Deficiency of the Spleen and Kidney; Failure of the Stomach to Propel Downward.

THERAPEUTIC PRINCIPLES: Treat the Biao (secondary and superficial) aspect for emergency, reconciliate the Stomach and suppress upward-reverse flow of Qi to nourish and activate the Blood and invigorate the Hollow Viscera.

PRESCRIPTION: Rhizoma pinelliae, 10 gm; Poria, 10 gm; Rhizoma zingiberis recens, 15 gm; Pericarpium citri reticulatae, 10 gm; Radix et rhizoma rhei, 8 gm; Radix angelicae sinensis, 10 gm; Radix salviae miltiorrhizae, 20 gm; Fructus amomi, 10 gm; Fructus ophiopogonis, 15 gm; Oryzae germinatae, 15 gm; and Ignited yellow earth, 60 gm. Decoct ingredients in appropriate amount of water. Dosage at 100 ml per day. Dosage can be reduced if frequency of administration is to be increased.

FOLLOW-UP/COURSE OF TREATMENT:

Second consultation: After five days, the patient's vigour returned and symptoms of nausea and vomiting decreased markedly and he could take a small quantity of liquid food. Bowel movement once a day. Appropriate vitamin and oral essential amino acids were prescribed.

Third consultation: Patient in good spirits and appetite good. He started to put on weight. Urine output and bowel movement normal. Same mode of treatment was followed from May 1987 to April 1988. Patient's condition remained stable. BUN, 42 mg%; creatinine, 7.2%; and hemoglobin, 7.09%.

DISCUSSION: Traditional Chinese medicine believes that a chronic progressive course of disease generally results in deficiency. This is a case of deficiency of both Spleen and Kidney Yang. Accumulation of Dampness blocks Spleen-Yang, the Spleen loses its normal transporting functions and fluid dampness stagnates and accumulates.

Disturbance of regulation of Water-flow as a digestive tract symptom in uremic patients is due to failure of the Sanjiao (Three Burners). In such a case, the Clear Yang fails to ascend and the Turbid Yin to descend resulting in the fluid Dampness not being able to be propelled downwards. Principles of treatment are dissolving turbidity, depressing the upward-reverse flow of Qi and warming Spleen Yang by giving a small dose of Pinellia tuberifera and Pathyma cocos decoction. Rhubarb has the function of eliminating Dampness by clearing Hollow Viscerae and relieving water accumulation through diuresis. Amomum echinosphaesa is able to regulate Qi with its aromatic property, activate the Spleen and militate the Stomach. Dried orange peel regulates the Qi and stops the vomiting. It also dries the Dampness and eliminates the Phlegm. The function of Terra flava usta is to warm the Zhongjiao (Middle Burner) and to stop vomiting.

1.15 INTRACTABLE HEART FAILURE (ANASARCA)

Guo Yungen, Wu Dehui and Chen Zeying
Fujian People's Hospital and the Fujian College of Traditional Chinese
Medicine Hospital, Fuzhou

L.M. Wang, 54, male, sewing machinist. Admitted on January 10, 1986.

CHIEF COMPLAINT: General edema for three years and exacerbated progressively in recent months.

HISTORY OF PRESENT ILLNESS: Three years ago, the patient noticed edema on his ankles and shortness of breath after physical exertion. Symptoms seemed to get more and more severe accompanied by palpitation, dyspnea on exertion and edema which advanced to involve the thighs and abdomen. For three years he had been consulting most of the doctors in all the big hospitals in Fuzhou City and had been hospitalized several times. He was treated with digitalis, diuretics and some other drugs; response to the treatment was transient. Relapses were so fast and frequent that he was not able to do any physical labour and was unable to take care of himself. During the eight days prior to admission, he had general edema, abdominal distention, oliguria, anorexia and respiratory embarrassment caused by even the slightest labour.

PAST HISTORY: Non-contributory.

PERTINENT PHYSICAL EXAMINATION & LABORATORY FINDINGS: Temperature, 36.4°C; pulse rate, 92/min; respiratory rate, 20/min; blood pressure, 120/70 mmHg. Moderate build, undernourished, chronic disease facies, stretcher-bound. He was sallow-complexioned. Significant engorgement of the neck veins. No neck rigidity and no thyroid enlargement. Dullness of right lung base on percussion with scattered moist rales over the base of both lungs. Percussion of the heart revealed a slight enlargement of cardiac dullness to the left. Heart rhythm showed atrial premature beats. There was a split P2 over the pulmonary valve area, and no murmurs appreciated on other valves. Distended abdomen, abdominal circumference 87 cm. Abdominal tonicity normal, shifting dullness (++), fluid wave (++). Right lobe of liver palpable. Spleen not palpable and no abdominal mass was palpated. There was marked edema of the scrotum (with phimosis) and on the lower extremities. Both knee jerks were hypoactive. Results of routine examination of blood and urinalysis were normal. Chest X-ray film showed a moderately enlarged heart and a small amount of fluid in the right thoracic cavity. ECG revealed sinus rhythm with occasional atrial premature systoles and strain of right ventricle. Two dimension echocardiogram showed normal movement of mitral valve and increase of the diameters of the left and right ventricular cavities and reduced systolic capacity of the ventricles. All these signs and symptoms agree with the manifestations of congestive myocardiopathy.

INSPECTION OF TONGUE: Swollen, dark-red colour and its coating white, which had partly peeled off revealing some petechia at the smooth surface of the tongue.

PULSE CONDITION: Deep and taut with irregular missing beats.

MODERN MEDICINE DIAGNOSIS: Dilated Primary Myocardiopathy; Atrial Premature Systoles; Refractory Biventricular Failure; Grade IV Heart Function (NYHA).

TRADITIONAL CHINESE MEDICINE DIAGNOSIS: Anasarca; Accumulation and Stagnation of Dampness and Heat; Deficiency of the Spleen and Kidney.

FOLLOW-UP/COURSE OF TREATMENT: After admission, the patient was managed with bed rest, low-salt diet with administration of full-dose digitalis including cedilanid intravenously and digoxin orally which was combined with intravenous injection of furosemide. In addition, Ji Sen Shen Qi Wan, one dose in two draughts daily, was prescribed. The prescription is composed of Radix codonopsis, 15 gm; Radix astragali, 15 gm; Fructus ligustri lucidi, 15 gm; Semen plantaginis, 15 gm; Radix achyranthis, 9 gm; Semen phaseoli, 30 gm; Rhizoma alismatis, 12 gm; Radix aconiti praeparatae, 5 gm; and Stigma maydis, 30 gm.

Second consultation on January 20, 1986: The patient complained of abdominal distention and dyspnea. The tongue proper was light-red in colour with white coating. Pulse was slippery, deep and taut. His major clinical manifestations all indicated Deficiency of the Spleen and Kidney but his cheeks were purplish red. Even though he had difficulty breathing, he spoke with a loud voice. In addition, the patient was constipated. Based on these manifestations, it was determined that this condition was a deficiency symptom-complex complicated by symptoms of excessiveness. The principle of treatment is to invigorate and to dissolve simultaneously. Modified the last prescription by replacing Pao Ke with Flos genkwa, 8 gm and Semen pharbitidis, 6 gm. One dose daily for three consecutive days.

Third consultation on January 24, 1986: After taking the decoctions, the patient's urine output increased significantly to 1,500-1,800 ml/24 hr. Bowel movement was two to three times a day. He reported that the symptoms of abdominal distention and dyspnea seemed relieved, though abdominal circumference was still 87 cm. Modified the prescription of second consultation by adding Semen pharbitidis, 6 gm, and Fructus ziziphi, 5 pieces. One dose daily for three consecutive days.

Fourth consultation on January 27, 1987: Abdominal distention, edema and other symptoms seemed relieved somewhat and the patient felt comfortable. The tongue was dark purplish in colour with thick coatings and the pulse was thready and taut with irregular missing beats. Prescription: Radix codonopsis, 15 gm; Radix astragali, 24 gm; Polyporus umbellatus, 9 gm; Poria, 9 gm; Semen plantaginis, 9 gm; Radix achyranthis, 9 gm; Rhizoma atractylodis macrocephalae, 6 gm; Ramulus cinnamomi, 6 gm; Rhizoma alismatis, 15 gm; Radix ranuculi ternati, 15 gm; and Stigma maydis, 30 gm.

Fifth consultation on February 18, 1987: At this stage, the patient's condition was taking a turn for the better in general with occasional relapse of symptoms. Though abdominal swelling was relieved, signs of ascites were still evident and abdominal circumference 85 cm. Feet edema (++). The patient had one bowel movement in two days. Eight more doses of the last prescription were prescribed as well as Radix Euphorbiae Powder, 2 gm, to be taken by mixing with lukewarm water. After taking this modified treatment, urine output was increased to 2,100 ml/24 hr and the patient passed three to four soft stools each day. He was more comfortable than before. The ascites and edema improved markedly and abdomen circumference reduced to 82 cm.

Sixth consultation on February 26, 1987: Tongue red with white and thin coating. Pulse slightly taut. Shi Pi Yin Decoction was prescribed with additional herbs added to activate the Blood and to remove Blood stasis. Rhizoma atractylodis macrocephalae, 10 gm; Radix paeoniae rubra, 9 gm; Rhizoma zingiberis recens, 3 gm; Pericarpium arecae, 12 gm; Cortex magnoliae officinalis, 6 gm; Radix aucklandiae, 9 gm; Radix salviae, 18 gm; one dose daily. The conditions improved henceforth.

Seventh consultation on March 17, 1987: Abdomen swelling and dyspnea relieved dramatically. Tongue red, coating thin and slippery and pulse smooth. Zhen Wu Tang decocted with Radix codonopsis, 15 gm, and Radix astragali, 15 gm, was prescribed. Prescription to be modified as necessary. After administration of a total of 60 doses, dyspnea was markedly relieved, abdominal and feet edema lessened and abdominal circumference reduced to 79 cm. He began to take a walk with the help of a walking cane. Chest X-ray examination on March 18 showed disappearance of fluid on the right chest. No premature beat was detected by ECG examination on March 9. He was discharged from hospital on May 30, 1986.

DISCUSSION: This patient had frequent attacks of dyspnea and edema for many years and the symptoms worsened progressively. No history of hypertension nor nephritis and no valvular murmur. Chest X-ray examination showed a generally enlarged heart shadow. The echocardiogram disclosed that the diameter of the left and right ventricular cavities was enlarged and aortic valve not involved.

A diagnosis of dilated primary cardiomyopathy was established in this case. The widespread pathological changes of myocardium resulted in extensive impairment of systolic function of the ventricles and led to the clinical manifestations of both left and right heart failure (whole heart failure). Over the past few years the condition has been deteriorating progressively. The patient sought medical advice and was given digitalis, diuretics and vasodilators repeatedly. However, the response to the therapies had not been well all along. Therefore, this was a case of refractory heart failure.

Based on its symptom-complex differentiation, this case was diagnosed as "Engorgement" and "Anasarca Syndrome," classified as "Pi Shen Yang Xu" (Deficiency of vital function of the Spleen and Kidney) with accumulation and stagnancy of Dampness and Heat. The patient was advanced in age and with Deficiency of functional activities of the Spleen and Kidney. Since he suffered from the illness for rather a long time, the persistence of this condition might have caused the appearance of "Ying Shui" (edema of Ying). For a long period of time the patient was given modern medicine therapy made up of powerful diuretic drugs which usually lead to imbalance in electrolytes, such as potassium and sodium loss. The more diuretics the kidney is exposed to, the more damage to the kidney and this condition will eventually lead to failure of the kidneys to respond to the diuretics at all, agreeing with the saying that "more diuretics make more oliguria."

During admission, administration of digitalis, a small dose of synthetic diuretic and vasodilator was continued. In accordance with the principle of invigorating the function of the Spleen and Stomach, reinforcing the Kidney, invigorating the Yang and vital function and transforming the vital activity, the patient was treated with a regimen to relieve Water and to clear up endogenous Heat. For this reason, he was given modified Ji Sheng Shen Qi Wan and Shi Pi Yin prescriptions. In the prescriptions, Radix codonopsis, Radix astragali, Poria and Rhizoma dioscoreae invigorate the function of the Spleen and Stomach and transform the vital activity leading to relief of water retention; Radix aconiti warms the Kidney and invigorates the Yang; Rhizoma zingiberis recens disperses the Cold and consequently relieves Water retention; Cortex magnoliae officinalis and Radix aucklandiae regulate the flow of vital energy and dispel Dampness. Polyporous umbellatus, Rhizoma alismatis, Stigma maydis and Semen plantaginis serve as diuretics to resolve Dampness. As this is a chronic case of a rather severe nature, the therapeutic effect, though it proved to be effective, was still not very pronounced.

Detailed observation of the manifestations disclosed that the deficiency symptom-complex was complicated by that of excessiveness. Such a case must be treated by tonifying the Spleen and Kidney together with medicinal herbs which are cathartic in nature. Shi Zao Tang was prescribed to dispel endogenous Heat and Water from lungs and to clear away excessive fluid from the intestine by its potent purgative action, in order to obtain a quick result. Yet, in consideration of its strong nature, Yuan Hua was administered from the beginning complemented by Fructus ziziphi to take advantage of its sweet nature. Moreover, Semen pharbitidis was added in order to enhance the efficacy of the diuretics and to dispel water accumulation.

Taking the mild catharsis therapy mentioned above for six days, the therapeutic effect increased significantly. In consideration of the fact that it might be over-treated with the same method in the long term, the patient was given tonifying herbs; herbs diuretic in nature were also administered to remove Dampness. The prescription was based on Ji Sheng Shen Qi Wan with some modifications. In this way, the patient could have ample time to restore his physical activities and to improve his condition progressively.

In order to keep abreast with the clinical situation, a further course of Radix euphorbia was added for a period of time and this proved to be effective in dispelling Water retention. Two things must be pointed out, however. First, in order to keep full efficacy of the purgatives and diuretics, Radix euphorbia must be pulverized and taken after mixing with warm boiled water lest its medicinal property be compromised during the process of decoction, and second, during administration of a herbal prescription containing powerful cathartics, close monitoring must be maintained so that appropriate treatment for possible side effects can be carried out promptly.

The patient has been in stable and good condition after taking Zhen Wu Tang combined with other medicinal herbs such as Radix codonopsis and Radix astragali. Full recovery is expected following this approach.

1.16 CONGESTIVE HEART FAILURE (PALPITATION AND DYSPNEA)

Gu Jingyan

Jiangsu Institute of Traditional Chinese Medicine, Nanjing

Li Yinlan, 44, female, Han nationality, married, worker. Admitted on December 16, 1987. Medical record number: 23237.

CHIEF COMPLAINT: Repeated attacks of palpitation and dyspnea for 13 years, worsened in the past month.

HISTORY OF PRESENT ILLNESS: The diagnosis of rheumatic heart disease with mitral stenosis was established years ago through repeated examinations by auscultation, ECG, echocardiogram and fluoroscopy of the chest. Medical treatment with digoxin and/or diuretics, sometimes with vasodilator, was given intermittently in the past. The patient had refused surgical treatment. Recently, the symptoms worsened gradually after a cold lasting for more than one month. Symptoms of dry cough and dyspnea on mild exertion bothered the patient so much that she could not lie flat at night. The cough was not productive and there was no fever. The patient also complained of weakness, fatigue and loss of appetite.

PAST HISTORY: Positive history of arthralgia of both knees in her 20's; frequent attacks of colds and sore throat. No history of rheumatic fever.

PERSONAL HISTORY: Non-contributory.

PERTINENT PHYSICAL EXAMINATION & LABORATORY FINDINGS: Pale with malar flush (mitral facies). Mild venous engorgement. Bilateral rough breath sounds, no rales. Cardiac dullness over left third intercostal space; slightly enlarged; apical first sound loud and snapping; a characteristic rumbling mid-diastolic murmur of moderate degree and opening snap heard over the apex, accompanied by a thrill; P2 accentuated; cardiac rate 96/min, with extrasystole at 3-4/min. Liver palpable 2 cm below the right costal margin on the right mid-clavicular line, consistency soft, non-tender, hepatojugular reflex (±). Laboratory findings essentially normal except for slight anemia. ECG finding: P wave $\geqslant 0.12$ sec, notched, peak interval, 0.04 sec, Ptfv 1.04 ms, with atrial extrasystole (indicating enlargement of left atrium). UCG findings: distinct enlargement of left atrium (50 mm.); no enlargement of ventricle; a peak on anterior mitral valve leaflet absent; decrease of EF slope to flat plateau configuration; homolateral movement of both leaflets, amplitude of opening between both leaflets decreased (8 mm). X-ray chest film finding: pear-shaped cardiac shadow, double density near cardiac border, filling out of middle segment of cardiac silhouette. Both lungs clear. Various non-invasive examinations of cardiac performance showed insufficiency of heart function (see Table 1 for detailed data).

INSPECTION OF TONGUE: Tongue proper purplish in colour with thin white coating.

PULSE CONDITION: Deep, small and rapid with occasional missing beats.

MODERN MEDICINE DIAGNOSIS: Chronic Rheumatic Heart Disease; Mitral Stenosis; Congestive Cardiac Failure, Grade I; Cardiac Arrhythmia (Atrial Extrasystole).

TRADITIONAL CHINESE MEDICINE DIAGNOSIS: Zhenchong (palpitation) and Dyspnea (Xu-type, due to deficiency).

Symptom-complex differentiation: Deficiency of Qi and Yin-Blood of the Heart, with stasis of Blood circulation, as well as disturbance of pure and descending actions of the Lung.

THERAPEUTIC PRINCIPLES AND PRESCRIPTIONS:

1) Using Shen Fu Tang (Ginseng and Aconitum Decoction) and Sheng Mai San (a powder made up of Ginseng, Radix ophiopogonis and Fructus schizandrae) to replenish Qi, to warm the Yang and also to refresh the Heart as the chief therapeutic measure.

2) Addition of other medications to promote Blood circulation, clear the Lung and descend the Qi.

Ingredients of the primary prescriptions are Radix astragali, 15 gm; Radix codonopsis pilosulae, 20 gm; Radix aconiti praeparatae, 6 gm; Radix ophiopogonis, 10 gm; Fructus schizandrae, 10 gm; Rhizoma polygonati odorati, 20 gm; Radix salviae miltiorrhizhae, 20 gm; Poria (with cortex), 30 gm; Semen lepidii seu descurainiae, 15 gm; Semen plantaginis, 20 gm; Cortex mori radicis, 15 gm; and Radix asteris, 10 gm.

FOLLOW-UP/COURSE OF TREATMENT: The patient was initially treated only by this composite prescription and symptoms were alleviated after eight doses. She could lie flat at night, thereby the same treatment was continued for about one month. Since then she felt quite well except for slight dyspnea on moderate exertion. The prescription was modified by replacing Radix asteris and Semen plantaginis with Radix angelicae sinensis and Radix paeoniae alba to nourish the Blood. This was prescribed as maintenance treatment.

Before being discharged from hospital, re-examination by auscultation and ECG showed normalization of heart rate (about 70/min) and disappearance of atrial extrasystole; non-invasive examinations for evaluation of cardiac performance also expressed improvement as seen by the increase in SV (stroke volume), CO (cardiac output) and CI (cardiac index), decrease in TPR (total peripheral resistance), PCWP (pulmonary capillary wedge pressure) and LVEDP (left ventricular end-diastolic pressure), shortening of PEP (pre-ejection period) and depression of PEP/LVET (pre-ejection period/left ventricular ejection time). See Table 1 for detailed data.

TABLE 1. RESULTS OF NON-INVASIVE EXAMINATIONS OF CARDIAC PERFORMANCE BEFORE AND AFTER TREATMENT

EXAMINATION	INDEX	BEFORE TREATMENT	AFTER TREATMENT
STI (Systolic Time Interval)	PEP (sec)	0.12	0.09
	LVET (sec)	0.27	0.29
	PET/LVET	0.44	0.33
EIC (Electrical Impedance Cardiogram)	Q-Z interval (sec)	0.19	0.14
	SV (ml/beat)	40.14	57
	CO (L/min)	3.171	4.218
	CI (L/min/m)	2.329	4.218
UCG (Echocardiogram)	SV	39	44
	CO	3.27	3.7
	CI	2.30	2.68
	EF(%)	0.55	0.56
	TPR (dyne sec/cm)	1981.56	1751.35
	C(ml/mmHg)	1.3928	1.1
	PCWP (mmHg)	33.57	30.94
	LVEDP (mmHg)	37.6	34.58

DISCUSSION: Based on the history, signs and symptoms and the positive findings of ECG, UCG and X-ray chest film, the diagnosis of chronic rheumatic heart disease and mitral stenosis with congestive cardiac failure is well established in this case. The diagnosis is further supported by results of various non-invasive examination of cardiac performance.

In traditional Chinese medicine, on account of the clinical manifestations, this case may be considered to belong to the category of Zhenchong (palpitation) and dyspnea of the Xu-type. In view of the past history of Bizheng (arthralgia), invasions by Wind, Cold and Dampness are considered the exogenous pathogenic factors in this case. TCM theories believe that the prolonged existence of these exogenous pathogenic factors inside the body may attack the Heart through the Channels, resulting in injury and defects in Qi and Yin-Blood of the Heart. Loss in support and nutrients due to deficiency of Yin-Blood causes uneasiness of the Heart and Mind, manifested as palpitation clinically; while depression of the action to promote the Blood circulation due to deficiency of Qi may lead to sluggish flow of Blood, even stagnation of Blood resulting in clinical signs and symptoms of purplish tongue proper, small pulse with missing beats and mass formation below the costal margin. TCM teaching states that the Heart controls the Blood and the Lung controls the Qi. Both these organs reside in Shangjiao (Upper Burner, the Chest) with their functions closely related to each other. So deficiency of Qi (and/or Yang) of the Heart will influence the function of the Lung which in turn results in insufficiency of the Upper Jiao's Qi-Yang, leading eventually to disturbance of Water-Dampness transportation. With the aqueous Qi affecting the Heart, symptoms such as palpitation, shortness of breath, distress sensation of the chest and severe cough may thus occur clinically. Furthermore, instability of the Wei-principle due to Lung insufficiency may explain the patient's vulnerability to colds, which could cause recurrence or exacerbation of the symptoms mentioned above. In short, based on symptom-complex differentiation, this case belongs to deficiency complicated with excess, affecting both the Heart and Lung, with deficiency of both Qi and Yin as the primary aspect of pathogenesis, while sluggish flow of Blood and loss of clearing and descending actions of the Lung are secondary aspects of pathogenesis. Therefore, using tonics to replenish the deficiency should be the most fundamental and important therapeutic measure. In addition, the combination of methods to activate the Blood flow, to dispel Dampness, to clear and descend the Lung, to release dyspnea and cough was also necessary. In view of the Yin-Yang teachings such as "independence of Yin and Yang," "a flourishing Yin based on a virilized Yang," "Yang generalized from Yin," "Yin flourishing smoothly and Yang dancing steadily," replenishing the deficiency must take into consideration both the Yin and the Yang, so the combination of Shen Fu Tang and Sheng Mai San is therefore the best choice for invigorating and warming the Qi and Yang, and at the same time for nourishing the Yin and tranquilizing the Heart. Rhizoma polygonati odorati is added to enhance the effect of nourishing the Yin by protecting the Yang. Radix astragali seu hedysari could potentiate the effect of Qi reinforcement and consolidate the exterior to help defend against exogenous pathogenic factors. Radix miltiorrhizae is used to nourish the Blood and accelerate the Blood circulation; Semen lepidis seu descurainiae possesses the action of purging the Lung as well as dispelling Water-Dampness, thus relieving dyspnea and cough; Poria can remove water too by strengthening the Spleen; Semen plataginis and Cortex mori radicis clear the Heat from the lung and remove the excess Water-Dampness; Radix asteris is added to relieve cough and eliminate Phlegm. As a whole, the composition of this prescription conforms with the concept of integration and comprehensiveness of the therapy. Satisfactory therapeutic effect is thus obtained as evidenced by the improvement of cardiac performance which could be illustrated by either the clinical condition of the patient or by the non-invasive examinations of heart function.

Mechanism of action of this prescription's therapeutic efficacy may be explained by pharmacological studies on the herbs used. Many reports in our country have recognized that Ginseng and Sheng Mai San have positive inotropic effect on the heart demonstrated by an increase in myocardial contractility, stroke volume, cardiac output and ejection fraction of the left ventricle on the one hand, and decrease of systemic circulation resistance, improvement of peripheral circulation and cardiac metabolism on the other hand. (The pharmacological mechanism of Radix codonopsis pilosulae is similar to that of Ginseng.) The active component of Radix aconiti praeparatae appears to act on the heart, too. It has also been reported that there are actually some types of cardiac glycoside in the root or stem of Rhizoma polygonati odorati and in Semen lepidis seu descurainiae. Cortex mori radicis, Poria and Semen plantaginis all can induce diuresis. These scientific evidences explain why this prescription displays such cardiokinetic and diuretic effects. Radix astragali seu heydysari not only reinforces the defensive mechanisms of the body, but also promotes diuresis. In addition, Radix salviae miltiorrhizae enriches the blood supply of myocardium by dilating the coronary artery and raising cardiac tolerance to ischemia. The effects of these medicinal herbs in regulating the nutritional and metabolic conditions of the heart are in many ways similar to cardiac medications of modern medicine with the added benefits of the absence of any significant toxic side effects.

Regarding our clinical experience, TCM therapy may be employed alone in the compensatory stage of cardiac failure, while a combined approach (with those drugs such as cardiac glycosides, diuretics, etc., in smaller daily dosage than usual) is in favour in the treatment of the decompensatory stage of cardiac failure. As to those severe conditions where the dosage of digitalis is hard to control, toxic effects occur easily and therapeutic effects are not justified, we usually use both Chinese herbal medicines and modern medicines including diuretics and/or vasodilators, accompanied by intermittent administration of small doses of fast-acting digitalis (such as cedilanid, IV, 0.13-0.20 mg per dose or oral digoxin, 0.125 mg per dose, one to two times every week). Such a regimen can result in further improvement of the clinical condition. It is our experience that the combination of traditional Chinese and modern medicine is the most valuable therapeutic regimen in the management of congestive heart failure, and it merits further study and investigation.

1.17 VIRAL MYOCARDITIS (PALPITATION OF HYPERACTIVITY OF FIRE DUE TO YIN DEFICIENCY)

Zou Ciqing
Shandong College of Traditional Chinese Medicine, Jinan

Zhang, 16, male, Han nationality, student. Medical record number: 24685. Date of first visit: September 12, 1986.
CHIEF COMPLAINT: Low-grade fever, palpitation and oppressive feeling in

chest for one week.

HISTORY OF PRESENT ILLNESS: Two weeks prior to consultation, the patient had fever of 39.6°C with general malaise, pain and itchiness in the throat and cough. He sought medical help and was told that he had a common cold. Treated by kanamycin injection and Chinese medicinal herbs, his temperature was lowered to 37.5°C. Then he experienced palpitation, chest distress and disorder of heart rate manifested as bigeminy-coupled rhythm. The patient was treated with penicillin and hydrocortisone for five days but to no avail. Signs and symptoms on admission were palpitation, chest distress, shortness of breath, dry throat with bitter taste and vexation. He had poor appetite, dyschesia, difficult and painful urination and no urinary urgency nor frequency.

PAST HISTORY: No history of palpitation, chest distress or rheumatic fever.

PERTINENT PHYSICAL EXAMINATION & LABORATORY FINDINGS: General condition fair. Pharynx red, congested tonsils without arthrocele. Temperature, 37.2°C; blood pressure, 130/80 mmHg; heart rate, 123/min. Secondary systolic murmur appreciated in apical region, first heart sound low and clear; irregular heart rate with bigeminy-coupled rhythm. Lung findings negative. ECG findings showed sinus tachycardia; low voltage; R+S in limb leads I, II, III, 0.4 mV; multiple ventricular bigeminy; incomplete right bundle-branch block; myocardial damage; T wave inversion in V_1-V_4. Chest X-ray did not show definitely enlarged heart borders. CBC showed WBC, 8,500/mm; neutrophil, 63%, and lymphocyte, 45%; mononuclear cell, 4%; SGOT, 46 units and CPK, 73 units. Routine urinalysis negative.

INSPECTION OF TONGUE: Red, dry and uncoated tongue.

PULSE CONDITION: Active and fast.

MODERN MEDICINE DIAGNOSIS: Pathologic Myocarditis.

TRADITIONAL CHINESE MEDICINE DIAGNOSIS: Palpitation; Hyperactivity of Fire Secondary to Yin Deficiency.

THERAPEUTIC PRINCIPLES: Clear up the Yin and detoxicate, and nourish the Yin to reduce pathogenic Fire.

PRESCRIPTION: Rhizoma coptidis, 6 gm; Radix scutellariae, 9 gm; Flos lonicerae, 30 gm; Fructus forsythiae, 12 gm; Cornu bubali, 6 gm; Radix ophiopogonis, 9 gm; leaf bud of Herba lophatheri, 6 gm; Radix salviae, 12 gm; Radix rehmanniae, 15 gm; Radix scrophulariae, 12 gm; Radix paeoniae alba, 12 gm; and Colla corii asini, 9 gm. Decoct in 500 ml water. One dose three times a day.

FOLLOW-UP/COURSE OF TREATMENT:

Second consultation: After administration of six doses, the patient's body temperature was lowered to 36.6°C, heart rate 118/min. He complained of palpitation, chest distress, vexation, acratia, dry stool, scanty and dark urine, red tongue with little fur, and occasional quick pulse. Fructus forsythiae removed from the prescription and six more doses prescribed.

Third consultation: Heart rate 116/min, occasional quick pulse. Other signs and symptoms are palpitation, chest distress, vexation and acratia, night sweating, dry mouth without craving for drink and dark urine. The patient did not have dry stool. ECG examination showed some improvement in sinus tachycardia, occasional ventricular premature beat, myocardial damage, low voltage and incomplete right bundle-branch block. SGOT, 32 units and CPK, 54 units. Prescription: Radix glycyrrhizae praeparatae, 12 gm; Radix rehmanniae, 15 gm; Radix paeoniae alba, 12 gm; Colla corii asini, 9 gm; Radix ophiopogonis, 12 gm; Fructus schisandrae, 6 gm; Radix ginseng, 9 gm; Plastrum testudinis, 15 gm; Concha ostreae, 30 gm; Carapax trionycis, 15 gm; and Semen biotae, 12 gm.

Fifth consultation: After 12 doses of the prescription, the patient's bowel movement was normal, sweat had disappeared and symptoms such as palpitation, chest distress, vexation and acratia were alleviated. Tongue appearance normal with slender and quick pulse. Heart rate, 92/min. ECG normal. The patient was discharged from hospital with medications. When last seen in follow-up a year later, he was in good health.

DISCUSSION: The diagnosis of this case relies mainly on ECG changes and symptoms of palpitation, chest distress, vexation and acratia. There was positive medical history of upper respiratory tract infection two weeks ago. Serum enzyme level was elevated and rheumatic myocarditis, toxic myocarditis and tuberculous pericarditis were ruled out. Finally, the diagnosis of pathologic myocarditis was established.

Symptom-complex differentiation of the case indicates hyperactivity of Fire due to Yin deficiency. This finding is based on signs of tongue, pulse, stool and visceral Yin-Yang dysfunction between the Heart and Kidney. Organic changes detected by ECG offer clues for the diagnosis to be established on first consultation and as a basis to select the proper therapeutic regimen.

Fluctuating low-grade fever, dry stool, scanty dark urine, red tongue with little fur and tremulous pulse with failure to send up Yin-Qi and suppress Yang-Qi, as seen on the first visit, reflect overwhelming presence of pathogen with a little Heat, weakened body resistance without impairment of the Kidney and flaring-up of Heart-fire. Treatment with Qing Yin Tang and Huanglian Ajiao Tang removed exogenous pathogens, suppressed the flaring-up of Heart-Fire, tonified the Kidney and relieved mental strain. The effect of this regimen was evident during the second visit. On the third visit, bowel movement and stool were normal but the patient manifested signs of dark urine, red tongue with little fur and occasional quick pulse. There was evident improvement of ECG findings with normal serum enzyme. Rapid therapeutic effect was evidenced by improvement of heart rate, pulse rate and alleviation of palpitation. This indicates that Yin deficiency due to hyperactivity of Fire had been transformed to hyperactivity of Fire due to Yin deficiency. Applied Huanglian Ajiao Tang and Sheng Mai San (Pulse-activating Powder) to replenish vital essence, strengthen the Qi, clear away the Heat and purge the Fire. The patient had taken six doses of the prescription at that time. It could have been better to take two to three doses and then to modify the prescription. This accounts for the rather slow progress of improvement of the symptoms of palpitation and rapid pulse which were sometimes more severe than before. In fact the sign of excessive Fire was changed to hyperactivity of Yang due to Yin deficiency. Administration of Sunjian Fumai Tang Zhi Tang (Decoction of Prepared Licorice) in this case nourished the Yin and suppressed the excessive Yang, nourished the Blood and effected a full recovery from the disease. In clinical practice, proper symptom-complex differentiation facilitates full comprehension of the pathological process and the mapping out of a proper treatment regimen. Otherwise, a prescription often loses its therapeutic efficacy through unnecessary modifications. In our case, therapeutic effect was stalled because of prescription modification during the third consultation.

1.18 CARDIAC NEUROSIS (PALPITATION SECONDARY TO KIDNEY-YANG INSUFFICIENCY AND FLARING HEART-FIRE)

Zou Ciqing

Shandong College of Traditional Chinese Medicine, Jinan

Zhang, 43, female, Hui nationality, married, teacher. Medical record number: 64825. Date of first consultation: March 26, 1985.

CHIEF COMPLAINT: Palpitation and "cardiac pain" of nine years duration, exacerbated in the past year.

HISTORY OF PRESENT ILLNESS: Nine years prior to admission, the patient suffered from severe emotional trauma because her husband had passed away and her daughter had fallen ill. She was severely depressed and had no food intake for a long time. Accompanying symptoms were hypertension and insomnia. She recovered from the symptoms gradually after treatment. Since then, the patient frequently experienced palpitation, chest pain, insomnia or dreamful sleep and anxiety. She had been treated in many hospitals as a case of cardiac neurosis. Relying purely on ECG examination, many doctors had been reluctant to give a definitive diagnosis of coronary heart disease. Throughout the years she took Librium, Miltown, Propanolol, Radix Salviae Tablets, Coronary Storax Pill and other Chinese medications to nourish the Heart and calm the Mind. Symptoms had been recurrent and she was never in a state of good health.

During the last year up to the time of consultation in our clinic, the patient noticed that palpitation was getting more severe and that chest pain and palpitation were easily induced by fright or emotional strain. Other signs were vexation with little sleep, feverish sensation in head and face, dizziness and tinnitus, dry mouth with a bitter throat, hyperhidrosis of the palms and coldness experienced on both lower extremities. She was intolerant to both cold and heat, with edema on the face and extremities, dry mouth, loss of appetite, scanty stool and frequent urination. Amount of menstruation had been scanty for the last six months and was usually delayed.

PAST HISTORY: Non-contributory.

PERTINENT PHYSICAL EXAMINATION AND LABORATORY FINDINGS: Low spirits, morbid facies, hyperhidrosis of palms and slight tremors of both hands. Temperature, 36.8°C; blood pressure, 145/92 mmHg; and heart rate, 106/min. Strong heart sounds, accentuation of apical impulse with secondary systolic murmurs. ECG revealed sinus tachycardia, occasional ventricular extrasystole, slow T waves in leads II, III and avF.

INSPECTION OF TONGUE: Red tongue with little fur.

MODERN MEDICINE DIAGNOSIS: Cardiac Neurosis.

TRADITIONAL CHINESE MEDICINE DIAGNOSIS: Palpitation Secondary to Kidney-Yang Insufficiency and Flaring of Heart-Fire.

THERAPEUIC PRINCIPLES: Warm the Kidney and reinforce Yang, purge the Heart of pathogenic Fire, and regulate the relationship between the Heart and Kidney.

PRESCRIPTION: Shangxia Liangjidan and Liangjiao Tang. Rhizoma rehmanniae praeparatae, 12 gm; Fructus corni, 12 gm; Radix angelicae sinensis, 9 gm; Semen ziziphi, 15 gm; Rhizoma coptidis, 3 gm; Rhizoma atractylodis macrocephalae, 9 gm; Radix ginseng, 9 gm; Radix ophiopogonis, 9 gm; Rhizoma anemarrhenae, 9 gm; Rhizoma alismatis, 15 gm; Semen sinapis albae, 6 gm; and Cortex phellodendri, 9 gm. Decoct in 500 ml of water. One dose three times every day.

FOLLOW-UP/COURSE OF TREATMENT:

Second consultation: After taking six doses of this prescription, symptoms were alleviated significantly, and feverish sensation and edema in face disappeared. The patient still complained of anxiety, sweating and numbness of limbs. Modified the prescription by removing Rhizoma anemarrhenae, 9 gm, and added Radix astragali, 15 gm, Fructus schisandrae, 6 gm, and Fructus ziziphi jujubae, 30 gm.

Third consultation: Completion of a 12-dose treatment course. Chest pain occurred only when induced by state of excitement and overworking which could be relieved by calming down the patient and rest. Another 12 doses of the same prescription were prescribed.

Fourth consultation: The patient's condition stable after finishing the last 12-dose treatment course. Prescription discontinued and the patient was shifted to a regimen of Oryzanol, Propanolol, Buxin Dan and Diazepam. Recently, some symptoms recurred such as palpitation, chest distress and pain and vexation with sweating induced by emotional strain and exposure to cold weather. Heart rate was 98/min and ECG showed occasional ventricular extrasystole. Tongue was slightly red with wiry pulse. Above formulae were prescribed again with the addition of Concha margaritifera usta, 30 gm, and Dens draconis, 30 gm. Decocted in water.

The patient felt better after taking the last prescription and continued taking it for over two months. She recovered fully and went back to work. There has not been any recurrence.

DISCUSSION: Though there is no organic pathological change, cardiac neurosis, with its long course of disease and many accompanying symptoms, if left untreated, could prove to be most distressing to the patient. Two effective therapeutic regimens were discovered through many years of clinical experience. One is soothing the Liver to reduce the Fire and nourishing the Heart to calm the Heart indicated in the 20 to 40 age group. The other is restoring normal coordination between Yin and Yang, the Heart and Kidney indicated in menopausal patients (over 40 years of age). This case belongs to the latter.

Disintegration of normal physiological coordination between the Heart and Kidney, which is often seen in neurosis and seldom seen in cardiac neurosis, leads to loss of normal relation between the Heart-Yang and Kidney-Yin, manifested in symptoms of vexation and insomnia, palpitation and dreams. Once cardiac neurosis is evident, through the long course of the disease, the main symptom-complex of Kidney dysfunction, e.g. shortness of breath, palpitation, chest pain and shortness of breath, appears with the symptom-complex of concurrent coexistence of Deficiency and Excess. Such a symptom-complex encompasses symptoms of concurrent exhibition of Cold and Heat, of vexation and insomnia, dizziness and sweating, feverish sensation in head and face, dry mouth with bitter taste, cold lower extremities, bowel movement deregulation, urinary frequency, edema of face and numbness of extremities. Since the syndrome is rather complicated, numerous unorthodox manifestations, such as insufficiency without reinforcement, excess without diarrhea, coolness causing Cold and warmth causing Dryness, are present during the course of treatment.

Initially, the effect of the medications administered is rather inconsistent. ST-T in ECG changes easily, which is normal at one time, heavy at another, and sometimes fast, slow or in pace with the change of the heart rate. All these signs pertain to the pathologic syndromes of Fire due to Yang insufficiency and imbalance of Yin and Yang. Hence, the treatment is to use Shangxia Liangjidan and Liangjiao Tang in which Ginseng, Rhizoma atractylodis and Rhizoma anemarrhenae are for warming the Yang and strengthening the Yin; Rhizoma rehmanniae, Fructus corni, Radix angelicae and Radix ophiopogonis for nourishing Yin and keeping the Yang; Semen sinapis albae and Rhizoma coptidis for clearing and activating the Channels and Collaterals; and Semen ziziphi for nourishing the Heart and calming the Mind. This prescription is for regulating Yin and Yang, Qi and Blood; tonifying the Kidney and relieving mental stress; restoring coordination between Water and Fire, Yin and Yang; and coordinating the body's functions. Once equilibrium of the inner environment is restored, the patient's condition will recover.

Treatment for this kind of disease requires a certain period of time. Both the physician and patient must have faith in the treatment. Otherwise, ill-planned and hastily administered therapeutic procedures, such as tonifying today and purging tomorrow, warming without effect of cold and cooling without effect of warmth, changing the treatment or attending physician randomly, will certainly lead to failure in obtaining a satisfactory therapeutic outcome.

2. RESPIRATORY DISEASES

2.1 RECURRENT COLD AND COUGH (DAMP-HEAT DISEASE)

Jean Yu

Santa Barbara College of Oriental Medicine, California, USA

Pearson, 77, female, white, widow, retired. Medical record number: 72. Date of first visit: February 11, 1986.

CHIEF COMPLAINT: Recurrent cold for one year.

HISTORY OF PRESENT ILLNESS: The patient had been having recurrent common cold for one year with sore throat, nasal congestion and a dry cough. The colds were recurring at a rate that was almost continual. She also had a continuous dry cough with some mucus in the morning that was yellowish, thick and easily expectorated. She was not bothered with headache. She complained of low energy and tiredness. She reported no sensations of heat or cold in her body, but was generally thirsty and drank much water. She had night sweats in the early stages of her common cold and had a decreased appetite when her colds were bad. Otherwise her digestion, stools and urination were normal. She reported sleeping well, but that sleeping was interrupted by coughing bouts.

PAST HISTORY: The patient has had no serious illness other than acute hepatitis in 1955 and arthritis twelve years ago. She is presently taking thyroid extracts and Premarin (estrogen). Several years ago she developed collapsed Eustachian tubes from airplane decompression.

INSPECTION OF TONGUE: Red tongue, reddish edges, thick dry yellow coat in centre of tongue.

PULSE CONDITION: Superficial and tight overall.

MODERN MEDICINE DIAGNOSIS: Recurrent Common Cold; Chronic Bronchitis.

TRADITIONAL CHINESE MEDICINE DIAGNOSIS: Heat in the Shangjiao with slight Dampness Accumulation.

THERAPEUTIC PRINCIPLES: Clear away Heat in the Lung and eliminate Dampness.

PRESCRIPTION: Yin Qiao San modified—three doses. Flos lonicerae, 9 gm; Fructus forsythiae, 12 gm; Radix platycodi, 9 gm; Fructus arctii, 9 gm; Flos magnoliae, 9 gm; Semen Plantaginis, 12 gm; Radix scutellariae, 9 gm; Radix clemitidis, 15 gm; and Radix glycyrrhizae, 6 gm.

FOLLOW-UP/COURSE OF TREATMENT:

Second consultation on February 18, 1986: The patient reported that his cough had eased but that she had dryness of the mouth. She had no sore throat and generally felt better. Energy was still low. There was still thirst. All other indicators were normal. Pulse was superficial and moderate and the tongue still had a thick, dry yellow coat but the body was less red. The formula was further modified to stop cough and dispel Phlegm and moisten Dryness. Modification: three doses. Constituents: Radix scutellariae, 9 gm; Flos lonicerae, 9 gm; Fructus xanthii, 9 gm; Cortex mori radicis, 9 gm; Radix stemonae, 9 gm; Radix peucedani, 9 gm; Radix trichosanthes, 15 gm; Radix clematidis, 9 gm; and Radix glycyrrhizae, 6 gm.

Third consultation on February 24, 1986: The patient reported that she was still coughing. She had been coughing up yellow and dark phlegm especially in the morning. Her throat was still dry but not sore. She was still thirsty and very tired. Her tongue still had a thick dry yellow coat which appeared to be peeling. Her pulse was thin and wiry. It had become obvious that the phlegm retained in the lung was persistent and phlegm-expelling herbs were needed in a further modification. Modification: five doses. Flos lonicerae, 9 gm; Cortex mori radicis, 9 gm; Radix peucedani, 9 gm; Radix stemoniae, 9 gm; Bulbus fritillariae cirrhosae, 9 gm; Semen sinapsis albae, 9 gm; and Radix scrophulariae, 15 gm.

Fourth consultation on September 21, 1987: The patient returned to the clinic one and a half years later complaining of shortness of breath and palpitation in stressful situations. She reported that she had not had a cold or cough since taking the doses of herbs prescribed on February 24, 1986.

DISCUSSION: The success of this treatment lay in the vigorous method of resolving persistent phlegm. Cortex mori radicis, Radix peucedani, Semen sinapsis albae and Radix scrophulariae are all herbs that have strong effects in helping the body to expel persistent phlegm. Care was taken in the design of this formula to nourish the Yin and preserve fluids. Radix scrophulariae, Bulbus fritillariae cirrhosae and Radix stemoniae all act in this regard.

(Collator: Brock Haines)

2.2 ACUTE BRONCHITIS
(IMPAIRMENT OF THE LUNG AND YIN
DUE TO WIND HEAT)

Lin Qiucheng and Lin Zhaohui

Fujian Institute of Traditional Chinese Medicine, Fuzhou

Lin Huasheng, 23, male. Date of consultation: April 20, 1987.

CHIEF COMPLAINT: Cough for three weeks.

HISTORY OF PRESENT ILLNESS: Three weeks prior to consultation, the patient felt discomfort in the throat accompanied by dry cough. Three days later the cough became worse and was accompanied by dyspnea. The amount of expectoration was very small. The cough was more severe at night and it disturbed the patient's sleep. He had chills and slight fever, thirst and flushed face, acratia and loss of weight, scanty dark urine and constipation. During the first four days he took SMZ, Bisolvon and Toclase without much effect. He then took She Dang Chuan Bei Mo and Expectoral Syrup of Phenergan for two days but still to no avail. The next four days he took erythromycin and Expectoral Syrup of Man Shan Bai without much relief of the symptoms. After these attempts, he was treated with amoxycillin and amikacin for four days, but the cough still did not abate. The patient subsequently came for TCM treatment.

PAST HISTORY: Non-contributory.

PERTINENT PHYSICAL EXAMINATION & LABORATORY FINDINGS: Blood pressure, 100/60 mmHg; throat congested, tonsils of normal size. Breath sounds coarse and there were some scattered dry rales. Auscultation of heart was normal. No abdominal tenderness, no palpable viscera or mass. Hemoglobin, 11 gm%; WBC, 11,000/mm^3; neutrophils, 75%; eosinophils, 5%; lymphocytes, 18%; monocytes, 2%. Eosinophilic granulocyte absolute count was 440/mm^3, 35 mm/hr; ASO test, 50 u. Chest X-ray findings of heart and lungs normal.

INSPECTION OF TONGUE: Tongue substance red and coated with a thin yellow fur.

PULSE CONDITION: Floating, slippery and rapid.

MODERN MEDICINE DIAGNOSIS: Acute Bronchitis.

TRADITIONAL CHINESE MEDICINE DIAGNOSIS: Cough with Dyspnea; Wind-Heat Violating the Lung; Deficiency of Lung-Yin.

THERAPEUTIC PRINCIPLES: Clear away Heat and relieve exterior syndrome; facilitate the flow of Lung-Qi to relieve asthma; and invigorate Qi and Yin.

PRESCRIPTION: Modified Decoction of Ephedrae, Apricot kernel, Gypsum and Licorice; Pulse-Activating Decoction. Ephedra, 9 gm; Apricot kernel, 9 gm; Gypsum herba ephedrae, 6 gm; Semen armeniacae, 9 gm; Gypsum fibrosum, 24 gm; Radix pseudostellariae, 15 gm; Flos lonicerae, 15 gm; Fructus forsythiae, 15 gm; Radix ophiopogonis, 19 gm; Radix glycyrrhizae, 15 gm; Radix adenophorae, 15 gm; Radix astragali, 15 gm; Radix stemonae, 15 gm; Herba taraxaci, 15 gm; and Herba houttuyniae, 30 gm. Give one dose immediately.

FOLLOW-UP/COURSE OF TREATMENT:

Second consultation: After administration of the prescription, the patient felt much better at night. The cough lightened, chills and fever subsided and he was able to lie flat in bed. Continued the same prescription for three more days.

Third consultation: The patient only had cough with dyspnea occasionally accompanied by a small amount of white, sticky expectoration as well as constipation. His tongue was red and was coated with a thin fur. Pulse thready and rapid. Modified the prescription to contain Radix pseudostellariae, 15 gm; Radix stemonae, 15 gm; Flos lonicerae, 15 gm; Fructus forsythiae, 15 gm; Herba taraxaci, 15 gm; Herba houttuyniae, 30 gm; Radix glycyrrhizae, 3 gm; Radix astragali, 15 gm; Fructus trichosanthis, 15 gm; Radix rehmanniae, 15 gm; Radix scrophulariae, 15 gm; and Herba violae, 15 gm. After taking three doses of this modified prescription, the patient was completely cured.

2.3 CHRONIC SINUSITIS AND BRONCHIAL ASTHMA (COLD-DAMPNESS IN THE LUNG)

Jean Yu
Santa Barbara College of Oriental Medicine, California, USA

Courtois, 70, female, white, single, retired. Medical record number: 894. Date of first visit: November 9, 1987.

CHIEF COMPLAINT: Coughing bouts for more than sixty years.

HISTORY OF PRESENT ILLNESS: The patient was diagnosed with bronchial asthma and had recurrent sinus infections. She complained of cough with copious white mucus. She had difficulty breathing when lying down and a tight chest. She had a runny nose with red eyes. She reported that she had cold and asthma attacks easily, normally following a common cold in the winter. She suffered from palpitation, from over-medication and from trouble going to sleep and awaking in the night as well as waking up with coughing bouts. She was taking the medications Proventrilo, Theodur, Prednisone and Thyroid. She complained of night sweats, poor hearing and ringing in the ears. She had cold hands and feet and caught cold easily. She did not complain of thirst but drank much water. Her appetite and energy were reported to be low. She had a chronic hiatal hernia. Her stools were dry and with a frequency of bowel movement at two to three times a day. She had frequent urination and woke up to urinate three to four times a night. She had slight edema in her ankles.

PAST HISTORY: Two months previously, the patient had a mastectomy followed by pneumonia. She had been diagnosed as having bronchial asthma at age nine.

INSPECTION OF TONGUE: Reddish body with a deep crack running down the centre and white, thick coat and peeled fur.

PULSE CONDITION: Forceful, slippery and rapid (100/min) in all positions.

MODERN MEDICINE DIAGNOSIS: Chronic Bronchial Asthma; Chronic Sinusitis; Recovery from Surgery and Pneumonia.

TRADITIONAL CHINESE MEDICINE DIAGNOSIS: Cold and Dampness accumulated in the Lung; Qi and Yin Deficiency.

THERAPEUTIC PRINCIPLES: Tonify the Qi and Yin, dry Dampness, and soothe asthma.

PRESCRIPTION: Two doses—each dose taken six times daily. Radix pseudostellariae, 9 gm; Fructus schisandrae, 6 gm; Radix ophiopogonis, 9 gm; Poria cocos, 12 gm; Rhizoma atractylodis macrocephalae, 9 gm; Semen armeniacae amarum, 9 gm; Cortex mori radicis, 9 gm; Radix scutellariae, 9 gm; Folium eriobotryae, 9 gm; Semen raphani, 6 gm; and Radix glycyrrhizae, 6 gm.

FOLLOW-UP/COURSE OF TREATMENT:

Second consultation on November 17, 1987: The patient reported that her sinus infection had improved and there was less nasal mucus and pressure. The cough and amount of phlegm had decreased, but she still had tightness and mucus in the chest. Her energy was still low. Both her appetite and digestion were good. All other symptoms were unchanged. Her tongue was red and peeled and her pulse was wiry and rapid. It was determined that the formula was fairly effective and was modified to dispel the phlegm in the Lung more vigorously and to cool the Liver. Modification: three doses. Folium mori, 9 gm; Flos chrysanthemi, 9 gm; Radix ophiopogonis, 9 gm; Radix glehnia, 9 gm; Semen armeniacae amarum, 9 gm; Poria cocos, 12 gm; Cortex mori radicis, 9 gm; Bulbus fritillariae cirrhosae, 9 gm; Pericarpium trichosanthes, 9 gm; and Radix glycyrrhizae, 6 gm.

Third consultation on November 23, 1987: The patient reported that the asthma had improved and phlegm had decreased. She was still coughing up white mucus in the morning. The patient's sinus infection had entirely cleared up. Her eyes were still red and she complained of palpitation. Her pulse was irregular and slippery and her tongue red on the sides and top and peeled.

DISCUSSION: The patient presented a large number of symptoms and as such was a complicated diagnostic case. In this case it was determined that the root and branch of the disorders be treated together. As the patient was recovering from surgery and pneumonia, it was important to nourish the Yin and Qi and to produce fluids in the body. At the same time, Dampness in the Lung system needed to be expelled. Radix glehnia nourishes the Yin and is an expectorant. Radix ophiopogonis and Fructus schisandrae also nourish the Yin. Radix ophiopogonis soothes the Lung and the Heart in addition. Fructus schisandrae nourishes Qi and nourishes the Lung and Kidney as well as produces fluids and astringes sweat. Semen armeniacae amarum and Folium eriobotryae are antiasthmatics and antitussives. Radix scutellariae and Semen raphani are antibacterial herbs with special effects on bacteria that invade the Lung. Poria and Rhizoma atractylodis macrocephalae tonify the Middle by drying or dispelling Dampness. Folium mori clears away Heat in the Liver and benefits the Lung. Obviously, this patient will need long-term nourishment of both her Qi and Yin as well as pacification of the spirit in subsequent treatments.

(Collator: Brock Haines).

2.4 RADIOACTIVE PNEUMONIA (COUGH)

Zhang Daizhao
Sino-Japanese Friendship Hospital, Beijing

Zhen, 49, female, Han nationality, married, engineer. Medical record number: 146913. Date of first consultation: May 25, 1981.
CHIEF COMPLAINT: Severe cough of two months duration.
HISTORY OF PRESENT ILLNESS: The patient discovered a 2 × 3 cm mass at

the upper part of her right breast which was later diagnosed to be adenocarcinoma of the breast. Radical mastectomy was performed on September 21, 1980. Histology report of the resected mass was "adenocarcinoma, right breast, with metastasis to five-eighths of lymph node in the right axilla." After the operation, the patient received 18-day radiotherapy course with a total amount of DT4,000, DT4,000 and DT5,800 rads to right clavicular, sternal and right axillary regions, respectively. She also had four courses of chemotherapy on January 9, 1981, including TSPA and Endoxan. A nodule with a diameter of 0.5 cm was noted later at the third intercostal space, right sternal border. In addition, a broad, bean-shaped lymph node, hard and fixed, was palpated on the right clavicular region. Considering this as lymph node metastasis, a second course of radiotherapy was administered from January 28 to March 17, 1981. During the course of radiotherapy, radiation at the dosage of DT6,000 and DT5,500 rads were delivered to the right clavicular region and the sternum, respectively. To each of the two nodules by the sternum, a dosage of DT4,000 rads was also administered. Upon completion of the radiotherapy course in mid-March, the patient began to experience severe bouts of unproductive cough accompanied by low-grade fever, fatigue and shortness of breath. Condition got worse in early May; the cough was more severe with a small amount of yellowish and thick sputum. The patient also felt thirsty and had a low-grade fever. X-ray examination of lungs done immediately in the hospital revealed radioactive pneumonia in both lungs, with the right lung more serious than the left one. The patient received a therapeutic regimen consisting of hormones and antibiotics (penicillin and erythromycin) which proved to be ineffective. She was subsequently referred to our clinic by the radiotherapist.

PAST HISTORY: Non-contributory.

PERTINENT PHYSICAL EXAMINATION & LABORATORY FINDINGS: Temperature between 37.5°C and 38°C; right chest wall s/p mastectomy; skin of the radiated region dry, brawny, indurated and with pigmentation. Increased breath sounds, overall dry and moist rales at the bases appreciated on both lungs. Chest X-ray examination indicated radioactive pneumonia in both lungs, of which the right lung was more serious. ESR, 74 mm/hr; WBC, 8,800/mm³; neutrophil, 78%.

INSPECTION OF TONGUE: Tongue proper deep red with yellow, thin and sticky coating.

PULSE CONDITION: Thready and rapid.

MODERN MEDICINE DIAGNOSIS: Adenocarcinoma of Breast; Partial Recurrence after Right Radical Mastectomy; Metastasis of Lymph Node on Right Clavicle; Radioactive Pneumonia.

TRADITIONAL CHINESE MEDICINE DIAGNOSIS: Right Breast Cancer; Nucleus of Spit; Cough.

Symptom-complex differentiation: The patient coughs with a little yellowish sputum. She experiences shortness of breath on minimum physical exertion. She often runs a fever between 38°C and 38.5°C. She also complains of pain in the right breast, thirst and sweating. Other accompanying symptoms are de-regulated pulse condition, deep-red tongue proper with yellowish and thin sticky coating. These clinical manifestations indicate progressive, excessive consumption of Yin of the Lung and Stomach after radiotherapy. Therapeutic principles would be to eliminate the Evil Heat and clear off the harmful pathogens by nourishing and reinforcing the Vital Energy and the Lung as well as restoring the taste. The most important therapeutic approach is to invigorate Blood circulation and to alleviate pain.

PRESCRIPTION: Lonicera japonica thunb, 30 gm; Coptis chinensis, 6 gm; Clelmia littoralis, 30 gm; Ophiopogon japonicus, 12 gm; Phragmites communis, 30 gm; Citrus reticulate blanco, 10 gm; Lilium lancifolium thunb, 12 gm (decocted in small package); Glycyrrhizae uralensis fisch, 6 gm; and Panas pseudo-ginseng powder, 3 gm (taken after mixing with water).

FOLLOW-UP/COURSE OF TREATMENT:

Second consultation on January 8, 1981: Symptoms of fever, severe cough, shortness of breath alleviated markedly. She had a better appetite, though still with symptoms of dry stool, yellowish tongue coating, deep-red tongue proper and thready and rapid pulse. Modified previous prescription by adding 30 gm of Trichosanthes Kirilowii Maxim. Fourteen doses. Yang Yin Qing Fei Extract was also prescribed (two tablespoonfuls per day, one in the morning and the other in the evening).

Physical examinations were done during the period from June 22 to July 22, 1981. Significant findings were disappearance of all rales and an ESR reading of 23 mm/hr.

Re-examination by X-ray showed that radioactive pneumonia in lungs had disappeared almost completely and the patient was near complete recovery. She occasionally complained of cough and felt thirsty. Red tongue proper with yellowish coating and rapid pulse was also noted. The prescription was to be continued in order to maintain the therapeutic effect.

As the incidence of breast cancer increases, so will cases of radiotherapy to breast leading to a concurrent increase in the incidence of radioactive fibrosis and radioactive pneumonia. Moreover, in recent years, some cancer patients are treated by both radiotherapy and chemotherapy which tend to damage the Lung. At present, the incidence of this illness is still regarded as one of the complications of radiotherapy of breast cancer which is difficult to control.

Nowadays, modern medicine usually treats the disease by means of antibiotics, antiprothrombin and other medicines. This leads to a less than satisfactory result since these medicines are used on a trial-and-error basis.

Chinese medicine determines the treatment according to various conditions, including pathogenesis and consequent symptoms. Those symptoms are interpreted as secondary to invasion by evil heat factor.

Disturbance of the Spleen and Stomach, stasis of Vital Energy and Blood and damage of body fluid, all lead to what modern medicine sees as fibrosis of lungs with exudative inflammation. Four therapeutic principles are employed to eliminate the Heat and clear away the harmful factors, namely, to nourish the Lung and Yin, to strengthen the Stomach and Spleen, to invigorate Blood circulation and to eliminate venous stasis.

The prescription is made up of these medicinal herbs: Lonicera japonica thunb, Scutellaria baicalensis georgi, Coptis chinensis, Houttuynia cordate thunb, Taraxacum mongolicum Hand and other herbs to eliminate Heat and clear away harmful factors;

Clelmia littoralis, Asparagus cochinchinensis, Phragmites communis, Eriogotrya ja-ponica, Lilium lancifolium thunb and others to promote body fluid and moisturize the dryness; Atractylodes macrocephalae, Gallus domesticus, Citrus reticulata blanco and others to regulate the function of the Spleen and Stomach; Panax notoginseng, Paeonia lacitiflora pall, Allium macrostemon bge and Gurcuma aromatica salisb to facilitate the elimination of venous stasis and relieve pain.

This prescription has been proven effective in clinical practice. In our experience, it is also effective in disease prevention. In other words, patients should take the prescription one or two months before undergoing radiotherapy. Should traditional medicine treatment be started only after the damage of radiation, i.e., when radioactive pneumonia has settled in, the therapeutic effect would not have been as remarkable as if the prescription were administered beforehand.

2.5 ACUTE EXACERBATION OF COR PULMONALE (GASPING COUGH)

Gao Chiyan, He Qichang and Lin Qingxing
Xiamen Traditional Chinese Medicine Hospital, Xiamen

Su, 63, male, Han nationality, married, cadre. Medical record number: 155. Date of first consultation: March 2, 1975.

CHIEF COMPLAINT: Chronic cough for more than 20 years, exacerbated in the last two weeks.

HISTORY OF PRESENT ILLNESS: The patient suffered from chronic cough for more than 20 years which worsened during cold seasons. Two months prior to admission, he sought medical advice because of common cold, fever and cough (about 60-70 ml of sputum were coughed up each day) and was treated with antibiotics (penicillin, streptomycin, erythromycin, doxycycline, TMP and gentamicin, etc.), cough mixture and corticosteroids but his condition did not improve. Two weeks prior to admission, these symptoms gradually took a turn for the worse. The cough was productive with yellowish and viscous sputum accompanied by panting, palpitation, low-grade fever, vertigo, abdominal distention, anorexia, scanty urine and urinary frequency, loose stools, edema of lower extremities and inability to lie flat. He was subsequently admitted to this hospital.

PAST HISTORY: The patient has been smoking about 20 cigarettes a day since his youth and often had symptoms of cough and shortness of breath lasting for several months which was not responsive to antibiotics treatment. Positive history of hyper-tension. Had typhoid fever when he was a boy.

PERTINENT PHYSICAL EXAMINATION & LABORATORY FINDINGS: Temperature, 37.8°C; pulse rate, 102/min; respiratory rate, 22/min; blood pressure, 170/120 mmHg. Fair development and nutritional status, exomorphic, conscious, shortness of breath aggravated by physical exertion, in semi-Fowler's position. Purplish lips. No enlarged lymph nodes. Slightly distended neck veins. Vague heart sounds, arrythmia with occasional premature beats; no murmur appreciated; A2 = P2. Diminished breath sounds with clear shrilling sounds; moist rales audible at bilateral lung bases. Abdomen soft; pulsation visible on upper abdomen. Upper limit of the liver on seventh intercostal space and lower limit 1.5 cm below right costal margin; medium-size liver without obvious tenderness and percussion pain. No ascites, slight edema of the lower extremities. Chest X-ray examination revealed hilar shadow on both lungs with accentuated lung markings; severe pulmonary emphysema; pendulous heart and slight protruding arch of aorta. ECG findings: low voltage on limb leads, clockwise, low and smooth T wave in V5. Pulmonary function test finding: severely reduced. Ultrasonic electrocardiogram shows flowing passageway of right ventricle; internal diameter of lift atrium = 1.4 Hemoglobin, 13.2 gm%; WBC, 5,100/mm^3; neutrophils, 73%; lymphocytes, 24%; eosinophils, 3%. Sputum culture shows positive growth of Bacillus aeruginosa, Neisseria coccus, Hemophilia bacillus and Staphylococcus. Bacteria sensitivity test: colonies insensitive or slightly sensitive to penicillin, streptomycin, chloromycetin, erythromycin, doxycycline, sulfa and gentamycin. Immunity test: Erythrocyte antibody complement rosette forming cell, 35.5% (normal value 56.2%); Lymphocyte changing rate, 48% (normal value 58.6%). Liver function test basically normal. Serum cholesterol, 302 mg%; triglycerides, 46 mg%; sputum examination: neutral white blood cell (+++). Degree of damage of ciliated epithelial columns (+). Special necrotic cells (+). DNA density 0.3104 mg/ml.

INSPECTION OF TONGUE: Dark and gloomy, enlarged with tooth marks; yellowish, glossy and thick coating.

PULSE CONDITION: Slippery and rapid.

MODERN MEDICINE DIAGNOSIS: Chronic Bronchitis with Pulmonary Emphysema; Acute Exacerbation of Cor Pulmonale.

TRADITIONAL CHINESE MEDICINE DIAGNOSIS: Gasping Cough (Deficiency of the Heart, Lung, Spleen and Kidney and External Affections of Heat, Edema Type).

THERAPEUTIC PRINCIPLES: Dissipate the Heat and detoxify, eliminate the Phlegm and control the panting, strengthen the Spleen and enhance diuresis, eliminate the stagnation and activate the Blood.

PRESCRIPTION: Modified Retan Tang. Flos lonicerae, 15 gm; Fructus forsythiae, 15 gm; Semen armeniacae, 10 gm; Rhizoma pinelliae, 9 gm; Radix paeoniae rubra, 9 gm; Radix salviae, 9 gm; Radix scutellariae, 9 gm; Herba houttuyniae, 15 gm; Folium isatidis, 9 gm; Semen plantaginis, 15 gm; Radix adenophorae, 15 gm; Poria, 15 gm; and Herba taraxaci, 15 gm. Five doses.

Concurrent administration of low flow O_2 and a small dose of regitine, IV drip for three days.

FOLLOW-UP/COURSE OF TREATMENT:

Second consultation on March 9, 1975: After being treated by the combination of traditional Chinese and modern medicine for five days, the patient's symptoms showed signs of improvement. Daily sputum production reduced to 40 to 50 ml and could be coughed up. Signs of panting also improved but the sputum was still viscous and purulent. The patient complained of restless sleep and increased urine output. Physical examination showed small amount of moist rales audible on the back lower side of the lungs. Lower limit of the liver is 1.5 cm below right costal margin. Edema on lower extremities relieved. Tongue proper red in colour, slightly dark purplish on two sides with yellowish and glossy coating. Rapid pulse. These symptoms indicated that the exterior syndrome has not been cleared. Continued applying the principles of eliminating the Phlegm and clearing away the Heat, strengthening the Spleen and controlling the panting. Prescription: Flos lonicerae, 15 gm; Rhizoma pinelliae, 9 gm; Radix scrutellariae, 9 gm; Radix salviae, 15 gm; Herba taraxaci, 15 gm; Herba houttuyniae, 15 gm; Poria, 15 gm; Radix stemonae, 15 gm; Radix isatidis, 15 gm; and Pericarpium citri reticulatae, 9 gm. Four decoctions.

Third consultation on March 14, 1975: Daily sputum output reduced to 30 ml but it was still yellowish and viscous. The signs of panting improved markedly and body temperature was normal. Neck vein distention reduced. Moist rales on the back lower side of the lungs and the edema of the lower extremities also reduced significantly. The patient's appetite was getting better and he could lie flat. His tongue was red with slightly yellowish coating and pulse changed from rapid to slow, which indicates that phlegm and heat had not been completely cleared away. Therapeutic principles to follow are those of eliminating the Phlegm and clearing away the Heat, strengthening the Spleen and dispelling the Dampness. Prescription: Flos lonicerae, 15 gm; Rhizoma pinelliae, 6 gm; Herba taraxaci, 15 gm; Herba houttuyniae, 15 gm; Radix scutellariae, 9 gm; Folium isatidis, 15 gm; Radix adenophorae, 12 gm; Pericarpium citri reticulatae, 6 gm; Semen persicae, 9 gm; and Radix glycyrrhizae, 3 gm. Four decoctions.

Fourth consultation on March 19, 1975: The cough was alleviated markedly and production of white, mucous phlegm was about 20 ml per day. Slight shortness of breath. Sound sleep and increased appetite. Neck veins no longer distended and pulmonary breath sounds only slightly lowered with occasional dry rales appreciated. Lower border of liver still 1.5 cm below the right costal margin. Light red tongue substance with white, thin coating and tooth marks. Pulse slow. Phlegm had not been cleared away completely though the transport function of the Spleen had recovered. Applied the principle of eliminating the Phlegm and clearing away the Heat, moisturizing the Lung and strengthening the Spleen. Prescription: Flos lonicerae, 15 gm; Herba taraxaci, 15 gm; Herba houttuyniae, 15 gm; Radix stemonae, 15 gm; Rhizoma dioscoreae, 15 gm; Fructus trichosanthis, 15 gm; Radix adenophorae, 12 gm; Bulbus fritillariae cirrhosae, 9 gm; Pericarpium citri reticulatae, 6 gm; and Radix glycyrrhizae, 3 gm.

Fifth consultation on March 24, 1975: The patient coughed only occasionally. Daily phlegm output reduced to less than 10 ml of white and viscous sputum which was coughed up easily. There were no signs of panting. Shortness of breath occurred only when the patient engaged in physical activity. Normal appetite and sound sleep. Slightly lowered breath sound, no rales appreciated. Lower border of the liver was 1.5 cm below the right costal margin without tenderness. No edema of the lower extremities. Chest X-ray examination showed increased lung markings with moderate degree of pulmonary emphysema and slightly protruding aortic arch. Pendulous heart. ECG showed clockwise configuration, low and smooth T wave in V_5 and lay-up position test of ECG negative. Pulmonary function tests: moderately reduced. Routine blood examination normal. Sputum culture showed positive growth of Neisseria coccus (+). Tongue substance light-red with thin, white coating. Pulse slow. The Biao (apparent manifestations) of this disease had been cured basically and the patient was treated with Gu Ben Pill (Ingredients: Radix aconiti praeparatae, Fructus psoraleae, Radix angelicae, Radix paeoniae rubra, Radix salviae, Radix adenophorae, Rhizoma ligustici, Fructus schizandrae, Radix rehmanniae, Cortex cinnamomi, Fructus lycii, Semen cuscutae, Radix astragali, Cortex phellodendri, etc.) for consolidation of therapeutic effects. The patient was back to work daily.

DISCUSSION: Respiratory tract infection is the primary cause of acute exacerbation of cor pulmonale. Severe cases of these acute episodes could be fatal. To treat it early with an anti-infection regimen is the key to increasing therapeutic efficacy and to decreasing mortality. In this particular case, in which the patient suffered from the illness for more than 20 years, his condition often broke out during cold seasons or secondary to sudden climate change. During the initial stage of the illness, he was treated with antibiotics and therapies for symptomatic relief for about two months, but no satisfactory results were obtained. Meanwhile, his condition worsened day by day and heart failure started to appear.

It is common knowledge that because of extensive application of antibiotics, many clinics are exposed to problems such as decreased therapeutic effect and occurrence of side effects. With long-term and extensive application of antibiotics, for instance, it becomes difficult to identify the pathogenic bacteria or virus of pulmonary infections, resulting in many cases where antibiotics have to be used in a blind attempt to control the acute attack of cor pulmonale. Such a practice will inevitably lead to dissociation of bacteria groups and cross infections making the infections more difficult to treat while the resistance of the bacteria to the antibiotics keeps getting stronger. In addition, most patients who suffer from cor pulmonale are of bad nutritional status. Extensive application of antibiotics may cause a decreased appetite and hinders the synthesis of body protein and metabolism of nucleic acids leading to lowered body immune defenses and, indirectly, to damage of the patient's Zheng Qi (Primordial Principal). These problems seriously affect the therapeutic effect and efficacy assessment of antibiotics that are being used for treating cor pulmonale nowadays. Such a situation was evident in our case. The patient was treated by various kinds of antibiotics for about two months with no satisfactory effects, while his condition worsened day by day.

Through deduction by the Four Methods of Diagnosis, the patient was diagnosed to have gasping cough (deficiency of the Heart, Lung, Spleen, Kidney, external affection of Heat, edema type). Putting the infection under control was the key to the success of treatment in this case. All antibiotics that had been used so far were discontinued after the patient was admitted and large amounts of herbal medications capable of dissipating Heat and detoxifying were used combined with regimens to control panting, eliminate Phlegm, strengthen the Spleen, dispel the Dampness, eliminate stagnation and activate Blood. In addition, short-term, low-volume O_2 administration coupled with systemic administration of vasodilator rigitine ensured a satisfactory outcome of the course of treatment.

In this case, the patient had deficiency of the Viscera and Primordial Principals and thus was extremely vulnerable to invasion by exogenous pathogens. Pathogens invading the Lung cause impaired circulation of pulmonary Qi and obstruction of the flow of Vital Energy. The result of this is gasping cough. Because of insufficiency of Primordial Principals and protracted existence of pathogens, the stasis was transformed into Heat and accumulation of this pathogenic Heat damaged the Jin Qi. This pathogenesis was manifested clinically as coughing up yellowish and turbid phlegm and inability to lie flat. This Heat also damaged the Spleen causing a deficiency of Splenic Qi which compromises its transportation functions.

Unable to be transformed into Jin, the stagnant material secondary to this transport dysfunction could be seen clinically as large amounts of phlegm, indigestion and loss of appetite, epigastric distress, abdominal distention and increasing internal accumulation of Dampness. Aqueous Qi affecting the Heart caused palpitation; water being transported downward was not able to be metabolized by the Kidney, leading to internal accumulation of water as manifested by scanty urine and progressive general anasarca. In view of these symptoms, Ben, which was in deficiency in this case, had to be reinforced and strengthened, while Biao needed immediate attention. Following the teaching of "cutting off all means of retreat," the priority of treatment was to control the internal transformation of pathogenic Heat and this was accomplished by applying herbal recipes which are capable of dissipating Heat and detoxifying the body. By selecting appropriate herbs based on analysis of the Four Methods of Diagnosis, the patient's condition improved day by day. The main symptom of gasping cough was put under control quickly. Finally, using Gu Ben Pill to reinforce body resistance from Yin to Yang, from excess to deficiency, the patient was able to recover his health and went back to his job.

The Heat-dissipating and detoxifying recipe used in this case was a kind of preparation for the treatment of fever toxins. Through clinical and laboratory experience in the past several years, it has been shown to have a very strong effect on combating bacteria and virus. At the same time, it is effective in improving blood circulation and increasing body resistance to disease. Therefore, it is appropriate to discontinue all antibiotics during the initial stage of the illness and apply large doses of Heat-dissipating and detoxifying medications. This was the key to the patient's speedy recovery.

It can be said here that application of large doses of Heat-dissipating and detoxifying medications is indicated in acute attacks of cor pulmonale, but one must also remember that these herbs are all bitter-cold in nature. They are not suitable for symptoms such as Cold and Dampness or deficiency of Yin and Yang. Cor pulmonale is classified as a disease entity with "excess of Biao and deficiency of Ben." These herbs are used primarily to treat the Biao and they play no role in reinforcing the Ben. Accordingly, they should be used in consideration of the patient's condition and supplemented by other medications such as expectorants and antitussives and herbs which replenish the Qi, control the panting, activate the Blood and tonify the Yin to increase therapeutic efficacy.

2.6 CHRONIC OBSTRUCTIVE PULMONARY DISEASE (ACCUMULATION OF PHLEGM AND HEAT IN THE LUNG, DEFICIENCY OF BOTH QI AND YIN)

Lin Qiucheng and Lin Zhaohui
Fujian Institute of Traditional Chinese Medicine, Fuzhou

Zhang Zuyan, 72, female. Date of first consultation: January 11, 1988.

CHIEF COMPLAINT: Chronic cough for 10 years, exacerbated in the last three months.

HISTORY OF PRESENT ILLNESS: For the past 10 years, the patient usually had productive cough in winter seasons. Sometimes it was accompanied by dyspnea. For the last three years prior to admission, the condition became progressively worse. She caught a common cold easily and experienced productive cough and dyspnea for a prolonged period of time. Three months prior to admission, she had a cold again and the cough and dyspnea became worse, the amount of expectoration increased, the sputum was white to yellow and sticky, and it was difficult to be expectorated. The cough was more severe at night and it prevented the patient from lying flat in bed. She also complained of dry mouth, constipation, scanty dark urine, palpitation, loss of appetite and weight, acratia, lassitude, weakness in loin and legs and cold extremities. She was treated by SMZ c.o., IV cephalosporin, gentamycin, medemycin, kanamycin, spiramycin, Expectoral Syrup of Phenergan, Bisolvon, Toclase, aminophylline and ketontiphen, but they afforded no relief. Modified Decoction of Three Kinds of Seeds for the Aged was used, but the patient still did not feel better.

PAST HISTORY: The patient was a smoker for twenty years and stopped smoking three years before being admitted. For the last year, the patient felt chest distress, palpitation and dyspnea; she sought medical advice in the Provincial Hospital and was diagnosed as having suspicious coronary heart disease.

PERTINENT PHYSICAL EXAMINATION & LABORATORY FINDINGS: Slightly cyanotic. Hyper-resonance on chest percussion. There were a few sticky rales appreciated at both lung bases, and some scattered wheezes. Hepatojugular reflex positive. Hemoglobin, 14 gm%; WBC, 8,000/mm³; neutrophils, 82%; lymphocytes, 16%; monocytes, 1% and eosinophils, 1%. Pulmonary function test: RV/LTC, 47%; FEV1/FVC, 50%; MBC, 54%. Chest X-ray examination showed pulmonary emphysema. ECG: frontal average electricity axis 100; voltage of P wave 2.5 mV.

INSPECTION OF TONGUE: Bright red tongue proper with thin, yellowish fur. Venous engorgement at the back of tongue.

PULSE CONDITION: Thready and rapid. Chi pulse weak.

MODERN MEDICINE DIAGNOSIS: Chronic Obstructive Pulmonary Disease.

TRADITIONAL CHINESE MEDICINE DIAGNOSIS: Cough with Dyspnea; Accumulation of Phlegm and Heat in the Lung; Deficiency of both Qi and Yin.

THERAPEUTIC PRINCIPLES: Remove Heat from the Lung and dissolve the Phlegm, replenish the Qi and nourish the Yin.

PRESCRIPTION: Modified Decoction for Keeping Pure the Lung and Dissolving Phlegm. Fructus trichosanthes, 15 gm; Rhizoma pinelliae, 6 gm; Pericarpium citri reticulatae, 5 gm; Radix astragali, 15 gm; Radix pseudostellariae, 15 gm; Radix salviae 15 gm; Radix scutellariae, 10 gm; Fructus forsythiae, 12 gm; Radix adenophorae, 15 gm; Herba taraxaci, 20 gm; Herba violae, 20 gm; and Herba houttuyniae, 24 gm.

FOLLOW-UP/COURSE OF TREATMENT: The patient felt much better after intake of this prescription; cough and dyspnea had obviously alleviated, amount of expectoration had reduced markedly, but she still had acratia and loss of appetite. Her tongue was red with little fur, pulse thready and weak. Continued the same prescription adding Fructus crataegi, 15 gm, and Fructus hordei germinatus, 15 gm. One dose every day for six days.

Third consultation: The patient recovered almost fully from the condition after taking the modified prescription. Administration discontinued for one week. Weather of the last two days was rather cold and the patient had chills, fever, nasal discharge, sore throat and slight cough again. Her tongue was red and was coated with a slightly yellowish fur. Her pulse was thready and rapid. Signs and symptoms indicated a common cold of Wind-Heat type. Modified Powder of Lonicera, Fructus forsythiae, 15 gm; Flos lonicerae, 15 gm; Herba lophatheri, 6 gm; Spica schizonepetae, 6 gm; Fructus arctii, 10 gm; Herba mentae, 3 gm; Rhizoma phragmitis, 30 gm; Radix glycyrrhizae, 3 gm; Radix astragali, 20 gm; Herba houttuyniae, 30 gm; and Rhizoma polygonati odorati, 15 gm. One dose every day for three days.

Fourth consultation: The cold was completely cured after taking the above prescription. The patient still complained of palpitation, dyspnea, acratia, loss of appetite, night sweating, spontaneous perspiration, dizziness and tinnitus. Her tongue was red with little fur, pulse thready and weak. TCM diagnosis was Qi and Yin Deficiency of the Lung, Spleen and Kidney. Prescription: Radix astragali, 20 gm; Radix pseudostellariae, 15 gm; Poria, 12 gm; Radix codonopsis, 15 gm; Rhizoma atractylodis macrocephalae, 9 gm; Radix glycyrrhizae, 3 gm; Radix ophiopogonis, 15 gm; Fructus schisandrae, 6 gm; Fructus psoraleae, 10 gm; Concha ostreae, 30 gm; and Semen cuscutae, 15 gm. One dose everyday for 10 days.

Follow-up three months after discharge showed no relapse of the symptoms.

2.7 LUNG CANCER
(FEIJI, COUGH)

Yu Rencun

Department of Oncology, Beijing Traditional Chinese Medicine Hospital, Beijing

Gao Wenbin, 58, male, married, cadre. Medical record number: Z167. Date of first consultation: September 6, 1976.
CHIEF COMPLAINT: Cough, chest pain and sweating one week after exploratory

thoracotomy.

HISTORY OF PRESENT ILLNESS: Three months prior to consultation, the patient experienced discomfort and had cough similar to that which accompanies a common cold. A shadow in the right lung was discovered by X-ray examination on July 19, 1976, and a middle lobar atelectasis of the right lung was seen by X-ray one week later. Bronchoscopy was performed the next day. Granulation tissues in the middle lobe of the right lung were detected and biopsy histology report was adenocarcinoma of the lung. Exploratory thoracotomy of the right lung was performed on August 31, 1976, at the PLA General Hospital. Operation findings were old TB foci in the apical segment of upper lobe of the right lung and middle lobe of the right lung adhesive to pericardium. Metastasis to the hilar lymph nodes (middle and lower lobes) evident. The mass was hard. After freeing the arteries and veins of the upper lobe, it was discovered that there were hard metastatic lymph nodes on retrotracheal bronchi and under the carina tracheae. They adhered tightly to the retrotracheal wall as well as extending to the left mediastinum, so it was difficult to determine the borders of the lesion. Because of extensive metastases of pulmonary hilar and mediastinum lymph nodes, surgical resection was abandoned since the lesion could not be removed completely. To prepare the patient for radiotherapy, stainless steel markers were placed on the surface of the lymph nodes.

Seven days after the operation, the patient developed cough, chest pain and profuse sweating during physical activity. Appetite was poor and he complained of pain on surgical wound.

PAST HISTORY: Stomach ailment of more than 20 years. Positive history of abdominal distention, hypotension, anemia, malnutrition and pneumonia, A smoker for more than 20 years, the patient gave up the habit in 1963. CRBBB was found by ECG in 1973.

INSPECTION OF TONGUE: Pale tongue proper with tooth marks, thin and whitish fur.

PULSE CONDITION: Thready, slippery and slightly rapid.

MODERN MEDICINE DIAGNOSIS: Bronchial Adenocarcinoma, Middle Lobe of Right Lung; Lymph Node Metastasis, Right Hilus and Mediastinum; Atelectasis, Middle Lobe of Right Lung; S/P Exploratory Thoracotomy, Right Lung.

TRADITIONAL CHINESE MEDICINE DIAGNOSIS: Feiji, Cough.

THERAPEUTIC PRINCIPLES: Replenish the Qi and consolidate the external resistance, reduce Phlegm and resolve masses.

PRESCRIPTION: Radix astragali, 30 gm; Rhizoma atractylodis, 10 gm; Radix ledebouriellae, 10 gm; Radix adenophorae, 15 gm; Os draconis, 30 gm; Concha ostreae, 30 gm; Radix peucedani, 12 gm; Folium eriobotryae, 10 gm; Fructus aristolochiae, 10 gm; Bulbus fritillariae, 10 gm; Fructus schisandrae, 10 gm; and Spica pranella, 15 gm.

FOLLOW-UP/COURSE OF TREATMENT:

Second consultation on September 13, 1976: After taking the first recipe the patient had less phlegm, less sweat, better appetite but with the same tongue and pulse conditions. Continued the same prescription. Removed Seng Ba Ye (loquat leaf) from the first recipe and added Zi Yuan (Root of tataruan aster), 12 gm; Ban Zhi Lian (Herb of barbed skullcap), 30 gm; and Bai Hua She Cao (Herb of spreading heduyotis), 30 gm.

Fourth consultation on September 27, 1976: The patient had received seven doses of radiotherapy. Each dose was 200 rads. His appetite was poor and he coughed a little. The tongue was reddish with tooth marks, tongue fur thin and white. Thready and slippery pulse. To act in synergy with radiotherapy, therapeutic principles employed were to strengthen the Spleen, replenish the Kidney, reduce the phlegm and resolve the masses. Prescription: Radix astragali, 30 gm; Radix codonopsis, 15 gm; Rhizoma atractylodis, 10 gm; Poria, 12 gm; Radix asparagi, 15 gm; Fructus ligustri, 15 gm; Semen cuscutae, 10 gm; Caulis spatholobi, 30 gm; Bulbus fritillariae, 10 gm; Folium pyrrosiae, 30 gm; Herba scutellariae, 30 gm; Radix peucedani, 12 gm; and Spica prunellae, 15 gm.

Seventh consultation on October 18, 1976: During the course of radiotherapy, the patient felt sensation of heat on the palms and increased frequency of nocturia. Bowel movement was normal. Light-reddish tongue with tooth marks. Thready, slippery and rapid pulse. Replaced Radix asparagi, Radix peucedani, Spica prunellae and Folium pyrrosiae with the following herbs: Radix adenophorae, 15 gm; Rhizoma rehmanniae et praeparatae, 10 gm; Radix salviae, 15 gm; Semen eryales, 12 gm; Caulis polygoni multiflori, 30 gm; and Fructus alpiniae oxyphyllae, 12 gm.

Consultation on November 15, 1976: Course of radiotherapy (Co_{60} with accelerator) was completed with a total dosage of 7,000 rads delivered. There were no severe side effects. The patient still experienced sensation of heat on palms and had restless sleep. Light-reddish tongue with tooth marks. Whitish and thin fur. Pulse deep, thready and slippery (left); taut and slippery (right). Since radiotherapy exhausts the Qi and Yin, therapy was modified to replenish the Qi and nourish the Yin and detoxicating together with measures to strengthen the body resistance and combat the cancer. Radix adenophorae, 15 gm; Rhizoma rehmanniae, 10 gm; Radix astragali, 30 gm; Caulis spatholobi, 30 gm; Fructus lycii, 12 gm; Fructus ligustri lucidi, 30 gm; Radix sophora subprostratae, 15 gm; Herba scutellariae barbatae, 30 gm; Bulbus fritillariae, 10 gm; Fructus trichosanthis, 30 gm; Semen persicae, 10 gm; Radix peucedani, 12 gm; Herba solani nigri, 30 gm; and Semen ziziphi spinosae, 15 gm.

From December 20, 1976, to April 1977, the patient had a cold with fever and radiation penumonitis which was successfully treated with antibiotics and traditional Chinese medications. A course of chemotherapy was started using 5-FudR, 1.0 gm, every other day for a total of 20 gm. In addition, 80 mg of CCNU were given orally. During the course of chemotherapy, the patient took traditional Chinese medications and the toxic effects of chemotherapy were not severe. The course of chemotherapy was uneventful.

The patient was re-examined on April 11, 1976. General condition was good. So were his appetite and spirits. Light reddish tongue with tooth marks. Thready, slippery and slightly rapid pulse. To consolidate the therapeutic effects, continued the principles of strengthening the Spleen and replenishing the Qi and detoxicating and resolving masses. Radix astragali, 20 gm; Radix codonopsis, 15 gm; Rhizoma dioscoreae, 18 gm; Rhizoma atractylodis, 10 gm; Rhizoma pinelliae, 12 gm; Sargassum, 10 gm; Bulbus fritillariae, 10 gm; Herba lobeliae radicantis, 30 gm; Herba oldenlandiae diffusae, 30 gm; Herba solani nigri, 30 gm; Radix adenophorae, 18 gm; Radix peucedani, 10 gm;

Fructus amomi, 6 gm; Prunellae, 15 gm; and Radix asteris, 10 gm.

Since May 1977, the patient has been practising the New Guolin's Qigong Exercises. He exercised four to five hours every day. He was in better spirits and had greater body strength and appetite. At the same time, he continued to take traditional Chinese medications daily. No recurrence or metastasis was found in annual X-ray examination of the chest. He was able to go back to work in early 1979. ECG examination showed disappearance of CRBBB. From 1980 to 1983, the patient's condition was stable and the same prescription was maintained with minor modifications. Radix astragali, 30 gm; Radix codonopsis, 15 gm; Rhizoma atractylodis, 10 gm; Rhizoma dioscoreae, 10 gm; Herba solani lyrati, 30 gm; Herba solani nigri, 30 gm; Rhizoma zingiberis, 6 gm; Fructus ligustri lucidi, 10 gm; Herba salviae chinensis, 30 gm; and Caulis paulis polygoni multiflori, 30 gm.

From April 1983 to July 1984, the patient experienced occasional increased heart rate and loose stool. Light reddish tongue with tooth marks. Thin and whitish fur. Thready and slippery pulse. Recipes to strengthen the Spleen, replenish the Qi, detoxicate and suppress the cancer were prescribed. Radix ginseng, 5 gm; Radix adenophorae, 30 gm; Radix astragali, 20 gm; Rhizoma atractylodis, 10 gm; Poria, 10 gm; Rhizoma dioscoreae, 10 gm; Bulbus fritillariae, 10 gm; Spica prunellae, 10 gm; Herba oldenlandiae diffusae, 15 gm; Flos chrysanthemi indici, 10 gm; Radix ophiopogonis, 15 gm; Radix thalictri baicalensis, 10 gm; Fructus schisandrae, 10 gm; and Radix pseudostellariae, 30 gm.

In January 1985, a general examination was performed on the patient. ESR, liver function test and renal function test were all normal. Blood glucose level was 132 mg%. C-tides insulin release elevated. He was diagnosed as having non-insulin dependent type of diabetes. X-ray chest examination showed increased bronchovascular shadow as well as pleural thickening of the right chest wall. No cancer cells were detected in sputum smear. Ig level was slightly lower. Ea rosette 24% (normal 46.6±7.6%); Et rosette 29% (normal 59.9±6.9%). ß-type ultrasonic examination showed no abnormality in the abdomen. CBC and routine urinalysis were normal. Twenty-four-hour Holter ECG monitoring detected 42 beats of supraventricular premature beat. The premature beat could be controlled by cardiac medications. The patient continued to take traditional Chinese medications and practised Qigong.

From May 1985 to March 1986, the patient had repeated common colds, cough and two episodes of pulmonary infection. Atelectasis in the middle lobe of the right lung was detected. Inflammation absorbed completely after treatment. Immunological examination: IgM level lowered; C23, 99 mg% (normal 114±54 mg%); total complement, 33.5 u/ml (normal 59.9±6.9%). Lymphoblast transformation rate 50% (normal 51-70%). Therapeutic principles: to strengthen the Spleen and replenish the Kidney, resolve phlegm and control the cough. After the treatment, follow-up showed improvement of immune functions and results of laboratory findings were all within normal limits. Prescription: Radix astragali, 30 gm; Radix pseudostellariae, 30 gm; Poria, 10 gm; Radix adenophorae, 30 gm; Rhizoma atractylodis, 10 gm; Radix asteris, 10 gm; Radix ophiopogonis, 15 gm; Radix codonopsis, 15 gm; Radix platycodi, 10 gm; Pericarpium citri reticulatae, 10 gm; Fructus ligustri lucidi, 15 gm; Fructus lycii, 10 gm; and Herba epimedii, 10 gm. One dose per day.

The last general examination was on October 25, 1986, 10 years and two months after the exploratory thoracotomy. The patient's condition was stable, so was his heart condition. Appetite, stool and urine were normal. Light reddish tongue with whitish and thin fur. Pulse was thready and slippery. No abnormality found in laboratory examinations. Traditional Chinese medicine prescriptions were discontinued.

After his last examination, the patient continued to visit the doctor regularly, once every several months. His general condition was good. His face reddish, his spirits and appetite were good. He insisted on doing Qigong exercises several hours a day. In recent years, because of the successful outcome of his condition, he had been visited by many people who were interested in him sharing his experiences. He has become a model and source of inspiration for people suffering from malignant diseases.

DISCUSSION:

1) The diagnosis of this case is definite bronchial adenocarcinoma in the middle lobe of the right lung. Lymph node metastasis in the right hilus and mediastinum was established by histological examination and surgical exploration. Resection could not be done.

2) The successful outcome of this case is mainly the result of the integration of modern and traditional treatment methods. The patient started to take traditional Chinese medications one week after the operation. The therapy of "strengthening Qi and consolidating external resistance, reducing Phlegm and resolving masses" made him recover from the operation quickly and prepared him for the radiotherapy later.

3) Radiotherapy in this case was successful. This outcome can be attributed to (1) metastatic mediastinal lymph nodes labeled by stainless steel markers during the exploratory thoracotomy which offer an accurate location for delivery of radiation; (2) the taking of traditional Chinese medications, allowing the patient to recover from the operation rapidly and enabling the radiation therapy to take place only two weeks after the operation; (3) the aid of traditional Chinese medications, which are effective in strengthening the Spleen and replenishing the Kidney, promoting blood circulation and replenishing Yin, so that the patient suffered minimum toxic side effects from radiotherapy and received the radical 7,000 rads dosage smoothly; and (4) the radiation acting in synergy with traditional Chinese medications. This proved the advantage of combined modern and traditional Chinese medicine approach. The patient had only one course of chemotherapy (5-FudR and CCNU), whose therapeutic effect in this case is considered to be minimal.

4) The patient is an avid follower of Guolin's Qigong Exercises. Qigong therapy is a whole body therapy and can regulate Yin and Yang, dredge the Channels, promote the exchange of Qi and Blood and promote the metabolic and immunological functions. Physically and psychologically, it played an important role in the patient's recovery. The patient believes, whole-heartedly through his own experience, that this therapy could cure diseases and lead to a long and productive life.

5) The patient insisted on taking traditional Chinese medications for 10 years. At every stage, a recipe was prescribed based on his condition and symptom-complex differentiation. Also in application is the TCM principle of Li Fa Fang Yao. It entails

integration of differentiation and diagnosis, integration of body resistance reinforcement and anti-cancer therapy and integration of local therapy (e.g., radiotherapy) and systemic therapy. Body resistance is strengthened mainly through strengthening the Qi and replenishing the Spleen, nourishing the Yin and replenishing the Kidney. Anti-cancer therapy is achieved by using traditional Chinese herbs which are capable of clearing the Heat and detoxicating, softening hardness and resolving masses, dissolving Phlegm and removing Dampness, promoting Blood circulation and removing Blood stasis, subduing swelling and counteracting toxic substance. For this particular case, traditional Chinese herbs which were used to strengthen the body resistance are: Radix astragali, Radix pseudostellariae, Radix codonopsis, Radix adenophorae, Rhizoma atractylodis, Radix ophiopogonis, Fructus ligustii lucidi, Fructus lycii, Rhizoma dioscoreae, Radix ginseng, Fructus schisandrae ootheca mantidis, Caulis polygoni multiflori, Radix paeoniae alba, Poria, Semen cuscutae, Radix rehmanniae et praeparatae, Herba lophatheri and Fructus apinasae oxyphyllae. Medicinal herbs which have the properties to clear away Heat and toxic materials are: Herba taraxaci, Herba scutellariae barbatae, Herba solani nigri, Flos lonicerae, Herba solani lyrati, Radix sophorae subprostratae, Bulbus fritillariae, Herba houttuyniae, Radix et rhizoma thalictri baicalensis and Radix duchesnear indicae. Those which have the effect of dissolving Phlegm and resolving masses are: Fructus trichosanthis, Rhizoma pinelliae, Semen armeniacae amarum, Pericarpium citri reticulatae, Radix peucedani, Radix asteris, Bombyx batryticatus, Sargassum, Concha ostreae, Radix platycodi, Fructus aristolochiae and Bulbus fritillariae. The herbs effective in promoting Blood circulation and removing Blood stasis are: Semen persicae, Radix paeoniae rubra, lumbricus, Radix salviae, Eupolyphaga seu steleophaga, Hirudo, Caulis spatholobi and Bufo siccus.

6) The patient has a scientific attitude towards the treatment and cooperates well with the doctors. He never uses those "oblique prescriptions" popular in the folklore but rather follows the advice of one doctor from the beginning to the end. He undertakes examinations periodically and strives to maintain bodily and psychological well-being and is rewarded by this most satisfactory outcome.

2.8 LUNG CANCER
(FEIJI)

Yu Rencun

Department of Oncology, Beijing Traditional Chinese Medicine Hospital, Beijing

Zhao, 57, male, Han nationality, married, cadre. Medical record number: Z387. Date of first consultation: March 10, 1981.
CHIEF COMPLAINT: Tiredness, acratia and sweating of one month duration.
HISTORY OF PRESENT ILLNESS: One year prior to admission, because of cold and fever, X-ray chest examination was done and a shadow was discovered. Lung

cancer was suspected but after several bronchoscopy and chest tomography the diagnosis of inflammatory mass was given. The patient was given anti-inflammatory treatment but follow-up X-ray chest examination on December 22, 1980, showed enlargement of the same lung mass. Lung cancer was confirmed after the case was referred to specialists. The patient agreed to undertake left upper lung lobectomy at the PLA General Hospital on January 10, 1981. The surgical procedure was uneventful and post-operative recovery was smooth. Histology of the resected tissues revealed squamous epithelial carcinoma. No metastatic lymph node was found in mediastinum and hilus. The patient started to take traditional Chinese medications prescribed by our clinic. At the time of consultation, the patient complained of fatigue, somnolence, sweating due to debility worsened by physical activity. His appetite was fair. Bowel movement once a day with loose stool. Urination was normal.

PAST HISTORY: A smoker for 40 years, two packs per day. Chronic bronchitis for many years. Positive history of pulmonary tuberculosis.

INSPECTION OF TONGUE: Red in the edges and tip, white fur.

PULSE CONDITION: Thready and slippery.

MODERN MEDICINE DIAGNOSIS: Squamous Epithelial Carcinoma of the Lung; S/P Upper Left Lobectomy; Chronic Bronchitis; TB.

TRADITIONAL CHINESE MEDICINE DIAGNOSIS: Feiji; Qi and Yin Deficiency; Endogenous Toxin and Heat.

THERAPEUTIC PRINCIPLES: Replenish Qi and nourish Yin, clear away endogenous Toxin and Heat.

PRESCRIPTION: Radix astragali, 30 gm; Rhizoma atractylodis macrocephalae, 10 gm; Radix pseudostellariae, 30 gm; Poria, 10 gm; Pericarpium citri reticulatae, 10 gm; Radix adenophorae strictae, 30 gm; Radix ophiopogonis, 10 gm; Fructus schisandrae, 6 gm; Radix arnebiae seu lithospermi, 10 gm; Rhizoma bistortae, 15 gm; Herba salviae chinensis, 20 gm; Herba typhae, 30 gm; Herba scutellariae barbatae, 20 gm; and Herba oldenlandiae diffusae, 3 gm. Fourteen doses.

FOLLOW-UP/COURSE OF TREATMENT:

Second consultation: After taking the above prescription, general condition was better, less sweating, less fatigue, stool was not loose. The patient complained of bitter taste, dry throat, red tongue with yellowish and thin fur. Thready and taut pulse. Therapy was the same as before. Prescription: Radix pseudostellariae, 30 gm; Rhizoma atractylodis macrocephalae, 10 gm; Charred treplet, 30 gm; Radix ophiopogonis, 15 gm; Radix adenophorae, 30 gm; Rhizoma rehmanniae, 15 gm; Herba dendrobii, 10 gm; Herba scutellariae barbatae, 30 gm; Herba oldenlandiae diffusae, 30 gm; Radix scutellariae, 10 gm; Herba salviae chinensis, 20 gm; Herba houttuyniae, 30 gm; and Radix arnebiae seu lithospermi, 10 gm. One dose every day.

June 6, 1981: The patient's general condition was better, but the tongue was still red and its fur yellow-white and greasy. Pulse was thready and slippery, indicating accumulation of endogenous Damp-Heat. Modified the prescription to one that primarily clears away Heat and eliminates Dampness, moisturizes the Lung and resolves the Phlegm. Prescription: Herba artemisiae scopariae, 15 gm; Radix scutellariae, 10 gm; Radix stemonae, 10 gm; Fructus aris tolochinae, 10 gm; Herba houttuyniae, 30 gm; Semen coicis, 15 gm; Herba agastachis, 10 gm; Semen armeniacae amarum, 10 gm; Exocarpium citri grandis, 10 gm; Bulbus fritillariae thunbergii, 10 gm; Radix ophiopogonis, 15 gm; Charred treplet, 30 gm; Rhizoma bistortae, 15 gm; and Herba oldenlandiae diffusae, 30 gm.

September to October 1981: The patient received one course of chemotherapy in the hospital. A regimen consists of CYC, 2,400 mg; MTX, 60 mg and VCR, 4 mg were given. During the course of chemotherapy, serum GPT was elevated. Treated with traditional Chinese medications, no severe toxic side effect of chemotherapy occurred. Upon discharge from the hospital, the patient had normal liver and kidney functions and normal blood picture. However, after chemotherapy, his tongue became red and its fur yellow, thick and greasy. Pulse was thready and slippery, indicating heavy Damp-Heat. As a result, prescription was modified with medicinal herbs which have the effect of removing Dampness by means of aromatic properties as well as addition of those bitter in taste and cold in nature also for the elimination of Dampness. Prescription: Herba artemisiae scopariae, 15 gm; Herba eupatorii, 10 gm; Herba agastachis, 10 gm; Exocarpium citri grandis, 10 gm; Semen armeniacae amarum, 10 gm; Radix scutellariae, 10 gm; Rhizoma coptidis, 3 gm; Radix gentiane, 10 gm; Herba solani nigri, 30 gm; Herba scutellariae barbatae, 30 gm; Radix sophora subprostratae, 10 gm; Rhizoma atractylodis, 30 gm; Rhizoma atractylodis macrocephalae, 30 gm; Charred treplet, 30 gm; Radix adenophorae, 30 gm; and Radix ophiopogonis, 15 gm.

The patient took a total of 120 doses of this prescription, some of them with minor modifications. The signs of Damp-Heat diminished significantly. The tongue turned reddish in colour and the fur changed from yellow-white, thick and greasy to thinner, lighter and less in amount. However, the tongue was still red, with whitish thin fur. Pulse was better too.

June to July 1982: Second course of chemotherapy administered. CYC 2.4 gm; MTX, 60 gm and VCR, 4 gm. No severe side effects. Appetite and spirits were good. Owing to the fact that chemotherapy consumes the Qi, during the period from November 9, 1982, to February 26, 1983, the patient was given traditional Chinese medications which have the main effects of nourishing Qi and strengthening the Spleen, clearing away toxic material and being anticancer in property. Prescription: Radix gentiane, 10 gm; Radix sophora flavescentis, 10 gm; Rhizoma bistortae, 15 gm; Exocarpium citri grandis, 10 gm; Caulis bambusae in taeniam, 10 gm; Charred treplet, 30 gm; Herba solani nigri, 30 gm; Semen coicis, 15 gm; Herba oldenlandiae diffusae, 30 gm; Radix pseudoscutellariae, 30 gm; Radix adenophorae, 30 gm; Rhizoma atrac-tylodis macrocephalae, 10 gm; Poria, 10 gm; Caulis spatholobi, 30 gm; and Semen armeniacae amarum, 30 gm.

No discomfort was experienced after taking this prescription. The appetite was good. The red colour of the tongue was markedly lightened, yellowish, thin fur only located at the root of the tongue. From March 1983 onward, the prescription was changed to one which moisturizes the Lung and resolves the Phlegm, detoxicates and is anticancer in property. The patient's condition was stable and he had no special complaints.

Four years after operation, in January 1985, the patient's tongue was a little red with thin white fur. Traditional Chinese medications were prescribed with the effect of nourishing Qi and strengthening the Spleen, detoxicating and suppressing the cancer. Radix sophora, Radix gentianae and Caulis bambusae in taeniam in previous prescription were replaced by Radix astragali, 15 gm; Bulbus fritillariae, 10 gm; and Herba scutellariae, 20 gm.

Follow-up in May 1985: No change on chest X-ray findings. However, having taken the prescription for three months, the patient displayed more severe signs of Damp-Heat accumulation such as cough and loose stool. The tongue became red, fur was yellow-white and greasy. Pulse thready and slippery. Taking into consideration that this might be related to the use of Root of Heterophylly Falsestarwort and Root of Mongolian Milkvetch, which are warm in nature, the prescription was modified mainly to clear away Heat and eliminate Dampness, resolve Phlegm and detoxicate. Herba artemisiae, 15 gm; Semen coicis, 20 gm; Semen alpiniae katsumadi, 8 gm; Rhizoma atractylodis, 10 gm; Charred treplet, 30 gm; Radix sophorae, 10 gm; Radix platycodi, 10 gm; Poria, 10 gm; Radix adenophorae, 30 gm; Bulbus fritillariae, 10 gm; Herba salviae chinensis, 20 gm; Herba scutellariae, 30 gm; and Herba oldenlandiae, 30 gm. The patient's serum CEA level increased to 23.33 ng/ml (normal 5 ng/ml). On November 12, 1985, colon fibroendoscopy found spasm in the areas of transverse colon and descending colon without other abnormalities. Up to January 1986, the CEA level was 25 ng/ml. CT scan impression: Upper right lobar old TB lesion with vesicular emphysema. Several small lymph nodes were discovered on the mediastinum which need to be observed further. Local bowel spasm was found in transverse colon during barium enema. Utrasonic examination demonstrated no abnormality in liver, gallbladder, pancreas and kidneys.

Because of elevated CEA (32.77 ng/ml), a course of chemotherapy was given in July 1986. At the end of chemotherapy course (MMC, 40 mg; 5FU, 2 gm and DDP, 60 mg), liver and kidney functions became normal. Blood picture was normal too. But picture of the tongue and pulse condition had not improved, still showing accumulation of Damp-Heat in the Lung and the Stomach.

From January to November 1987, the patient experienced no obvious symptoms. No abnormality was seen in chest X-rays taken on several occasions. Serum CEA was 32.5 ng/ml; ESR, 2 mm/hr; serum albumin and liver function were normal. The tongue was dark and red with yellow-white greasy fur. TCM prescription was administered continuously to moisturize the Lung, resolve the Phlegm, clear away Heat and detoxicate.

In September 1987, chest X-ray showed a shadow in the upper lobe of the right lung. Squamous epithelial carcinoma was confirmed by fibrobronchoscopy and biopsy. This was not metastasis from the previous cancer and a repetitive primary cancer was considered. The radiotherapy was given with electronic accelerator 6600Gy. After treatment, the mass disappeared and local radiopneumonitis remained. In February 1988, administration of traditional Chinese medicine was resumed. The tongue still tended to be dark-red in colour with thin and yellowish fur. Pulse was thready and slippery. Prescriptions were mainly those to moisturize the Lung, dissipate the Phlegm, resolve the hard lumps and consolidate the therapeutic effectiveness. The prescription given was composed of Spica prunellae, 15 gm; Bulbus fritillariae, 10 gm; Radix salviae, 30 gm; Caulis spatholobi, 30 gm; Herba scutellariae, 30 gm; Herba oldenlandiae, 30 gm; Radix adenophorae, 30 gm; Radix ophiopogonis, 15 gm; Semen armeniacae, 10 gm; Herba dendrobii, 10 gm; Radix peucedani, 10 gm; Semen coicis, 15 gm; Fructus amomi, 8 gm; and Poria, 10 gm.

DISCUSSION:

1) This is a case of squamous epithelial carcinoma of the lung. The survival period of this patient is more than seven years. He benefited from a treatment combining modern and traditional Chinese medicine. Six and a half years after the lobectomy, in September 1987, a second, primary cancer was found on the contralateral side.

2) After resection of lesion, patients usually have signs of Qi and Lung deficiency. But in this case, the sign of Damp-Heat in the Lung and Stomach persisted for several years. The patient had productive cough, red to dark-red tongue substance, yellow-white, thick and greasy fur. His appetite was good. He looked well and had no symptoms of Qi deficiency. All of these indicated that there remained certain pathogenic factors which might recur easily. Consequently, traditional Chinese medications with the effects of clearing away Heat and toxic material, moistening the Lung and resolving Phlegm were indicated. The treatment was based mainly on traditional Chinese medicine.

3) Within two years after the operation, two courses of chemotherapy were given and five and a half years after the lobectomy, the third course of chemotherapy was given. It appears that they did not bring about much benefit to the patient. The cancer cells of squamous epithelial carcinoma were not sensitive to chemotherapy and the tongue became bright red and crimson in colour with yellow-thick greasy fur after chemotherapy. This indicated a morbid state of retention of Damp-Heat in the interior and that the accumulation of noxious Damp-Heat was progressive. Accordingly, therapeutic approach was changed to that which eliminates Dampness with aromatics and clears away Heat and toxic material. After taking these traditional Chinese medications, the crimson colour of the tongue lightened and the fur became thin. Noxious Damp-Heat condition ameliorated markedly. The state of disease was relatively stable. However, when some medicinal herbs such as Radix astragali, Radix pseudostellariae, Rhizoma atractylodis macrocephalae, Poria, etc., which have warming and tonifying properties, were given, the Damp-Heat became heavier. The appearance of the tongue and the pulse condition returned to the original state. The lesson here is that one must determine the mode of therapy based on differentiation of the signs and symptoms. The importance of Bian Zheng Shi Zhi (determination of treatment based on symptom-complex differentiation) according to the basic theories of traditional Chinese medicine cannot be over-emphasized here.

4) In this case, Chinese medicinal herbs have been taken for a long time without toxic side effects. This shows that the application of herbal medicine is a safe mode of treatment.

5) After the surgical operation, the patient was subjected to regular annual examinations. In the first five post-operation years, no apparent abnormality was discovered. In the fifth year, serum CEA level was noted to have increased significant-

ly. It was one and a half years after this finding was noted that a contralateral, primary lung cancer was discovered. It seems that the CEA assay has a significance in monitoring the occurrence and development of cancer in the human body. CEA value is closely related to carcinoma of the colon. However, according to the theory of traditional Chinese medicine, the Lung and the Large Intestine are intrinsically related. It's a challenging objective of research to determine whether or not CEA level can reflect carcinogenesis in the lungs.

6) The characteristic of this case was an absence of deficiency syndrome after surgical operation. Taking into consideration the appearance of the tongue and pulse condition as well as the clinical experience, it indicates that pathogenic factors had not been totally removed and there existed the possibility of recurrence of cancer. Though the original cancer did not recur, a second primary cancer developed. It seems apparent that all those therapies had no effect on preventing carcinogenesis. The inception of this second cancer might be the result of absence of medicinal herbs with the properties of strengthening the body resistance, restoring normal body functions, consolidating the constitution, nourishing the Qi and replenishing the Kidney. These Chinese medicinal herbs are known to promote body immunity functions. This is a problem worthy of further investigation.

3. DIGESTIVE DISEASES

3.1 HICCUP
(ADVERSE RISING OF THE STOMACH)

Liu Shenqiu

Department of Traditional Chinese Medicine, Beijing Hospital, Beijing

Li Daquan, male, 69, Han nationality, married, cadre. Medical record number: 60539. Date of first consultation: July 13, 1978.

CHIEF COMPLAINT: Persistent hiccup for one day.

HISTORY OF PRESENT ILLNESS: During the period from 1974 to 1976, the patient had three attacks of "acute appendicitis" which were relieved by medical treatment. He was admitted on July 10, 1978, because of right lower abdominal discomfort with 38°C fever of one day duration. WBC count was 19,100/m³ with 84% neutrophils. He was treated with antibiotics without improvement and appendectomy was performed the next day. Operation and post-operative recovery were smooth. The patient started to experience hiccup after taking some liquids on July 12 which lasted into the next day. He complained of irritability, thirst and slight abdominal fullness. Temperature was normal. Acupuncture treatment failed to stop the hiccup. The patient was referred to us for TCM treatment.

PAST HISTORY: He has smoked 40 cigarettes daily for 40 years.

PERTINENT PHYSICAL EXAMINATION & LABORATORY FINDINGS: The patient's condition essentially normal except for the surgical condition. Blood pressure was 130/70 mmHg. Hemoglobin, 13.5 gm%; WBC, 8,500/m³. BUN, 10.9 mg%; SGPT level normal. HbsAg negative. Blood cholesterol, 201 mg%; triglyceride, 164 mg%; TTT, 2 u; lipoprotein, 563 mg% and FG examination negative. Routine urinalysis negative. X-ray chest examination showed accentuated markings of lungs, tortuous aorta and normal heart size. ECG showed bradycardia and coronary ischemia.

INSPECTION OF TONGUE: Pink tongue with thin white fur.

PULSE CONDITION: Deep, taut and fine pulse.

MODERN MEDICINE DIAGNOSIS: Hiccup; Acute Exacerbation of Chronic Appendicitis; S/P Appendectomy.

TRADITIONAL CHINESE MEDICINE DIAGNOSIS: Adverse Rising of Stomach-Qi.

THERAPEUTIC PRINCIPLES: Warm the Stomach-Qi and put down the adverse rising of Stomach-Qi.

PRESCRIPTION: Modified Xuan Fu Dai Shi Zhe Tang plus Ding Xiang Shi Di

San. Flos inulae, 9 gm; Ochra, 12 gm; Syzygii aromatici, 5 gm; Calyx kaki, 9 gm; Radix heterophylly falsetarwort, 12 gm; Cortex magnoliae officinalis, 9 gm; Radix saussurerae, 6 gm; Aurantii immaturus, 9 gm; and Dao Dou Zi (sword bean), 9 gm. Two decoctions.

FOLLOW-UP/COURSE OF TREATMENT:

Second consultation on July 15, 1978: Four days after operation, the hiccup persisted. The patient continued to take liquid diet. Abdominal fullness was relieved after passing of gas (flatus). Tongue with yellowish, thick and greasy fur. Pulse taut and moderate.

Symptom-complex differentiation: This was a case of disturbance of upward and downward movements of Qi. Despite the thick, greasy coated tongue, there was no accumulation in the large intestine and no materials to purge. The same principle of treatment was maintained, using moderately active drugs for lowering the adverse rising energy.

Prescription: Flos inulae, 9 gm; Ochra, 15 gm; Rhizoma pinelliae, 12 gm; Exocarpium citri grandis, 12 gm; Cauli bambusae in taeniam, 9 gm; Radix paeoniae, 15 gm; Cortex magnoliae officinalis, 9 gm; Rhizoma zingiberis, four pieces; Fructus amomi, 5 gm; and Radix panacis quinquefolli, 6 gm. One dose.

Third consultation on July 16, 1978: The patient's appetite improved but he had been constipated for five days. He took half a cup of honey as well as diazepam and Hoffman's mixture but without effect. Tongue with thick, white and greasy fur. Taut, fine, deep right bar pulse. Because of Qi deficiency in Middle Burner and disturbance of upward and downward movement of functional activities, hiccup could not be stopped. Ju Pi Zhu Ru Tang was given for the time being mainly to restore functional activities of the Stomach. Should constipation be relieved without purgatives and waste materials in Fu (Bowel) organ be discharged downward, then the hiccup might stop spontaneously. Since Stomach-Qi was of primary importance, purgatives should not be given indiscriminately. Prescription: Exocarpium citri grandis, 12 gm; Caulis bambusae in taeniam, 9 gm; Rhizoma zinaipha, 5 pieces; Fructus ziziphi jujubae, 10 pieces; Radix glycyrrhizae, 3 gm; Radix panacis quinquefolli, 9 gm; and Calyx kaki, 3 gm. Two doses.

Fourth consultation on July 18, 1978: The surgical wound healed up well and sutures were removed. Food intake increased and the patient was put on regular diet. Bowel movement twice. Hiccup was slightly decreased in frequency during sleep. Histological report of the resected specimen was acute exacerbation of chronic appendicitis. Tongue coated with thick greasy fur. Pulse was taut, fine and moderate. After operation, damage of Qi and stagnation of Blood are usually unavoidable. Accordingly, herbs for invigorating Blood circulation and eliminating Blood stasis were added to the last prescription. Exocarpium citri grandis, 9 gm; Caulis bambusae in taeniam, 9 gm; Rhizoma pinelliae, 12 gm; Radix glycyrrhizae, 3 gm; Fructus ziziphi, 10 pieces; Calyx kaki, 8 gm; Folium perillae, 6 gm; Semen persicae, 6 gm; Cortex magnoliae officinalis, 9 gm; Flos carthami, 3 gm; Radix paeoniae, 15 gm; and Radix panacis quinquefolli, 9 gm. Two doses.

Fifth consultation on July 20, 1978: Frequency of hiccup decreased slightly but did not stop completely. Tongue with thick and greasy fur. Pulse fine and moderate. At this stage, it was ineffective to use the common principle of treatment. Medicinal herbs with ascending properties were added to the prescription in order to regulate the ascending and descending functions of the Spleen and Stomach. Huang Qi (Root of Mongolian Milkvetch) was also added to reinforce the Qi. Prescription: Flos inulae, 9 gm; Calyx kaki, 6 gm; Folium eriobotryae, 12 gm; Radix platycodi, 8 gm; Rhizoma cimicifugae, 3 gm; Exocarpium citri grandis, 9 gm; Caulis bambusae in taeniam, 9 gm; Radix astragali, 15 gm; Semen amomi cardamomi, 3 gm; Rhizoma zingiberis, four pieces; and Radix panacis quinquefolli, 6 gm. Two doses.

Sixth consultation on July 22, 1978: Occurrence of hiccup stopped yesterday. No more greasy fur on the tongue. Pulse was fine and moderate. The last prescription was given for four more doses to stabilize the therapeutic effect. Hiccup did not recur and the patient was discharged in fairly good condition.

DISCUSSION: Hiccup, either in traditional Chinese or modern medicine's point of view, may be a minor symptom of transient duration or an extremely grave complication of a serious illness. In hypersensitive subjects the reflex may be initiated by temperature changes, i.e., sudden chilling, cold shower, rapid ingestion of ice-cold or very hot drinks or food. Hiccup may occur as an exceedingly grave complication of many surgical procedures. In our case, hiccup occurred together with mild abdominal distention after appendectomy. It lasted for a long time and was not responsive to acupuncture and modern medical treatment.

Hiccup is also known as Yue in TCM. Occurring in normal subjects, hiccup may stop spontaneously. It could be stopped instantaneously by induction of sneeze or holding the breath for a while ("Yi Bian"). If hiccup is caused by organic disease, it is essential then to differentiate the character, be it deficiency, excessiveness, Cold or Heat, before making a prescription. Persistent hiccup in an aged, debilitated patient or a patient after delivery is a sign of serious illness. Patients suffering from hiccup with running pulse can be cured, but those with regular intermittent pulse are difficult to treat ("Zheng Zhi Hui Bu").

Our case, a 69-year-old man, suffered from coronary and cerebral arteriosclerosis, chronic bronchitis, emphysema and other ailments for a long time. He contracted adverse rising of Stomach-Qi, and the hiccup persisted for 10 days unresponsive to treatments using diazepam and other drugs as well as acupuncture. It was evident that the hiccup would not stop spontaneously.

The first prescription was to warm up the Stomach and to put down the adverse rising Qi but it did not afford much relief. Later on, prescription of Ju Pi Zhu Ru Tang was administered to normalize the function of the Stomach and to regulate the adverse rising Qi. It proved to be ineffective, too. As the Spleen keeps upward and the Stomach sends the Qi downward, these two processes oppose and also complement each other. Therefore Rhizoma cimicifugae and Radix platycodi (herbs with effect of uplifting) were added to the previous prescription. Huang Qi was also added to reinforce American ginseng's strength to invigorate Qi. In so doing, this measure caused Spleen-Qi to travel upward and promoted the adverse rising stomach-Qi to move downward. This eventually relieved the patient from hiccup.

Thereafter, the author treated three more cases of persistent hiccup with the same principle of treatment. All proved to be effective. Experimental studies have shown that Huang Qi and other Qi-replenishing drugs could influence the tonus and contractility of the isolated small intestine of rabbits. Probably this plays an important role in the recovery from hiccup.

3.2 CONSTIPATION SECONDARY TO ACUTE MYOCARDIAL INFARCTION (CONSTIPATION AS A MANIFESTATION OF VARIOUS SYMPTOM-COMPLEXES)

Chen Keji

Xiyuan Hospital, China Academy of Traditional Chinese Medicine, Beijing

Constipation Secondary to Qi-Deficiency

Zhao, 46, male, Han nationality, married, cadre. Admission number 13732. Admitted on February 2, 1976, because of sudden acute epigastric pain and vomiting of five-hour duration. Symptoms started after eating lunch, which was accompanied by alcohol intake, first as sudden acute epigastric pain followed by vomiting, pallor and profuse perspiration with cold and damp extremities. ECG examination showed acute inferior wall myocardial infarction, blood pressure recorded as 130/100 mmHg. Cardiac rhythm regular, heart rate 90/min, no murmurs appreciated; both lungs negative; liver and spleen unpalpable; SLDH, 610 units, and SGOT, 330 units. Three hours after admission, the patient's blood pressure dropped to 80/50 mmHg with irregular cardiac rhythm. He was in a high state of agitation. ECG taken revealed migratory sinus rhythm and transient idiopathic premature contractions, pulse deep and thready, tongue substance dark and tongue fur thin. Traditional medicine symptom-complex differentiation classified it as Qi deficiency and Yang depletion with accompanying Blood stasis. He was given parenteral Anti-Shock Compound Prescription II (composed of Radix ginseng, Radix aconiti praeparatae, Rhizoma zingiberis, Radix ophiopogonis, Fructus schisandrae, Rhizoma atractylodis, Radix astragali, Cortex cinnamomi and Caulis spatholobi) 25 ml t.i.d. In consideration of the unstable blood pressure, the patient was given in addition Aramine, dopamine, hydroxycortisone, parenteral ginseng, lidocaine, etc., and was able to maintain the blood pressure at around 110/80 mmHg and the general condition was rendered stable. Signs of constipation started on the fifth day of hospitalization which forced the patient to strain strenuously on relieving himself. This exercise induced sudden onset of palpitation, shortness of breath, dizziness and profuse perspiration. Blood pressure reading 90/60 mmHg, cardiac rhythm regular, heart rate 92/min with systolic murmur appreciated on the left parasternal line on the third and fourth intercostal space; rales heard on bilateral lung bases; pulse was of thready and weak types, sometimes intermittent or uneven; tongue substance dark, tongue fur yellowish and thick with tooth marks on sides. Modern medicine diagnosis was interventricular septal perforation with cardiogenic shock. Traditional medicine diagnosis: Deficiency of Heart-Yang; Qi-Yang prostration. The patient's condition rendered stable after successful resuscitation. He still complained about shortness of breath and general body weakness as well as constipation, a general state caused by deficiency syndrome of Central Qi and dysfunction of colon movement. Applying the therapeutic principle of "tonifying the Qi and moistening the colon," the patient was given modified Buzhong Yiqi Decoction composed of Radix ginseng, 3 gm; Radix ophiopogonis, 9 gm; Fructus schisandrae, 9 gm; Radix astragali, 30 gm; Radix angelicae sinensis, 12 gm; Fructus aurantii immaturus, 12 gm; Rhizoma cimicifugae, 3 gm; and Radix bupleuri, 6 gm. This was able to relieve the constipation and the patient had bowel movement once a day regularly. Symptoms of general body weakness and palpitations were alleviated as well. The patient was observed for a period of 21 days during which the general condition was stable and there was no sign of constipation. Therapeutic regimen was changed to Buzhong Yiqi Pill to complete the treatment course. The patient was subsequently discharged after results of various examinations were found to be within the normal limits.

Constipation Secondary to Yin Deficiency

Na, 37, male, Hui nationality, married, labourer. Admission number 18631. Admitted on January 1, 1980, to the emergency room because of sudden, severe and unrelenting post-sternal area pain for three hours which was not relieved by taking nitroglycerine. On admission, he appeared agitated, complained of shortness of breath, sensation of asphyxiation, distention of the epigastric area and had profuse perspiration. Blood pressure 110/80 mmHg; irregular cardiac rhythm, heart rate 80/min; fourth heart sound appreciated on the apical area; bilateral pulmonary auscultation negative; pulse with occasional uneven and intermittent beats; and tongue substance umber. ESR, 49 mm/hr; SLDH, 880 units; ECG confirmed the diagnosis of recurrent acute inferior wall myocardial infarction. Traditional medicine symptom-complex differentiation classified it as deficiency of both Qi and Yin as well as Blood stasis. Therapeutic principles applied was that of "replenishing the Qi and nurturing the Yin, revitalizing the Blood and regulating the flow of Blood." The patient was initially given IV infusion of Shengmai Compound Solution and Guanxin II once a day. Six days later, the occurrence of chest pain was reduced to minimum but the patient complained of mouth dryness, general state of anxiety, lack of sleep, sometimes accompanied by heavy perspiration, stomach distention and constipation of five-day duration. No bowel movement was possible without using a glycerine enema. Tongue substance was changed to a healthy rosy colour with slightly yellowish tongue fur. Pulse examination showed both bars taut and cubits weak. Though the symptom of Blood stasis showed signs of remission, the discrepant pulse picture indicated a state of deficiency of Yin Fluid, the lack of which led to the inability to nurture the colon with resulting derangement of the Fu-Qi. The therapeutic principle to counter this phenomenon would be to "nurture the Yin and moisten the colon" and at the same time to regulate Fu-Qi. The prescription employed accordingly was to use Zhengye Chengqi Decoction as base with supplementary medicinal herbs of Radix scruphulariae and Radix ophiopogonis, 15 gm each; Radix rehmanniae, Radix rehmanniae praeparatae, Fructus aurantii immaturus and Cortex magnoliae officinalis, 10 gm each; and Fructus trichosanthis, 20 gm. On the same night of the administration of this decoction, the patient was able to pass the bowel content with instant relief of abdominal distention. He claimed to have a great sense of well-being and appetite was improved correspondingly. The patient was kept on this prescription thereafter and the symptom of constipation did not recur. The ECG picture improved and the condition rendered completely under control.

Constipation Secondary to Dampness and Heat

Zhao, 33, male, Han nationality, married, teacher. Admission number 18951. The patient was admitted on March 12, 1980, to the emergency room because of continuous chest wall dull pain accompanied by dizziness, nausea, profuse perspiration, palpitation and shortness of breath. ECG confirmed the diagnosis of acute high lateral wall myocardial infarction. With application of Qi-replenishing and Blood-revitalizing therapeutic principles, the pain was completely alleviated on the third day of confinement with significant relief of the symptoms of shortness of breath and palpitation. Other symptoms, e.g., dizziness, nausea and asphyxiating sensations, disappeared on the seventh day of confinement though he was not able to move his bowel for the duration. He complained of abdominal distention, excessive belching and acidic regurgitation. Application of bisatin did not afford relief from the constipation, though a large amount of flatus was passed and the patient showed signs of losing his appetite. Pulse examined to be smooth and thready, tongue fur slimy. Traditional differentiaton had it as "lingering of Dampness and Heat which congested at the Zhong Jiao (Middle Burner) leading to disorganization of Fu-Qi." Qi-replenishing and Blood-revitalizing herbs were prescribed to which was added "Heat- and Dampness-removing" composition Xianghuang Gao (Herba agastachis, 30 gm, and Radix et rhizoma rhei, 15 gm). One hour after the intake, the patient started to feel increased bowel motility which enabled him to pass out some desiccated stool. Within 24 hours, the patient moved his bowels six times which relieved him from all the abdominal discomforts. Dahuang Radix et rhizoma rhei was subsequently reduced to five gm. Thereafter, the patient had regular bowel movement once a day, pulse became thready and taut while tongue fur turned thin. Signs of constipation returned when Huoxiang Herba agastachis and Dahuang Radix et rhizoma rhei were discontinued from his prescription but the condition was corrected promptly with re-administration of Xianghuang Gao. Course of treatment uneventful thereafter.

Constipation Secondary to Qi-Stasis

Li, 55, male, Han nationality, married, cadre. Admission number 18810. Admitted to the emergency room on February 1, 1980, because of sensation of "chest obstructiveness" of seven hours duration. Accompanying symptoms were post-sternal area dull pain radiating to the back, shortness of breath, warmth seeking and frequent passage of flatus. Pulse taut and smooth, tongue substance dark, tongue fur yellowish; cardiac rhythm regular, heart rate 80/min; first heart sound dull, fourth heart sound appreciable on apical area; bilateral lungs negative; SLDH, 828 units; SGOT, 314 units; SGPT, 278 units and ESR, 65 mm/hr. ECG confirmed the diagnosis of acute generalized anterior wall myocardial infarction. The patient had been inclined to eat fatty food, consuming about six to 10 gm of fat-laden meat each meal and three to six *liang* of alcohol. He also smoked about 15 to 20 cigarettes a day. TCM differentiation classified the case as true Heart pain, deficiency of Heart-Qi accompanied by stasis of Qi-Blood. One week after application of the traditional therapeutic principle of "replenishing the Qi and invigorating the Blood," dull chest pain essentially disappeared and the patient felt better generally. At this stage, lower abdominal gas pain developed, with increasing amount of flatus passing frequently and the patient complained of constipation of five days duration. Medical applications of bisatin, Fanxieye Decoction and Maren Pill were not able to afford any relief; re-examination of the pulse revealed deep and taut beats, tongue substance dark and tongue fur yellowish. Consideration was given to the fact that the patient had been accustomed to a high alcoholic content diet resulting in considerable damage to the Spleen and Stomach, leading to derangement of Qi circulation. Subsequent Qi stasis led to congestion. Therapeutic consideration in such a case would be to promote digestion and to remove food stagnation and regulate the vital function of the Stomach in order to revert the derangement. Therapeutic regimen consisted of modified Muxiang Binglang Pill and Baohe Pill with additional herbs of Pericarpium citri reticulatae, 12 gm; Rhizoma pinelliae, 15 gm; Fructus crataegi, 20 gm; Massa fermentata medicinalis, 30 gm; Fructus forsythiae, 6 gm; Semen raphani, 15 gm; Pericarpium arecae, 6 gm; Cortex magnoliae officinalis, 15 gm; Radix aucklandiae, 12 gm; and Radix astragali, 15 gm. Application of this prescription enabled the patient to move his bowels once a day regularly and the symptom of general abdominal distention disappeared completely. The pathological course of the acute myocardial infarction was under control as well.

DISCUSSION: Traditional Chinese medicine believes that constipation is related to the functions of the Viscerae and the Bowels, and in particular, bears a close association to the Six Fu's (Bowels). The characteristics of the Six Fu's are that "they are hollow, discharging their content but not installing it" and that "they are made up of solid matter but are not full"; it is essential to digest and to remove the stagnation. Following this line of reasoning, it is imperative in all illnesses, be it of acute or chronic nature, to pay particular attention to the regular movement of bowels. In mapping out a therapeutic course, one must take into consideration the fact that various types of constipation secondary to acute myocardial infarction are not in consonance with traditional medical diagnostic "Yang-Ming" differentials; patients are usually of the older age group, with generally poorer health constitution and derangement of fluid transport. The main objective of the treatment should be based on the observation that the most frequently encountered types of constipation are the ones secondary to Qi-Deficiency, Yin-Deficiency, Qi-Stasis and Phlegm-Dampness. The cases cited here illustarte that to have a correct diagnosis and treatment based on an overall analysis of symptoms and signs according to basic TCM theories can successfully help the clinicians in accurately differentiating various types of constipation and treat them accordingly and in so doing, expedite the patient's recuperation.

3.3 STUBBORN CONSTIPATION
(STUBBORN CONSTIPATION)

Kang Ziqi

Department of Medicine, Peking Union Medical College Hospital, Beijing

Wang, 25, male, worker.

CHIEF COMPLAINT: Dry stool for over two years.

HISTORY OF PRESENT ILLNESS: The patient suffered from dysentery two years ago and recovered after two months of treatment by conventional medicine. Since then he had been passing dry, spheroid stool, once every two days. Each bowel movement would take him 30 to 40 minutes to complete, with bleeding and prolapse of anus from excessive straining. Other accompanying signs and symptoms were dry mouth, dry nose and pharynx, cracking and bleeding lips, diminished appetite, abdominal distention, fatigue and progressive loss of weight.

PAST HISTORY: Non-contributory.

INSPECTION OF TONGUE: Tongue proper red with thin coatings and cracks.

PULSE CONDITION: Deep, thready and rapid.

MODERN MEDICINE DIAGNOSIS: Stubborn Constipation.

TRADITIONAL CHINESE MEDICINE DIAGNOSIS: Stubborn Constipation.

Symptom-complex differentiation: Depletion of "Yin fluid," insufficiency of water leading to impairment of normal body functions.

THERAPEUTIC PRINCIPLES: Nourish the Yin and moisturize the dryness, supply the water to activate body functions.

PRESCRIPTION: Fructus cannabis, 10 gm; Gypsum fibrosum, 30 gm; Radix ophiopogonis, 10 gm; Semen armeniacae amarum, 10 gm; Folium mori, 10 gm; Herba dendrobii, 10 gm; Radix adenophora strictae, 10 gm; Radix angelicae sinensis, 12 gm; Radix paeoniae alba, 15 gm; Radix et rhizoma rhei, 10 gm; Fructus trichosanthis, 15 gm; Radix codonopsis pilosulae, 10 gm; and Natrii sulfas, 10 gm.

FOLLOW-UP/COURSE OF TREATMENT:

Second consultation: The patient still had dry stool once every two days. Abdominal distention reduced; lip rending diminished and lip bleeding stopped.

Prescription: Modify the prescription with Radix et rhizoma alba, 3 gm, and Fructus trichosanthis, 24 gm.

Third consultation: The patient's stool was normal, bowel movement once a day. No abdominal distention. Appetite and spirit were good. He was fully recovered.

DISCUSSION:

1) This case is characterized by dryness and accumulation of Heat in the Large Intestine. Prolonged existence of this condition affects the Lung, producing dryness of the Lung manifested by symptoms of dry throat, dry mouth and nasal dryness. The Lung is extrinsically and intrinsically related to the Large Intestine (Each Zang Organ is linked with a Fu Organ by a Channel, a situation known as the extrinsic-intrinsic relation). To treat this condition, the main prescription would be to correct the

impairment of Lung-Qi to dispel the dryness and to activate the dispersing function of the Lung and nourish the Yin in order to moisturize the bowels.

2) The Lung is the upper source of fluids while the Kidney is the lower source. According to the principle of treating the Lung and Kidney simultaneously (the therapy commonly used in treating Yin and Qi deficiencies of the Lung and Kidney), Radix rehmanniae and Radix scrophulariae are used to nourish the Kidney Yin and thus to expedite a full recovery.

3) Radix angelicae sinensis and Radix paeoniae are effective in nourishing Yin and Blood which in turn reinforce the body resistance.

4) The patient is young and presence of Excessiveness and Heat symptoms in this case is prominent (e.g., bleeding after defecation, prolapse of anus). Large dose of Radix rhizoma alba and sodium sulphate are given to eliminate dryness in the Large Intestine. This case took obvious effect by application of the therapeutic principle of simultaneous elimination and reinforcement.

3.4 CHRONIC GASTRITIS (EPIGASTRALGIA)

Zhang Jingren

Shanghai First People's Hospital, Shanghai

Feng, 59, female, Han nationality, married, cadre. Medical record number: 9810. Date of first consultation: November 30, 1983.

CHIEF COMPLAINT: Stomachache for more than 10 years, aggravated in recent weeks.

HISTORY OF PRESENT ILLNESS: The patient has had repeated attacks of stomachache for more than 10 years. In spite of various kinds of therapies, her condition was unstable, sometimes mild and sometimes severe with marked deterioration in recent weeks. Gastroscopy done on November 17, 1983, showed chronic atrophic gastritis which prompted her to come to our clinic for consultation. She complained of persistent stomachache, usually in the mid-upper abdominal region, accompanied by sensation of fullness, bitter taste in the mouth, eructation, anorexia and listlessness. Her bowel movement, urination and sleep were all normal.

PERTINENT PHYSICAL EXAMINATION & LABORATORY FINDINGS: Gastroscopy showed that there was a bean-sized polyp on the greater curvature side of the gastric antrum which was cauterized during gastroscopy. Antral mucosa was slightly coarse with fine-granular hyperplasia. Gastric body mucosa was thin with visible network of submucosal vessels. A diagnosis of chronic atrophic gastritis was given. Histology report showed (1) gastric antral mucosal papillary hyperplasia on the greater curvature side accompanied by moderate non-typical hyperplasia of epithelial cell and intestinal metaplasia; and (2) partial intestinal epithelial metaplasia of the mucosal polyp on the gastric antrum.

INSPECTION OF TONGUE: Red tongue with thin and greasy coating.

PULSE CONDITION: Wiry.

MODERN MEDICINE DIAGNOSIS: Chronic Atrophic Gastritis.

TRADITIONAL CHINESE MEDICINE DIAGNOSIS: Loss of Coordination between the Liver and Stomach; Accumulation and Obstruction of Stagnant Heat.

THERAPEUTIC PRINCIPLES: Coordinate the function of the Liver and Stomach and clear away the stagnant Evil-Heat.

PRESCRIPTION: Radix bupleuri, 6 gm; Radix scutellariae, 9 gm; Rhizoma atractylodis macrocephalae, 9 gm; Radix glycyrrhizae, 3 gm; Radix paeoniae alba and rubra, 9 gm; Cycas revoluta, 15 gm; Flos inulae, 9 gm; Ochra, 15 gm; Rhizoma cyperi, 9 gm; Fructus citri sarcodactylis, 6 gm; Fructus aurantii, 6 gm; Herba scutellariae barbatae, 30 gm; Herba oldenlandiae profusae, 40 gm; Fructus mume, 5 gm; and Fructus oryzae germinatus, 12 gm. These herbs were decocted with water and taken orally.

FOLLOW-UP/COURSE OF TREATMENT:

Second consultation on December 14, 1983: After being treated with this prescription, fullness and pain of the stomach were alleviated. Eructation became mild and appetite improved slightly. But two hours after meal, the patient had gastric discomfort with acid regurgitation. The pulse was thready and wiry, and tongue colour normal with thin coating. This indicated that the Liver and Stomach had started to coordinate gradually, but Spleen Qi was still weak. In addition to the original treatment, principles of strengthening the Spleen and regulating the Stomach were also implemented. Prescription: Radix bupleuri, 6 gm; Radix scutellariae, 9 gm; Rhizoma atractylodis macrocephalae, 9 gm; Rhizoma dioscoreae, 9 gm; Semen dolichoris, 9 gm; Rhizoma cyperi, 9 gm; Fructus citri sarcodactylis, 6 gm; Fructus aurantii, 6 gm; Radix glycyrrhizae, 3 gm; Gycas revoluta, 15 gm; Fructus oryzae germinatus, 12 gm; Herba oldenlandiae, 30 gm; and Radix paeoniae alba and rubra, 9 gm. Decoct for oral ingestion.

After taking the prescription persistently for more than one year, the pain and fullness of the stomach were basically relieved and epigastric discomfort appeared only after taking improper or unusual diets. The patient's appetite increased and her spirits rose.

Gastroscopy taken on December 6, 1984, in the same clinic showed a superficial antral gastritis and atrophic inflammation of the body of the stomach.

Histopathological report: (1) mild chronic mucosal inflammation with mild intestinal metaplasia of antral region; and (2) moderate chronic inflammation and mild intestinal metaplasia on mucosa of the body of the stomach. Both the gastroscopic inspection and histological findings indicated that after TCM treatment, intestinal metaplasia and non-typical hyperplasia of the gastric mucosa could be transformed or reduced and atrophic changes of the glands of gastric mucosa could also be reversed.

DISCUSSION: In chronic gastritis cases, pathological examination often revealed that the glands are atrophied and reduced associated with intestinal metaplasia of gastric mucosa. Some clinicians considered cases of atrophic gastritis with intestinal metaplasia in gastric mucosa as a high-risk group of gastric carcinoma and some even considered this pathological change a transition stage between atrophic gastritis and gastric cancer. So special attention should be paid to atrophic gastritis especially when it is associated with intestinal metaplasia.

Traditional Chinese medicine believes that chronic gastritis belongs to the category of epigastralgia with pathogenic Cold factor as its cause. Zhang Jingyue, a physician from the Ming Dynasty, pointed out that "in stomachaches, eight to nine tenths of the cases are due to Cold with one to two tenths due to Heat." However, our clinical observations showed that most cases of chronic gastritis belong to Heat syndrome. As to the pathogenesis, emotional upset, over-ingestion of alcoholic beverages and tobacco, as well as eating fatty and greasy diet, may lead to stagnation of Heat in the Liver and Gallbladder which attacks the Stomach and injures gastric mucosa. As time goes on, other pathologies such as Spleen asthenia with deficiency of Energy and stagnation of Blood which impede the circulation, may also occur. Thus the atrophy of gastric mucosa develops gradually. Based on this analysis, Radix bupleuri, Radix scutellariae and seeds of five leaf akebia in the prescription are used for soothing and purging the Liver and Gallbladder; Rhizoma atractylodis, Semen dolichoris and Rhizoma dioscoreae for relieving spasm and pain; Radix paeoniae, Rhizoma cyperi and Fructus aurantii for removing depression; Flos inulae and Ochra for lowering the adverse flow of Qi and promoting normal function of the Spleen and Stomach; Herba scutellariae and Herba oldenlandiae for clearing away Heat and eliminating ulcer; and Sago cycas leaf and Ardisia crenata sims for activating Blood circulation and eliminating Blood stasis. In addition, by combining sour Fructus mume and Fructus oryzae as modified Si Shi Wan Pill, the production of Yin (essence and fluid) may be enhanced and appetite improved. As a result, a favourable therapeutic effect was obtained.

3.5 GASTRIC ULCER, CHRONIC ATROPHIC SUPERFICIAL GASTRITIS (STOMACHACHE,LIVER DEPRESSION AND STOMACH-HEAT)

Wei Beihai and Chen Feisun
Beijing Traditional Chinese Medicine Hospital, Beijing

Li Wantian, 48, male, married, actor. Medical record number: 112829. Date of first consultation: October 14, 1984.

CHIEF COMPLAINT: Recurrent stomachache for more than 20 years, exacerbated during the past month.

HISTORY OF PRESENT ILLNESS: Twenty years prior to consultation, the patient began to experience stomachache caused by irregular diets. After treatment by gastric antacids and antispasmodics in a period of two or three weeks, his stomachache was completely eliminated. Several years later, the same stomachache recurred repeatedly due to stress, overwork and dietary disorder. One month prior to consultation, he again felt a burning stomachache, radiating towards the chest, which was often worse after eating. This symptom was accompanied by sour regurgitation, belching, dry mouth and bitter taste, anorexia, dry stool and constipation.

PAST HISTORY: Serum SGPT level abnormal in 1979.

PERTINENT PHYSICAL EXAMINATION & LABORATORY FINDINGS: Abdomen flat with slight tenderness over the right upper quadrant without rebound tenderness. Test for occult blood negative. SGPT, 40 King's units; SGOT, 50 King's units. Stomachgram: gastric body, 2.9 times/sec, amplitude, 30 μV; antrum, 30 times/second, amplitude 15 μV. Endoscopy: chronic inflammatory infiltration, intestinal metaplasia, glandular epithelium and thinning of the mucosa, superficial and atrophic gastritis.

INSPECTION OF TONGUE: Red tongue with yellowish fur.

PULSE CONDITION: Rapid and taut.

MODERN MEDICINE DIAGNOSIS: Chronic, Superficial and Atrophic Gastritis in Pyloric Antrum.

TRADITIONAL CHINESE MEDICINE DIAGNOSIS: Stomachache; Heat Depression of the Liver and Stomach.

THERAPEUTIC PRINCIPLES: Soothe the Liver, regulate the vital function of the Stomach and remove the Evil Heat.

PRESCRIPTION: Huagan Decoction (Soothing the Flow of Liver Vital Energy) combined with Zuojin Pills. Pericarpium citri reticulatae and viridea, 12 gm; Rhizoma coptidis, 3 gm; Cortex moutan, 12 gm; Fructus gardeniae, 6 gm; Radix paeoniae alba, 15 gm (decocted first); Cuttle fish bone, 20 gm (decocted later); Rhei, 3 gm; Bulbus fritillariae, 9 gm; and Rhizoma alismatis, 6 gm. Method of preparation: place ingredients in adequate amount of water, boil and retain a final decoction of 350 ml. Divide the liquid into three parts, three times a day. One prescription per day. Adjuvant treatment: massage the points Taichong (Liv. 3), Zhongwan (Ren. 12) and Zusanli (St. 36), twice a day. Soft and regular diet only, avoid stimulating food.

FOLLOW-UP/COURSE OF TREATMENT:

Second consultation on October 19, 1984: Stomachache and flatulence greatly relieved. The patient did not complain of constipation, sour regurgitation and belching. Dry mouth and bitter taste still present. Tongue substance red with yellowish fur, taut and slightly rapid pulse. Continued the same prescription but with Rhei being prepared separately, which means that the function of Rhei is changed from one of purging to dispersing.

Third consultation on October 24, 1984: Stomachache occurred abruptly after eating. There was no dryness of mouth and no bitter taste. Reddish tongue with thin coat, taut pulse. Prescription: Xiaoyao San (Xiao-Yao Powder) with Xiangsha Liujunzi Tang (Decoction of Xiangsha Six Nobles). Radix bupleuri, 12 gm; Rhizoma atractylodis macrocephalae, 12 gm; Poria, 12 gm; Rhizoma zingiberis, 3 gm; Herba menthae, 6 gm; Medicated learen, 15 gm; Fructus crataegi, 18 gm; Radix angelicae, 9 gm; and Radix paeoniae alba, 12 gm. concurrent administration of Xiangsha Liujunzi Pills, 9 gm, b.i.d.

Fourth consultation: All symptoms had disappeared. Endoscopic examination showed remission of ulcers and chronic inflammatory phenomena, signs of intestinal metaplasia and glandular epithelium alleviated. The patient was in convalescent stage. Decoction was discontinued and he was prescribed only Xiangsha Liujunzi Pills.

Follow-up visit: The patient was in good health three years later (on April 8, 1987). He did not complain of any gastric discomfort. Endoscopic examination showed full recovery from the inflammatory process. He has been taking Xiangsha Liujunzi Pills after supper ever since.

DISCUSSION: Traditional Chinese medicine considers stomachache as the chief complaint of diseases of the Stomach. The stomach and Spleen are intrinsiclly and extrinsically related with a connection between their coordination and functions. In addition, they are closely related to the Liver. The Liver possesses the functions of soothing and regulating the flow of Vital Energy and Blood in the Stomach and Spleen. It is also the viscus of Temperament. If the Liver falls ill, it would make one liverish, i.e., easily excited, fiery in temper and hard to be put under control or restrained. Blockage of the flow of Liver Vital Energy leads to stomachache because functions of the Spleen and Stomach are affected by the Liver. This malfunction could be manifested clinically as epigastric pain, belching, vomiting and acid regurgitation. These symptoms are attributed to Liver disturbance, which is also known as disharmony of the Liver and Stomach. This pathological process could then be transformed into stagnant Heat in the Liver and Stomach. If this condition exists long enough, deficiency of the Spleen and Stomach ensues manifested clinically as fatigue, sallow face, indigestion, abdominal distention and anorexia. This condition is often seen in cases of peptic ulcer, chronic gastritis and gastric neurosis. Pathogenesis of this disease entity usually has the following characteristics. Initially, presence of Liver Qi disorder affects transversely the Stomach followed by loss of coordination between the Liver and Stomach; Qi stagnation and Blood stasis result in accumulation of Heat in the Liver and Stomach. After a long period of existence, this pathological process disables the Spleen so that it cannot transport and transform the nutrients. If this deficiency turns to Coldness, then insufficiency of Spleen-Stomach Yang develops; and should this deficiency turn into Evil Heat, then insufficiency of the Spleen and Evil-Heat in the Stomach follows. Therefore, Spleen deficiency syndrome is usually seen in patients with gastric ulcers and chronic gastritis.

In a clinical study series, the International Peace Hospital reported on 600 cases of chronic gastritis and ulcers. Among them, 90% showed symptoms of Spleen and Stomach deficiency. Satisfactory therapeutic effects were obtained when they were treated by the principles of invigorating the Spleen, replenishing the Qi and regulating the Liver. According to the literature, about 60 to 70% of all the patients suffering from ulcers can be classified as either having Spleen and Stomach deficiency or insufficiency of Spleen-Stomach Yang.

In our case, decoction of Huagan and Zuojin Pills were used initially to coordinate the function of the Liver and Stomach, to soothe the Liver, to regulate Stomach Vital Energy and to dispel the stagnant Heat. Xiangsha Liujunzi Pill was subsequently added to invigorate, warm and tonify the Spleen and Stomach. A satisfactory outcome was obtained through these measures. This illustrates that Spleen-invigorating and Qi-replenishing principles can really strengthen and regulate the functions of the digestive system. Shijunzi decoction can promote the absorptive and secretory functions of the gastrointestinal tract, raise the absorptive rate of xylose, adjust pancreatic secretory functions, regulate secretion of gastric juice and relax gastrointestinal spasms, especially those of smooth muscles. Radix glycyrrhizae is effective in promoting the healing process of ulcers, absorption of gastric acid, induction of pepsin activity and in so doing protects the gastric mucosa from damage.

3.6 DUODENAL ULCER AND CHRONIC SUPERFICIAL GASTRITIS (STOMACH-HEAT AND INSUFFICIENCY OF THE SPLEEN, DISCORD BETWEEN WOOD AND EARTH)

Lin Qiucheng and Lin Zhaohui
Fujian Institute of Traditional Chinese Medicine, Fuzhou

Zhen Shaoxing, 40, male. Date of first consultation: December 20, 1985.

CHIEF COMPLAINT: Dull pain in upper abdomen for six years, becoming worse during the last two months.

HISTORY OF PRESENT ILLNESS: The patient has had chronic, periodic hunger pain in the upper abdomen for six years. It was noted to be better in summer and worse in winter and often occurred at the time about three hours after meals accompanied by acidic regurgitation and belching. Symptoms could be relieved by intake of food. The patient had hematemesis and melena last winter and was diagnosed as having a bleeding gastric ulcer. In the two months prior to admission, because of over-fatigue and improper diet, the pain became worse and lost its periodicity. The pain was persistent and was described as burning or dull in character. It could not be relieved by intake of food any more. Symptoms were accompanied by dryness of mouth, dysphoria, nausea, loss of appetite, insomnia, constipation and loss of weight. He had been treated by Probanthine, Ulcermin and Cimetidine but to no avail. He was subsequently referred to our clinic.

PAST HISTORY: Non-contributory.

PERTINENT PHYSICAL EXAMINATION & LABORATORY FINDINGS: The abdomen was soft and there was tenderness at the middle and right side of the epigastrium. Barium UGIS revealed duodenal ulcer. Gastroscopy showed duodenal ulcer and chronic superficial gastritis. Hemoglobin, 11 gm%; WBC, 8,300/mm^3. Occult blood test (+).

INSPECTION OF TONGUE: Tongue substance red with yellow and sticky fur.

PULSE CONDITION: Wiry and rapid.

MODERN MEDICINE DIAGNOSIS: Duodenal Ulcer; Chronic Superficial Gastritis.

TRADITIONAL CHINESE MEDICINE DIAGNOSIS: Epigastralgia; Stomach-

Heat and Insufficiency of the Spleen; Discord Between Wood and Earth.

THERAPEUTIC PRINCIPLES: Soothe the Liver and regulate the circulation of Qi, purge the Heat and regulate the Stomach.

PRESCRIPTION: Modified Bupleurum Powder for Relieving Liver-Qi and Sichuan Chinaberry Powder. Radix bupleuri, 6 gm; Radix paeoniae alba et praeparatae, 9 gm; Rhizoma cyperi, 15 gm; Pericarpium citri reticulatae, 6 gm; Radix scutellariae, 10 gm; Rhizoma coptidis, 9 gm; Fructus euodiae, 9 gm; Rhizoma corydalis, 10 gm; Fructus meliae toosendam, 10 gm; Fructus trichosanthis, 15 gm; and Radix glycyrrhizae, 9 gm. One dose per day.

FOLLOW-UP/COURSE OF TREATMENT:

Second consultation: After taking this prescription for six days, the patient felt much better. Epigastralgia obviously relieved. His tongue was red and coated with a slightly yellowish fur. Pulse was wiry. Modified the prescription by replacing Fructus trichosanthis with Radix pseudostellariae, 15 gm; Rhizoma atractylodis macrocephalae, 9 gm; and Poria, 10 gm. One dose daily for five days.

Third consultation: Epigastralgia almost completely remitted. The patient still complained of acratia, loss of appetite and tastelessness. His tongue was slightly red and coated with a thin and white fur. Pulse was thready and wiry. Prescription: Radix bupleuri, 6 gm; Radix paeoniae alba et praeparatae, 9 gm; Rhizoma cyperi, 15 gm; Radix salviae, 15 gm; Radix codonopsis pilosulae, 15 gm; Rhizoma atractylodis macrocephalae, 9 gm; Poria, 10 gm; Fructus amomi, 3 gm; Radix aucklandiae, 6 gm; Radix glycyrrhizae, 6 gm; Rhizoma pinelliae, 6 gm; and Pericarpium citri reticulatae, 6 gm. One dose daily for 10 days.

Epigastralgia did not recur during one year of follow-up.

3.7 DUODENAL BULBO ULCER (WEI WAN TONG, EPIGASTRALGIA)

Zhang Xiaoxing

Hubei College of Traditional Chinese Medicine Hospital, Wuhan

Yan, 32, male, Han nationality, married, driver. Medical record number: 85123.
Date of first consultation: September 11, 1987.

CHIEF COMPLAINT: Epigastric pain for about 16 years, pain becoming worse during the last month.

HISTORY OF PRESENT ILLNESS: The patient had epigastric pain since 1977, but had never received any treatment. He had always eaten irregularly and had injured his stomach through overeating, drinking and excessive hunger. In the winter of 1981, he passed tarry stool for two days and was admitted to hospital. Barium UGIS showed duodenal bulbo ulcer. Since then he often felt pain in the epigastrium just below the xyphoid process. The pain was described as sharp or prickly in character. The pain often occurred when the stomach was empty and could be relieved by taking food or medications such as gastropine, Busur, Roter, etc. Epigastric pain was less severe in summer and autumn but became aggravated in spring and winter. One month prior to admission, the patient experienced severe epigastric pain after taking a large amount of wine. The pain occurred in the epigastric region, three to four times a day, each time lasting for two to three hours. He felt better when he ate or drank something or when he massaged the epigastric region. He had a declining appetite and felt tired and dizzy, but he did not experience any vomiting, nausea or belching. He emptied his bowel one or twice a day and noticed black stools one day prior to admission. The urine was normal and sleep was good except when attacks of epigastric pain occurred.

PAST HISTORY: Exposed to water in schistosomiasis epidemic area; denied having hepatitis or other infectious diseases. He has been smoking for about 10 years.

PERTINENT PHYSICAL EXAMINATION & LABORATORY FINDINGS: Normal physique. There was no flushing colour on the face and no icterus of sclerae. Presence of halitosis. His teeth were irregular in arrangement with two teeth lost. Thyroid gland was normal in size. Auscultation of heart and lungs negative. Abdomen soft and flat. There was slight tenderness on the right epigastrium, stomach empty without any sign of retention. Liver palpable 4 cm below the xyphoid process, soft in consistency. Spleen not palpable. No malformation of the extremities and no pathologic reflexes elicited. CBC: Hemoglobin, 10.6 gm%; RBC, $3.99M/mm^3$; WBC, $4,300/mm^3$; polymorphs, 77%; lymphocytes, 23%. Blood HBsAg (RPHN method) negative. Total serum protein, 7.28 gm%; albumin, 4.3 gm%; globulin, 2.9%; A/GM = 1.5:1. Stool brownish black in colour; occult blood test (++). ELISA of schistosomiasis enzyme labelled antibody negative. Gastroscopy: hyperemia of gastric antral and pyloric mucosa, minimal congestion at the lesser curvature of the stomach with slight edema, peristalsis good. There was malformation and hyperemia of duodenal bulbus mucosa, a round ulcer was seen at the lesser curvature of the duodenal bulb about 0.6 × 0.6 cm in area. The surface of the ulcer was covered with white mucosa with obvious congestion at its edges. Diagnosis by gastroscopy was bulbar ulcer (active) and chronic superficial antral gastritis.

INSPECTION OF TONGUE: Tongue substance red with thin, yellow fur on its anterior part which was thicker on the root.

PULSE CONDITION: Soft-string pulse, regular, 84/min.

MODERN MEDICINE DIAGNOSIS: Duodenal-bulbo Ulcer (Active) with Hemorrhage; Chronic Superficial Antral Gastritis.

TRADITIONAL CHINESE MEDICINE DIAGNOSIS: Epigastralgia.

Symptom-complex differentiation: The Spleen and Stomach have been injured by eating and drinking irregularly leading to epigastric pain. Recent bouts of over drinking and over eating resulted in retention of Heat in the Stomach. Channels were subsequently injured which impeded the flow of Blood. The primary pathology of this disease is deficiency of the Spleen and Stomach and the secondary aspect is the combination of Heat retention in the Stomach and Blood stasis. So the principal manifestation of this case was deficiency while the secondary aspect was one of excess.

THERAPEUTIC PRINCIPLES: Apply pungent herbs for dispersion and bitter herbs for purgation, activate Blood circulation to dissipate Blood stasis, remove obstruction in the Channels, and regulate the flow of Qi to stop the pain.

PRESCRIPTION: Modified Wei Kui Lin. Rhizoma atractylodis macrocephalae, 10 gm; Rhizoma pinelliae, 10 gm; Radix salviae miltiorrhizae, 15 gm; Rhizoma coptidis, 6 gm; Rhizoma bletyillae gelatin, 10 gm; Radix rubiae, 10 gm; Fructus aurantii immaturus, 10 gm; and Ophicalcitum, 15 gm. Decocted in water for oral ingestion, one dose daily. The patient was told to eat a semi-liquid diet.

FOLLOW-UP/COURSE OF TREATMENT:

Second consultation on September 18, 1987: After taking the prescription for one week, epigastric pain was relieved and foul breath disappeared. The brownish-black colour of the stool turned yellow. The patient still complained of anorexia. Tongue proper slightly red and thick, yellow fur on the base of the tongue became thin. Pulse thready and slow. These findings indicated that Stomach-Heat had been dissipated but Spleen insufficiency still existed. Modified the prescription by replacing Ophicalcitum with Radix pseudostellariae, 10 gm; Endothilum corneum gigeriae, 10 gm; and Fructus amini, 10 gm.

Third consultation on September 28, 1987: After taking 10 doses of the modified prescription, epigastric pain disappeared and appetite improved. Stool and urine were normal. The patient's health was improving progressively. The tongue was covered with white and thin fur and the pulse still thready and slow. These signs indicated that stagnant Heat in the Stomach had been eliminated. Therefore, the therapeutic efficacy should be consolidated by reinforcing the Spleen and regulating the Stomach through promotion of Qi circulation and removal of stagnation. Ping Wei San and Si Jun Zi Tang were prescribed. Radix pseudostellariae, 10 gm; Atractylodis macrocephalae 10 gm; Poria, 9 gm; Os sepiella seu sepiae, 20 gm; Radix aucklandiae, 6 gm; Fructus amomi, 5 gm; Pericarpium citri reticulatae, 10 gm; Fructus oryzae germinatus, 12 gm; and Fructus hordei germinatus, 12 gm.

Fourth consultation on October 11, 1987: Upon completion of the 10-dose course of this prescription, stomach pain was gone and did not recur. The patient recovered his appetite and physical strength. Stool and urine were normal. Condition of the tongue fur and pulse was the same as before. His pale face turned slightly red and flushed. Minimal tenderness on the epigastrium. Continued the same prescription.

Fifth consultation on October 17, 1987: The patient's condition essentially the same as seen during the last consultation. Re-examination by gastroscopy showed gastric body and antral mucosa smooth, but there were several areas of slight congestion at the antrum. The pyloric mucosa was not as smooth or irregular in arrangement, and there was slight hyperemia. Duodenum was still deformed and mucosa of the ulcerated area had become more level than before. Surface of the ulcerated area was red in colour without any exudation. These gastroscopy findings indicated that (1) the duodenal ulcer was in a recovery phase, and (2) the chronic gastritis had improved. CBC: Hemoglobin, 11.5 gm%; RBC, 3.9M/mm^3. Occult blood test negative.

The patient's condition had improved greatly. He was discharged from hospital on October 28, 1987, and advised to continue taking the prescription given on the third visit.

3.8 UPPER GASTROINTESTINAL HEMORRHAGE (BLOOD SYMPTOM-COMPLEX, MELENA)

Zhang Wenliang

First Affiliated Hospital of Wenzhou Medical College, Wenzhou

A 34-year-old male, Han nationality, married, worker. Admitted to hospital on March 20, 1984.

CHIEF COMPLAINT: Melena of five-day duration.

HISTORY OF PRESENT ILLNESS: The patient usually experienced pain and fullness in the epigastrium after meals when he ate carelessly. Five days prior to admission, he worked very hard with much sweating and had a feeling of fatigue and weakness. Wanting to have a nutritious meal, he ate some pig kidneys. He developed diarrhea that night and passed tarry stool at six o'clock the next morning. The following days he passed black stool and when he was in toilet, he felt vertiginous and fainted. He was resuscitated and was sweating profusely. He was brought immediately to the emergency room in our hospital where he fainted once again. The patient was admitted to TCM ward with a working diagnosis of upper gastrointestinal hemorrhage.

PAST HISTORY: History of stomachache for about 10 years; denies history of hepatitis or tuberculosis.

PHYSICAL EXAMINATION & LABORATORY FINDINGS: Temperature normal, pulse rate, 100/min; respiratory rate normal; blood pressure, 100/60 mmHg. Conscious, pale. EENT examinations normal. Thyroid, heart and lungs essentially normal. Abdomen flat and supple. Liver and spleen not palpable. There was slight tenderness in the epigastric region. No deformation of extremities and spinal column. Neurological examination normal. Hemoglobin, 7.0 gm%; WBC count, 5,000/mm3; CP, 63%; platelets, 182,500/mm3; bleeding and clotting time normal. Liver function test and urinalysis normal. Tarry stool.

INSPECTION OF TONGUE: Coating of tongue white and thin.

PULSE CONDITION: Small and weak.

MODERN MEDICINE DIAGNOSIS: Upper Gastrointestinal Hemorrhage.

TRADITIONAL MEDICINE DIAGNOSIS: Blood Symptom-Complex, Melena.

THERAPEUTIC PRINCIPLES: Treat the Biao aspect for emergency first, eliminate the stagnation and hemostasis.

PRESCRIPTION: Hai Huang San Capsule (consisting of Sepiellae seu sepiae and Radix et rhizoma rhei), 0.5 gm per capsule, four to six capsules every four to six hours with cold, boiled water. In addition, 500 ml of 10% glucose in water, 500 ml of 5% glucose in normal saline, vitamin C and 10% potassium chloride solution were administered by intravenous route once a day. Liquid diet per orem.

FOLLOW-UP/COURSE OF TREATMENT: As soon as the patient was admitted on the afternoon of March 20, 1984, Hai Huang San was administered at the dosage described. The colour of stool turned to brown. The patient did not feel dizzy, but he was still weak and tired. He was advised to take Hai Huang San for another three days to stabilize the therapeutic effect.

Second consultation on March 23, 1984: General condition of the patient was fair. Intake of food was normal. He did not feel pain in the abdomen, neither was he thirsty, though occasionally he experienced dizziness. He had passed yellow and soft stools twice or three times a day for two days. Stool occult blood test became negative. Pallor still prominent and his tongue coating was thin and white. The pulse was weak. At this stage, it was believed that the bleeding had stopped but the patient was having deficiency of Blood. By TCM teaching, this clinical manifestation is classified as weak Spleen syndrome with deficiency of both Blood and Vital Energy. Hai Huang San was discontinued at this juncture, and the patient was treated in accordance with the principles of invigorating the Spleen and strengthening the Vital Energy. Prescription: Radix codonopsis 15 gm; Poria, 10 gm; Rhizoma atractylodis macrocephalae, 10 gm; Radix glycyrrhizae, 6 gm; Radix angelicae sinensis, 10 gm; Radix astragali, 30 gm; Fructus lycii, 12 gm; Cortex cinnamomi, 3 gm; Semen ziziphi spinosae, 12 gm; Radix aucklandiae, 6 gm; Pericarpium citri reticulatae, 6 gm; and Fructus jujubae, 6 gm. Three doses.

Third consultation on March 27, 1984: The patient's condition was stable. He had a normal appetite his epigastric pain had disappeared and his dizziness subsided. He passed yellow-colour stool once a day. Hemoglobin level was raised to 8.5 gm%. He was advised to take seven more doses of the same prescription.

Fourth consultation on April 3, 1984: The patient resumed normal activity. Appetite normal. He slept soundly every night. Stool and urine normal. X-ray examination of GI tract showed thick and convoluting gastric antral mucosa folds of the gastric antrum with occasional spasm. The body of the stomach and duodenum were normal. X-ray diagnosis was antral gastritis. Hemoglobin 9.5 gm%. Stool occult blood test negative. The patient had fully recovered and was discharged soon after.

DISCUSSION: Upper gastrointestinal hemorrhage (UGIH) is a disease commonly encountered by physicians and surgeons in the emergency room. We have used Hai Huang San (HHS) made from Os sepiellae seu sepiae and Radix et rhizoma rhei to treat UGIH for many years and have obtained considerable results. According to TCM teaching, all the blood which is out of the vessels is called stasis of stagnant blood. Eliminating the stagnation and hemostasis is the first step of treatment in UGIH. The effect of Rhubarb among HHS is to dissipate the internal Heat and to keep the Bowel open. Radix et rhizoma rhei had been repeatedly reported to be effective in treating UGIH. Recent pharmacological studies indicate that its main components—anthraquinone, free anthraquinone derivative and ellagitannin—can stimulate the intestinal wall to increase its peristalsis, thus reducing absorption of water which produces mild diarrhea. In addition, it reduces the permeability of capillaries and improves their fragility, thus diminishing exudation from lesion surfaces. Hai Huang San may also raise the number of platelets which facilitates blood clotting. It may also make the vessels constrict.

Os sepiellae seu sepiae is mainly composed of calcium carbonate, crystalline material, a little calcium phosphate, sodium chloride and magnesium salt, which have vasoconstricting effect to stop the bleeding and prevent damage from gastric acids. It is indicated in treatment of peptic ulcer, excessive acidity of gastric juices and gastric hemorrhage. These two drugs are henceforth chosen and made into powder form, which may be more effective in treating upper gastrointestinal hemorrhage.

We believe that the efficacy of Hai Huang San in treating upper gastrointestinal hemorrhage is derived from its components of anthraquinone derivative, ellagitannin and calcium ion. Specifically, the powder acts directly on the inflammatory, ulcerous and bleeding local mucosal lesion, thus bringing into play its hemostatic properties. Having had HHS, the patient was able to pass stool in a short time with a frequency of as high as three to five times a day. In this way, we can judge correctly whether UGIH had stopped or not and can spot any re-bleeding in time to institute the treatment. It is our clinical experience that side effects to this medicine are very uncommon, and if present, they are usually manifested as abdominal pain which can be relieved by bowel movement. Side effects of nausea and vomiting can be relieved by administration of atropine. The source of HHS is wide and it is easy to process HHS at a very low cost which would translate into a lighter financial burden on the patient. HHS stops upper gastrointestinal bleeding fast and its clinical importance has repeatedly been demonstrated. HHS's efficacy is not restricted by the age, pathogenesis or other conditions of the patient. It is suitable for wide application in the vast rural areas of China.

In our case, the bleeding stopped 12 hours after the patient took Hai Huang San. The stool occult blood test became negative after two days. In view of deficiency of both Qi and Blood, Gui Pi Tang was prescribed as an agent to tonify the Blood and Qi and to strengthen the Spleen. Recovery in this case was swift and the patient's hemoglobin level rose rapidly. In a situation like this, the TCM principle of treatment would be to treat the acute or emergency secondary aspect (Biao or manifesting symptoms) first, followed by treatment of the chronic, primary aspect (Ben or root of the disease).

3.9 CHOLECYSTITIS, CHOLELITHIASIS (HYPOCHONDRIAC REGION PAIN, JAUNDICE)

Hong Yongshen and Tian Yi
Hangzhou Red Cross Hospital, Hangzhousegment>

Fu Yixian, 48, female, Han nationality, married, worker. Medical record number: 85420. Date of first consultation: October 14, 1986.

CHIEF COMPLAINT: Recurrent pain in the right upper abdomen with fever and jaundice for two years, getting worse the past two days.

HISTORY OF PRESENT ILLNESS: Two years prior to admission, the patient experienced discomfort in the right hypochondriac region after eating some greasy food. Paroxysmal pain in the same region followed soon. The pain was described as too severe to tolerate and radiating to the right shoulder accompanied by fever

(38.6°C), chills, nausea and vomiting. Yellowish discolouration of sclerae, skin and urine was noted. Symptoms were getting worse progressively and the patient was in low spirits. She sought medical advice and was diagnosed to have cholecystitis and cholelithiasis. Symptoms were relieved with antibacterial and antispasmodic management, including ampicilline, gentamycine and "654-2." Since then, the symptoms relapsed frequently when she got tired or had improper diet. Three days ago, the patient was in emotional depression caused by a quarrel. The next day, she felt paroxysmal pain in the right upper abdomen getting worse progressively. She tossed and turned in bed and was restless when the pain was severe. She experienced bitter taste in the mouth, nausea and vomiting. She had fever and her body temperature was 37.7°C. She has not had any bowel movements for three days. She was admitted as a "cholecystitis and cholelithiasis" patient. The patient had neither hematemesis nor melena; the stool turned to ceramic earth colour when the symptoms became severe. Her appetite was fair.

PAST HISTORY: Non-contributory.

PERTINENT PHYSICAL EXAMINATION & LABORATORY FINDINGS: Temperature, 38.8°C; pulse rate, 100/min; blood pressure, 120/70 mmHg. Acute facies, conscious, low in spirits, mesomorphic in build. No edema, no purpura, nor ecchymosis. Superficial lymph nodes not enlarged. No puffiness of the eyelids, sclera jaundiced, no congestion of bulbar conjunctivae, pupils with normal light reflex. No discharge from external auditory meatus, no tenderness of the mastoids. Nose clear without discharge. No cyanosis noted on lips. Pharynx without congestion and tonsils normal in size. Neck supple. Heart and lung findings negative. Abdomen slightly protruding with extreme tenderness on the upper right quadrant accompanied by slight rebound tenderness and localized muscle rigidity. Liver and spleen not palpable. No mass. Murphy's sign (+). Pain on percussion on hepatic region. Shifting dullness test (-). Pain on percussion on kidney areas. No edema of lower extremities. No pathological reflex elicited. CBC: WBC count, 11,000/mm^3; neutrophils, 80%; SGPT, 18 u; ZnTT, 6 u; A/GM = 4.2/2.1; II, 18 u; bilirubin, 2.6 mg%; blood amylase, 32 u. Urinary amylase, 64 (Winslow's method). Ultrasonic examination: common bile duct 1.2 cm in diameter with a 1.5 × 2 cm^2 stone in it.

INSPECTION OF TONGUE: Red tongue substance, yellow and greasy tongue coating.

PULSE CONDITION: Wiry and fast.

MODERN MEDICINE DIAGNOSIS: Cholecystitis; Cholelithiasis.

TRADITIONAL CHINESE MEDICINE DIAGNOSIS: Hypochondriac Region Pain; Jaundice; Stagnation of Bile caused by Depression of Liver.

THERAPEUTIC PRINCIPLES: Soothe the Liver and promote bile secretion.

PRESCRIPTION: Radix bupleuri, 12 gm; Radix curcumae, 10 gm; Radix scutellariae, 15 gm; Radix aucklandiae, 9 gm; Rhizoma corydalis, 12 gm; Herba lysimachiac, 30 gm; and Fructus meliae, 10 gm. Three doses, one dose a day. Place ingredients in 600 ml of water and boil them for an hour until 200 ml of decoction remain. Take 100 ml each time, twice a day.

Other management: Acupuncture points Yanglingquan (GM.B), Dannang (Extra

34) and Qimen (Liv. 14) for relief of severe pain; and Neiguan (P. 6) and Hegu (L.I. 4) to relieve vomiting. Needles were retained for half an hour, twice a day. Semi-liquid and low-fat diet; 1,500 ml of intravenous fluid daily.

FOLLOW-UP/COURSE OF TREATMENT:

Second consultation: The patient had recurrent pain in the right upper quadrant with jaundiced sclerae. Body temperature was 38°C. The stool was dry. Tongue substance red with yellow and thick coating. Continued the original prescription; 30 gm of Herba lysimachiae boiled in water to be taken ad libitum; 30 gm of Radix et rhizoma rhei boiled in 200 ml of water for five minutes, twice daily. Acupuncture applied with stronger stimulation. The stool was examined daily.

After treatment, the patient had 500 ml of watery stool every day. Three days after treatment, abdominal pain was relieved markedly. Two gallstones were found in the stools, one 2.5×1.5 cm^2 in size, the other 1.5×1.0 cm^2.

Third consultation: Temperature 37.0°C, pain in the right upper quadrant alleviated and jaundice on sclera had disappeared. Abdomen flat and soft with slight tenderness in right upper quadrant. No rigidity. No masses. Murphy's sign (-). Tongue light red in colour with thin, yellow coating. Pulse normal.

Herba lysimachiae, 15 gm; Radix bupleuri, 10 gm; Radix curcumae, 10 gm; Radix paeoniae alba, 15 gm; Poria, 15 gm; Semen coicis, 15 gm; and Pericarpium citri reticulatae, 6 gm. Seven doses.

After taking this prescription, all symptoms were gone. The patient had recovered fully and was discharged.

DISCUSSION: This case has the following clinical features:

(1) Recurrent pain in right upper abdomen caused by unusual diet, emotional excitement, anger and fatigue;

(2) Pain often accompanied by fever, jaundice, bitter taste, nausea and vomiting;

(3) Tongue body red with yellow, greasy tongue coating, pulse wiry and fast.

This case was diagnosed as "hypochondriac pain, jaundice" and the locus of pathology was in the Middle Jiao. The Liver and Gallbladder have an intrinsic-extrinsic relationship. The Liver generates Visceral Energy, while the Gallbladder descends Visceral Energy. The Gallbladder is a hollow organ containing clear juice. Emotional problems, improper diet and Dampness stagnated in the Middle Jiao are the etiological factors which cause stagnation of Qi in the Liver and Gallbladder and retention of Dampness and Heat and make the Liver unable to promote the Gallbladder and the Gallbladder subsequently unable to descend and discharge bile. Long-standing depression of Liver Qi develops. The ensuing Fire and Dampness mixes with Heat and ultimately transforms into stones. When there is stasis, there is pain. This is the pathology of our case. Treatment of choice in modern medicine is to remove the stones by surgical operation. However, it is difficult to remove sandy stones, thus surgery was ruled out in this case as a definitive therapeutic measure.

Selection of the recipe in treating this case was based on TCM teachings. Radix bupleuri calms the Liver and relieves stasis; Radix curcumae activates bile secretion and eliminates jaundice; Radix scutellariae clears away Heat and toxins; Rhizoma corydalis, fructus meliae and Radix aucklandiae regulate Vital Energy and alleviate the pain; and Herba lysimachiae clears away the Dampness and Heat and eliminates the stone.

This prescription performs the functions of calming the Liver, activating bile secretion, clearing away heat and alleviating pain. But it did not work well. Traditional Chinese medicine states that "when there is stasis, there is pain" and "the six Hollow Organs must keep their dredging function." The signs and symptoms of this case were dull abdominal pain, abdominal distention, dry stool and yellow tongue coating. So the measure of purgation was adopted at the second consultation. Radix et rhizoma rhei and Herba lysimachiae were added to the regimen; they were boiled in water to be taken ad libitum. In addition, acupuncture was applied to relieve spasm, alleviate pain, and stop the nausea and vomiting. The symptoms disappeared three days after treatment, and the stones were discharged. This successful outcome prevented the patient from undergoing a surgical operation.

3.10 GALLBLADDER STONE WITH CHOLECYSTITIS (DAMPNESS AND HEAT IN THE LIVER AND GALLBLADDER)

Li Mingzhen

Institute for the Integration of Traditional and Western Medicine, Tongji Medical University, Wuhan

Kang Taizhang, 71, male, married, pensioner. Medical record number: Dan-88. Date of first consultation: July 12, 1976.

CHIEF COMPLAINT: Severe, recurrent pain in his upper abdomen for three months.

HISTORY OF PRESENT ILLNESS: Severe pain in his upper abdomen occurred about once each month accompanied by fever but no jaundice. At the time of consultation, the patient still experienced distending pain in the right upper quadrant of this abdomen, radiating to right back. He had difficulty falling asleep. He experienced mild fever, bitter taste, thirst and halitosis, fullness in the stomach and anorexia. His urine was scanty and dark. He also experienced constipation.

PAST HISTORY: Positive history of hypertension and coronary heart disease which are currently under treatment. Often discomfort in the epigastrium.

PERTINENT PHYSICAL EXAMINATION & LABORATORY FINDINGS: Temperature, 38°C; a 6 × 4 cm mass can be palpated in the right upper quadrant of his abdomen under the costal margin with tenderness and positive Murphy's sign. Ultrasound examination: Gallbladder measuring 6 × 6 cm, hydrops of the gallbladder. Oral cholecystography (X-ray No. 95970) indicated non-disappearance of the gallbladder, increased density shadow about 2 × 3.2 cm in size may be seen in gallbladder area, the centre of which was transparent and the edges clear with a circle of sclerosis. X-ray diagnosis: Gallbladder stone and chronic cholecystitis.

INSPECTION OF TONGUE: Dark and purplish tongue with yellow and greasy fur.

PULSE CONDITION: Taut and slippery pulse.

MODERN MEDICINE DIAGNOSIS: Gallbladder Stone Combined with Subacute Onset of Chronic Cholecystitis.

TRADITIONAL CHINESE MEDICINE DIAGNOSIS: Dampness and Heat in the Liver and Gallbladder; Excess of Yang Ming Fu Organ; Stagnation of Qi and Blood Stasis.

THERAPEUTIC PRINCIPLES: Clear away Heat and promote diuresis, keep the Bowels open by purgation, promote the circulation of Qi to remove Blood stasis.

PRESCRIPTION: Modified Yinchenhao Tang. Herba artemisiae capillaris, 30 gm; Herba lysimachiae, 30 gm; Radix curcumae, 15 gm; Herba taraxaci, 30 gm; Fructus trichosanthis, 9 gm; Radix aucklandiae, 9 gm; Pericarpium citri reticulatae, 9 gm; and Rhei, 15 gm. Decocted in water and divided into two parts for oral ingestion, one dose per day. Also Lidan Huayu Tablet (consisting of Artemisiae capillaris, Lysimachiae, Rhizoma zodoariae and Rhei, etc., a patent medication prepared by our hospital) four to five tablets, three times per day.

FOLLOW-UP/COURSE OF TREATMENT:

Second consultation on July 21, 1976: After taking three doses of the decoction, abdominal pain diminished and the patient was able to sleep well at night. Pain in the chest and hypochondrium may now be alleviated by belching. Body temperature decreased to about 37.5°C. Tongue fur changed a bit, pulse still taut and slippery. Modified the prescription. Herba artemisiae capillaris, 30 gm; Herba lysimachiae, 30 gm; Herba verbenae, 30 gm; Rhizoma curcumae longae, 9 gm; Rhizoma cyperi, 9 gm; Folium citri, 9 gm; Flos inulae, 9 gm; Radix aucklandiae, 9 gm; Lignum dalbergiae odoriferae, 9 gm; and Rhizoma polygonati, 12 gm. One decoction per day together with administration of Lidan Huayu Tablets.

Third consultation on July 24, 1976: All symptoms continued to improve. The patient still had a feeling of fullness in the stomach and decreased intake of food, with bitter taste and halitosis. Accordingly, Dampness removal was incorporated into the present treatment. Prescription: Herba artemisiae, 30 gm; Loosestrife, 30 gm; Herba lysimachiae, 12 gm; Radix bupleuri, 12 gm; Radix scutellariae, 12 gm; Rhizoma curcumae longae, 15 gm; Herba eupatorii, 9 gm; Semen coicis, 24 gm; Pericarpium trichosanthis, 9 gm; Bulbus allii macrostemi, 9 gm; Rhizoma pinelliae, 9 gm; Lignum dalbergiae odoriferae, 9 gm; and Fructus aesculi, 9 gm. One decoction per day accompanied by Lidan Huayu Tablets.

Fourth consultation on July 31, 1976: The patient's condition continued to improve. Food intake increased and temperature became normal. Greasy fur of tongue diminished and pulse became taut. The mass in the upper right quadrant of his abdomen had shrunk. Mass painful only when palpated. Continued the decoction with minimal modification and continued Lidan Huayu Tablets.

After administering the prescription continuously for more than a month, the patient experienced only mild pain in the right quadrant of his abdomen. Appetite was normal and he had only a little bitter taste in the mouth. Tongue fur became thin and pulse strong and slow. The mass on the right upper quadrant of his abdomen continued to shrink progressively. Prescription was discontinued and only patent traditional Chinese medicines prepared by our hospital were prescribed. In addition to Lidan Huayu Tablets, Kang Yan Tablets (consisting of Herba taraxaci, Rhei, etc.) were prescribed, three tablets, three times a day, for relief of constipation. When liberal bowel movement was achieved, Lidan Hewei Tablets (consisting of Herba capillaris artemisiae, Rhizoma atractylodis, Pericarpium citri, Fructus crataegi, etc.) were added, four tablets, three times per day.

After administration of these patent Chinese medicines for three months, the pain in this abdomen continued to be alleviated and finally vanished. Distending gallbladder shrank to such an extent that it was not palpable in the right costal margin.

Repeated oral cholecystography was done in 1978 and 1979; the shadow of the stone was similar to that at the first cholecystography. The patient's condition was stable with no severe abdominal pain, and he was able to take some greasy food. He occasionally experienced dullness in his upper abdomen which was relieved by the patent medications. Generally, the patient did not need to take medication any longer.

In 1981, the patient had right colectomy because of colon carcinoma. And without taking the Chinese drugs, the patient had some greasy foods and experienced no discomfort in the abdomen. He has been in good health ever since.

DISCUSSION:

1) The incidence of gallbladder stone increases as a patient's age increases. In the past, gallbladder stone was usually treated surgically. However, this therapeutic measure is not feasible in the aged because their conditions are often complicated with cardiovascular disorder or other organic diseases. Presently, litholytic and lithagogue therapies are only suitable for small cholesterol calculus and not effective in treating those more than 1 cm in size or calcium-containing calculus. The patient, who had to resort to traditional Chinese medicine, may be a typical case.

2) Generally, based on TCM symptom-complex differentiation, gallbladder stone without complication of cholecystitis is characterized as Dampness and Heat or excessive Heat in the Liver and Gallbladder. The patient has fever, abdominal pain, undeveloped cholecystography which indicate that gallbladder stone is complicated by subacute onset of chronic cholecystitis. According to symptom-complex differentiation, fullness and pain in the right hypochondrium suggest the site of illness to be in the Liver and Gallbladder. Epigastric fullness, decreased intake of food, decreased amount of urine, yellow and greasy tongue fur, taut and slippery pulse, are all signs of presence of Dampness and Heat. Abdominal pain and fullness, bitter taste and halitosis and constipation are signs of excess of Yang Ming Fu Organ. Pain and fullness in the hypochondrium and abdomen with a fixed site and dark and purple colour of the tongue are signs of Qi-stagnation and Blood stasis. Therefore, the conclusion of symptom-complex differentiation of this case is Dampness and Heat in the Liver and Gallbladder, excess of Yang Ming Fu Organ, Qi-stagnation and Blood stasis. The patient should be treated in light of the principles of clearing away Heat and promoting diuresis, keeping the bowels open and purgation and promoting the circulation of Qi to remove Blood stasis.

3) With regard to prescriptions, cases of gallbladder stone classified under Dampness and Heat or excess of Heat in the Liver and Gallbladder are often treated with modified Yinchenhao Tang (Oriental Wormwood Decoction), or Da Chaihu Tang (Major Bupleurum Decoction) or Xiao Chaihu Tang (Minor Bupleurum Decoction). If the sign of Heat is dominant, Fructus gardeniae, Radix scutellariae, Herba taraxaci, Herba verbenae, Cortex phellodendri and Rhizoma coptidis are added to clear away Heat and toxic material. If Dampness is the prominent pathogenic factor, Capillaris artemisiae, Lysimachiae, Semen plantaginis, Herba eupatorii, Trichosanthis and Semen coicis may be selected to eliminate Dampness or to remove Dampness by diuresis. If there is abdominal fullness due to Qi-stagnation, Rhizoma curcumae, Radix aucklandiae, Pericarpium citri reticulatae and viridae, Rhizoma cyperi, Radix saussureae, Flos inulae and Fructus aesculi may be added to promote circulation of Qi to relieve flatulence. For abdominal pain due to Blood stasis, Radix salviae, Cortex moutan radicis, Rhizoma zedoariae, Semen persicae and Feces trogopterorum can be used to promote Blood circulation, remove Blood stasis and treat the excess of Yang Ming Fu Organ. In addition to raw Rhei (decocted separately), Compound of Glauber-salt and Liquorice may be taken following its infusion to purge the Bowel. A patient, in whom Damp-Heat has been removed but who still manifests deficiency syndrome, should be given prescriptions which replenish the Qi and nourish the Blood and Yin according to the site of the lesion. For this case recipes and drugs chosen had obvious efficacy because they agreed with TCM symptom-complex differentiation. It has been 12 years since the patient first consulted us. Now he is 83 years old and still in good health.

3.11 INFECTION OF THE BILIARY TRACT (DAMPNESS AND HEAT IN THE LIVER AND GALLBLADDER, DEFICIENCY OF BOTH QI AND BODY FLUID)

Lin Qiucheng and Lin Zhaohui

Fujian Institute of Traditional Chinese Medicine, Fuzhou

Huang Xiuqin, 30, female. Date of first consultation: July 11, 1987.
CHIEF COMPLAINT: Alternate attack of chills and fever for four months.
HISTORY OF PRESENT ILLNESS: The patient has had chills and fever in the afternoon and paroxysmal pain in the right upper quadrant of her abdomen for four months. She was hospitalized with a diagnosis of biliary tract infection and septicemia. She was treated with erythromycin, chloromycetin, cephalosporin, gentamycin and kanamycin. The fever did not subside until Dexamethasone was used and returned when Dexamethasone was discontinued. Chills and fever abated at night accompanied by excessive sweating, palpitation, flushed face, tiredness, thirst and loss of appetite. She was subsequently transferred to the affiliated People's Hospital of the Fujian College of Traditional Chinese Medicine. The patient was treated initially by Modified

Sweet Wormwood and Scutellaria Decoction for Clearing Damp-Heat from the Gall-bladder which contains Herba artemisiae Qinghao, 12 gm; Caulis bambusae in taeniam, 12 gm; Rhizoma pinelliae praeparatae, 6 gm; Poria, 15 gm; Radix bupleuri, 6 gm; Radix scutellariae, 12 gm; Cortex magnoliae officinalis, 9 gm; Herba artemisiae capillaris, 12 gm; Fructus gardeniae, 12 gm; Radix glycyrrhizae, 3 gm; and Rhizoma coptidis, 5 gm. One dose daily. Concurrently, the patient was treated by modern medicine, but she did not feel better. In the last four days, chills and fever got worse.

PAST HISTORY: The patient had same attack last December and was diagnosed as having septicemia.

PERTINENT PHYSICAL EXAMINATION & LABORATORY FINDINGS: Temperature, 39.5°C. Throat congested. Abdomen soft and there was tenderness in the right upper quadrant. WBC count, 29,800/mm^3; neutrophils, 87%; lymphocytes, 12%; monocytes, 1%; hemoglobin, 10.8 gm%. Eosinophillic granulocyte absolute count 20/mm^3. Routine urinalysis negative. Duodenal drain examination: pyocyte (++) in the fourth tube. Positive Staphylococus albus growth in bacterial culture and highly sensitive to erythromycin and penicillin; resistant to gentamycin, streptomycin and chloromycin. ASO test<500 u; ESR, 80 mm/h; RF, (-); blood bacterial culture, (-); Widal's test negative; GPT, 31 u; TTT, 3 u; ZnT, 12 u; HBaAg, (-); serum amylase, 122 u; urine amylase, 40 u. Chest X-ray finding of heart and lungs negative. Abdominal ultrasonic diagnosis: (1) liver size normal; (2) cholecystitis and intrahepatic cholangitis; and (3) reactive pancreatitis.

INSPECTION OF TONGUE: Tongue substance red and coated with a thin, yellow and sticky fur.

PULSE CONDITION: Thready, wiry and rapid.

MODERN MEDICINE DIAGNOSIS: Biliary Tract Infection.

TRADITIONAL CHINESE MEDICINE DIAGNOSIS: Hypochondriac Pain; Shaoyang Syndrome; Summer-Heat Touches Off Incubative Pathogen; Dampness and Heat in the Liver and Gallbladder; Deficiency of both Qi and Yin.

THERAPEUTIC PRINCIPLES: Treat the Shaoyang disease by mediation; clear away Heat and toxic material; clear away the Gallbladder Heat and eliminate the Dampness; nourish the Yin to promote production of body fluid.

PRESCRIPTION: Modified Decoction for Clearing Away Summer-Heat and Reinforcing Qi and Minor Decoction of Bupleurum. Radix bupleuri, 6 gm; Herba artemisiae Qinghao, 15 gm; Rhizoma coptidis, 6 gm; Radix scutellariae, 15 gm; Rhizoma pinelliae, 6 gm; Petiolus nelumbinis, 10 gm; Herba dendrobii, 12 gm; Rhizoma anemarrhenae, 10 gm; Gypsum fibrosum, 30 gm; Flos lonicerae, 30 gm; and Fructus forsythiae, 15 gm. Two doses per day. Radix panacis quinquefolli added separately.

FOLLOW-UP/COURSE OF TREATMENT:

Second consultation: The patient had taken the prescription for six days; fever had got lower progressively and was normal at this stage. She still complained of sensation of oppression in the chest, and vexation. Tongue red and coated with a thin yellow fur; pulse thready. Prescription: Radix bupleuri, 5 gm; Flos lonicarae, 30 gm; Fructus forsythiae, 12 gm; Petiolus nelumbinis, 9 gm; Rhizoma aremarrhenae, 15 gm; Herba lophatheri, 12 gm; Bulbus allii macrostemi, 9 gm; and Radix curcumae, 6 gm. Two doses daily for two days.

Third consultation: The patient had no complaint except for pain on her left knee. Bulbus allii macrostemi in the last prescription was replaced by Radix pseudostellariae, 24 gm. One dose every day for three days.

Fourth consultation: The patient complained of acratia. Her tongue tip red and coated with a thin yellow fur; pulse thready. Prescription: Radix pseudostellariae, 30 gm; Petiolus nelumbinis, 8 gm; Herba lophatheri, 9 gm; Radix scutellariae, 9 gm; Radix curcumae, 9 gm; Radix adenophorae, 24 gm; Flos chrysanthemi, 9 gm; Rhizoma atractylodis macrocephalae, 9 gm; Poria, 12 gm; Rhizoma dioscoreae, 15 gm; Radix paeoniae alba, 15 gm; and Radix glycyrrhizae, 3 gm. One dose every day for three days.

The disease did not relapse during the one-month period of follow-up visits.

3.12 BILIARY ASCARIASIS (SYNCOPE DUE TO ASCARIASIS)

Guo Yungen, Wu Dehui and Zhou Damei
Emergency Clinic and Medical Department of the Fujian Provincial People's Hospital and the Fujian College of Traditional Chinese Medicine Hospital, Fuzhou

This patient was a 28-year-old woman worker who suffered from sudden spasmodic and lacerating pain over the epigastric region while working on October 6, 1984. No reason could be attributed to the inducement of this attack. Both the time of onset and the duration of attack were irregular. When the attack occurred, she screamed and writhed in pain. She almost fainted from the extreme pain which occurred five to six times within the span of an hour. The patient was subsequently sent to the hospital where the attack occurred again. There were no accompanying tremors or coma.

Physical examination revealed a body temperature of 37.0°C; pulse 68/min, relatively feeble and smooth. The patient was moderately nourished and with normal development. On admission, she appeared acutely ill and drowsy. She cooperated well during the physical examination except at times when the epigastric pain occurred, whereby she would toss restlessly and turn repeatedly. During these attacks, the patient was not able to maintain a supine position. There were no jaundice, edema or enlargement of superficial lymph nodes. The tongue was red, with thin and white coating. Neck supple and thyroid not enlarged. Heart and lungs essentially normal. Abdomen soft and mild tenderness on the epigastric region without rebound tenderness. Murphy's sign negative and no abdominal mass palpable. Liver and spleen not palpable and peristaltic sounds normal. No deformations on the extremities and no pathological reflexes elicited. Hemoglobin, 12.5 gm%; WBC count, 6,000/mm^3; neutrophils, 70%; eosinophils, 2%; serum amylase, 50 u (Somogyi's method); urine amylase, 300 Somogyi's units. Routine chest fluoroscopy showed normal signs of the heart and lungs and no air under the diaphragm. Ultrasound examination of the abdomen showed two ascarides in the biliary tract.

FOLLOW-UP/COURSE OF TREATMENT:

When the epigastric pain occurred again, the patient was treated on time by acupuncture and moxibustion. Inserted the needle into Point Ren 12 (Zhongwan) and passed through Point Ren 13 (Shangwan), then retained the needle for 15 minutes. Bilateral points of St 36 (Zusanli) were punctured with twisting method and needle inserted until the "Qi" or the flushing, tingling sensation was obtained, whereby the abdominal pain disappeared right away. Removed the needles after five minutes followed by acupuncture of the above-mentioned points in turn. Repeated this manipulation two to three times in half an hour. The patient has not experienced the pain since. As soon as the pain was under control, levamisol, 150 mg, was given per orem as well as IV infusion of 10% glucose solution. The patient's condition was maintained well throughout the day and she passed out 20 ascarides the next morning. At this stage, all symptoms had disappeared. Re-examination by ultrasound showed no shadow of ascarides in the biliary tract.

She was discharged in that afternoon. Two weeks later, she was re-examined at the OPD and no remarkable clinical finding was found.

DISCUSSION: Biliary ascariasis is a common emergency disorder which has been recorded long ago in traditional Chinese medical classics. In the Han Dynasty, Zhang Zhongjing, a famous physician of traditional Chinese medicine, described this disease and defined it as "syncope due to ascariasis."

To this author's knowledge, the therapeutic regimen combining analgesic and antispastic effects of acupuncture with administration of antihelmintics is the treatment of choice for this kind of case. Up to this date, it remains the most economical, easiest to handle, prompt-acting, and extremely effective mode of treatment.

For a very long time, biliary ascariasis has been considered a surgical emergency. The rationale of this thinking is that, first, the ascaride is adept in boring ahead and it could not move back once it gets into the biliary tract. Second, should ascarides remain inside, it would easily cause pyogenic infection of the hepatic biliary tract; and third, administration of antihelmintics may prompt the ascarides to bore further. Therefore, it has been firmly believed that antihelmintics is absolutely contraindicated in treating biliary ascariasis and that surgical operation is the appropriate mode of treatment to remove ascarides from the biliary tract. However, surgery itself can be a great trauma and risk to the patient, and it would not prevent the ascarides in the small intestine from getting into the biliary tract again. In the late 1950's, clinicians in China reported good results from applying Zhang Zhongjing's Wumeiwan to relieve the acute symptoms of biliary ascariasis and from that time on, surgical therapy of biliary ascariasis had been replaced, gradually, by non-surgical measures. It was advocated then, however, that antihelmintics should be applied two to three weeks after the pain had ceased. For the next 25 years, in our country measures quite elaborate and extensive were taken in stabilizing the behaviour of ascarides during the acute stage of biliary ascariasis. Herbs acidic in nature such as Fructus mume, the main component of Wumeiwan, vinegar or aspirin were administered in order to keep the ascarides from being agitated. TCM believes that acidic substances could calm down the ascarides and move them downstream. Such measures were combined with administration of atropine and vitamin K_3 to relieve smooth muscle spasm of biliary tracts so as to effect a remission from the pain. However, it was unanimously agreed, at that time, that antihelmintics must be administered two weeks after all the symptoms had subsided. It was believed that by this practice, incidence of surgical intervention would be kept low. This author, with his long experience in clinical practice, maintained that such a practice had several shortcomings: (1) this course of treatment entails administration of antihelmintics at a later stage, two weeks or sometimes later, which is definitely too long and often the clinicians forget about the antihelmintics all together; (2) the antispastic and stabilizing measures during the acute stage fail in many cases, and the pain may last several days, resulting in complications such as biliary tract infection and acute pancreatitis which make the clinical picture worse; and (3) in the latter stage of the course of the disease, the ascarides might die inside the biliary tract, antihelmintics would be completely ineffective in removing the remains and this may turn into foci of cholelithiasis formation in the future. For these reasons, the author believes that the key to a successful outcome would be to shorten the course of treatment, to reduce the incidence of complications and to administer effective antihelmintics promptly. In 1982, the author reported a series of cases where antihelmintic therapy was applied in the early stage with high and prompt curative rate, and there was not a single complication of pyogenic biliary infection, acute pancreatitis or ascariasis intestinal obstruction. On the other hand, however, the antispasmodics were still extensively applied in order to stop the severe pain in the course of the therapy. Later on, this was substituted by acupuncture analgesia combined with administration of medications. The rate of analgesia induced by acupuncture was nearly 100%. Such a successful rate of response could not be matched by administration of analgesics. The acupuncture points adopted are only Ren 12 and St 36, which are safe, straightforward, simple and convenient to use. In addition, the new generations of antihelmintics are of high potency and low side effects and are not contraindicated in patients with liver or kidney insufficiencies or during pregnancy. This kind of antihelmintics has a common property, i.e., to paralyse the muscle of ascarides and render them unable to wiggle and bore. This makes the ascarides easy to be passed out in pace with biliary tract motility without the danger of them boring further ahead. Such administration is extremely safe. Recently, it has been reported that ascarides in the biliary tract could be removed under direct vision by fiberduodenoscope. Despite its quick result, this mode of treatment requires special equipment and is not very convenient to operate and consequently not feasible to be recommended for extensive application in the future. Besides, there is always the complication that the operation would not be completely successful and that ascarides be only partially removed. Another point is that its clinical value is not equal to that of antihelmintics.

In short, application of acupuncture and moxibustion and administration of antihelmintics in the acute stage of biliary ascariasis is the quickest, safest, most reliable, simplest and most convenient mode of treatment with no harmful reactions. It's highly recommended for extensive application.

3.13 SUBACUTE NECROSIS OF THE LIVER
(ACUTE JAUNDICE)

Qing Li

Zhang Zhongjing University of Traditional Chinese Medicine, Nanyang

Zhou, 24, male, Han nationality, married, worker. Date of first consultation: November 2, 1967.

CHIEF COMPLAINT: Frequent nausea and vomiting, unconscious for four hours prior to admission.

HISTORY OF PRESENT ILLNESS: In June 1967, the patient had acute icteric hepatitis and was hospitalized in a county hospital. After four months of both modern and traditional Chinese medicine treatment, his condition did not get better but actually worsened. TT, 180 u and temperature, 39°C. Examination of abdomen showed shifting dullness and fluid thrill. Glucosuria (+). He was transferred to another hospital in Zhengzhou on October 20 where he was diagnosed as having subacute necrosis of the liver. After ten days of treatment the condition became worse. At the time of admission, the patient was noted to have dark eyes and complexion; dry mouth with purplish and cracking lips; nausea and vomiting. Comatose and restless. Occasional bowel movement with scanty amount and offensive stool. Oliguria with reddish urine. Fever scalding to touch. Temperature, 40.8°C; TT, 230 u. Ascites absent. (History related by relatives).

INSPECTION OF TONGUE: Crimson tongue substance, yellow, thick and dry fur.

PULSE CONDITION: Smooth and rapid.

MODERN MEDICINE DIAGNOSIS: Subacute Necrosis of the Liver.

TRADITIONAL CHINESE MEDICINE DIAGNOSIS: Acute Jaundice.

THERAPEUTIC PRINCIPLES: Cool the Blood and remove toxic material, clear away the Evil Heat and promote diuresis to eliminate jaundice.

PRESCRIPTION: Modified Yin Chen Hou Tang. Herba artemisiae capillaris, 45 gm; Radix et rhizoma rhei, 10 gm (to be put in later); Fructus gardeniae, 15 gm; Flos lonicerae, 60 gm; Fructus euodiae, 30 gm; Radix isatidis, 30 gm; Herba taraxaci, 30 gm; Radix bupleuri, 30 gm; Rhizoma coptidis, 15 gm; Cortex moutan radicis, 20 gm; Rhizoma alismatis, 15 gm; Herba eupatorii, 20 gm; Radix curcumae, 10 gm; Radix salviae miltiorrhizae, 60 gm; and Rhizoma imperatae, 60 gm. Place ingredients in adequate amount of water and simmer down to 300 ml. One dose per day.

FOLLOW-UP/COURSE OF TREATMENT:

Second consultation on November 3, 1967: Temperature had fallen to 38.6°C. The patient was slightly responsive. Other signs and symptoms same as before. Continued taking TCM prescription. Herba artemisiae capillaris, 45 gm. Radix et rhizoma rhei, 10 gm (to be put in later), Fructus gardeniae, 15 gm; Flos lonicerae, 60 gm; Fructus euodiae, 30 gm; Radix isatidis, 30 gm; Radix bupleuri, 20 gm; Rhizoma coptidis, 10 gm; Cortex moutan radicis, 15 gm; Rhizoma alismatis, 15 gm; Herba eupatorii, 20 gm;

Radix curcumae, 15 gm; Radix salviae miltiorrhizae, 45 gm; Rhizoma acori graminei, 10 gm; Fructus aurantii immaturus, 10 gm; Rhizoma imperatae, 30 gm; and Radix canna indica, 60 gm. Three doses.

Third consultation on November 6, 1967: Temperature had fallen to 37.5°C. Yellowish and soft stool, yellowish urine. Ascites reduced. The patient was conscious and able to answer questions and tolerated a small quantity of liquid diet. Tongue proper reddish with yellowish fur. Wiry and rapid pulse. TT, 110 u. According to his symptoms and signs, there was still Heat stagnant in the interior, so continued the Heat-clearing therapy. Prescription: Herba artemisiae capillaris, 30 gm; Radix et rhizoma rhei, 12 gm (to be put in later); Fructus gardeniae, 12 gm; Flos lonicerae, 60 gm; Fructus euodiae, 20 gm; Radix bupleuri, 20 gm; Radix salviae miltiorrhizae, 30 gm; Rhizoma alismatis, 10 gm; Radix paeoniae, 10 gm; Poria, 15 gm; Cortex magnoliae officinalis, 10 gm; and Semen plantaginis, 12 gm (wrapped with gauze). Six doses. Decoct Radix canna indica, 60 gm, in water to be taken ad libitum.

Fourth consultation on November 12, 1967: Jaundice regressing gradually. There was evident diminishment of ascites. The patient was able to take 100 ml of liquid diet each meal. There were slight pains on lateral sides of the thorax. Slightly yellowish urine. Modified the previous prescription. Herba artemisiae capillaris, 12 gm; Fructus gardeniae, 9 gm; Flos lonicerae, 15 gm; Radix isatidis, 30 gm; Radix bupleuri, 15 gm; Rhizoma cyperi, 9 gm; Radix paeoniae alba, 15 gm; Radix salviae, 30 gm; Cortex magnoliae officinalis, 9 gm; Pericarpium arecae, 20 gm; Rhizoma alismatis, 9 gm; Radix aucklandiae, 6 gm; and charred Rhizoma atractylodis macrocephalae, 15 gm. Six doses. Decoct Radix canna indica, 60 gm, in water to be taken ad libitum.

Fifth consultation on November 18, 1967: Body temperature normal. Minimal amount of ascites. The patient was ambulatory but with listlessness, shortness of breath and weakness of body. Wiry, small and rapid pulse. Prescription: Herba artemisiae capillaris, 10 gm; Radix isatidis, 30 gm; Radix bupleuri, 10 gm; Radix curcumae, 9 gm; Herba lysimachiae, 20 gm; Rhizoma pinelliae, 9 gm; Pericarpium citri reticulatae, 9 gm; Poria, 15 gm; Rhizoma atractylodis macrocephalae, 15 gm; Pericarpium arecae, 15 gm; Radix codonopsis pilosulae, 6 gm; and Radix glycyrrhizae, 6 gm. Six doses.

Sixth consultation on November 24, 1967: Slight sallow eyes and body with occasional abdominal distention. Slight pain on the right hypochondrium. Bitter taste in mouth, poor appetite, fatigue and yellowish urine. Tongue and pulse condition same as last consultation. Prescription: Herba artemisiae capillaris, 20 gm; Radix isatidis, 20 gm; Herba lysimachiae, 20 gm; Poria, 15 gm; Rhizoma atractylodis macrocephalae, 15 gm; Pericarpium arecae, 15 gm; Radix aucklandiae, 6 gm; Pericarpium citri reticulatae viride, 12 gm; Rhizoma cyperi, 15 gm; Semen persicae, 9 gm; Radix glycyrrhizae, 6 gm; and Radix canna indica, 30 gm. Decoct in water and to be taken continuously at one dose a day for two weeks.

Seventh consultation on December 10, 1967: Disappearance of jaundice. There was no pain experienced on both sides of the hypochondrium. Appetite was still poor and there was slight abdominal distention at night. The patient was to be treated by modified Xiaoyao Powder to coordinate the function of the Liver and Spleen. Radix angelicae, 12 gm; Radix paeoniae alba, 9 gm; Radix bupleuri, 12 gm; Poria, 15 gm; Rhizoma atractylodis macrocephalae, 15 gm; Radix aucklandiae, 6 gm; Pseudostellaria heterophylla, 9 gm; Fructus schisandrae, 9 gm; and Radix glycyrrhizae, 6 gm. Decoct in water, one dose per day for 20 days.

Eighth consultation on December 22, 1967: Aside from the complaints of listlessness, weakness and tiredness, almost all other symptoms had gone. TT and liver function tests were all normal. In order to consolidate the therapeutic effect, the patient was advised to take the prescription at home. He was also advised to have a suitable diet and to take good care of himself during the convalescent period. Prescription: Radix codonopsis pilosulae, 12 gm; Rhizoma atractylodis macrocephalae, 12 gm; Poria, 10 gm; Pericarpium citri reticulatae viride, 9 gm; Herba artemisiae capillaris, 6 gm; Radix bupleuri, 6 gm; Fructus schisandrae, 9 gm; stir-fried Rhizoma dioscoreae, 20 gm; stir-fried Semen coicis, 15 gm; Radix salviae miltiorrhizae, 15 gm; Rhizoma cyperi, 9 gm; and Radix glycyrrhizae, 6 gm.

The patient sent us a letter later saying that he had fully recovered from the condition after taking the prescription for two weeks continuously. The author visited the patient in 1971. He was healthy and the symptoms had not recurred.

DISCUSSION: Subacute necrosis of the liver can be classified in TCM as "jaundice," "epidemic jaundice," "acute jaundice," "hypochondriac pain," etc., which are characterized by acute onset, rapid development and high mortality. It is stated in *General Treatise on the Causes and Symptoms of Disease: Acute Jaundice Symptoms* that Spleen and Stomach disorders cause smoldering of food and Wetness-Heat in the Spleen, Stomach, Liver and Gallbladder. In addition, the patient was attacked by virulent Heat Evil. So the illness had a sudden onset manifested by fullness over the chest and hypochondria and dyspnea. His condition was critical. It was therefore called acute jaundice. The pathogenesis of this condition starts with Heat-Evil domination in the body, virulent Heat-Evil in the Blood and mental confusion. Heavy doses of Modified Herba Artemisiae Capillaris Decoction should be used promptly to cool the Blood and to remove the toxin, clear away the Heat-Evil and promote diuresis and eliminate jaundice. After Heat-Evil began to be reduced gradually, the prescription was modified based on the patient's signs and symptoms so as to eliminate the residual Heat-Evil. In order to get rid of the disease completely, the principles of coordinating Liver and Spleen functions should be applied during the convalescent period. From the author's vast clinical experience, here are some essential points in treating these cases:

1) At the initial stage of the critical state, the principles of treatment should be to relieve the primary and secondary symptoms simultaneously, which means to clear away the Heat and toxic materials, activate Blood circulation to dissipate Blood stasis, promote diuresis and eliminate jaundice. Taking into consideration the teachings of "Spleen disorder arises from Liver disorder" and "Liver bears the dispersing functions," the Liver and Spleen should be coordinated to avoid the decline of Spleen function and the hyperactivity of Wood and to avoid further deterioration of the condition. It is of utmost importance whether the function of dispersing the stagnant Liver energy can be kept in order. Thus, in addition to a heavy dose of herbs which act to eliminate

Heat-Evil, Wetness and jaundice, other medicinal herbs such as Radix bupleuri and Radix curcumae for dispersing the stagnant Liver energy and protecting the Liver, Rhizoma atractylodis and Poria to invigorate the Spleen and eliminate the Wetness, should be included in the prescription.

2) Though ascites was present, the therapeutic regimen of diuresis should not be used only to eliminate the ascites. The diuretic herbs should be taken to treat the symptom at its origin lest the disease recur or deteriorate.

3) Radix et rhizoma rhei can be administered in a large dosage in the prescription in the early stage of the disease. In this way, it not only purges the Fire-Evil and cools the Blood, it brings back consciousness and eliminates jaundice, and it can also get rid of the evil causes of the disease by relieving intestinal stasis.

4) Patients with elevated TT levels should be cared for by dispersing the stagnant Liver energy and promoting the subsidiary Channels in the body through which Vital Energy, Blood and nutriment circulate and through which Evil Wetness is eliminated. Radix canna indica can either be added to the prescription or decocted separately and be taken as a daily drink ad libitum. The therapeutic effect of this herb is most remarkable.

5) After disappearance of jaundice, prescription should not be discontinued at once. Taking into consideration the patient's condition, herbs for clearing away Heat-Evil and promoting diuresis should be taken for an additional period of time. And in order to consolidate the therapeutic effects and to strengthen its roots, the main thrust of treatment at this stage should be to coordinate the functions of the Liver and Spleen. To avoid recurrence of the disease, suitable exercise or exercise combined with rest should be instituted.

3.14 CIRRHOSIS OF THE LIVER WITH ASCITES (ACCUMULATION OF HEAT AND BLOOD STASIS WITH RETENTION OF WATER AND DAMPNESS)

Jiang Chunhua

Zhongshan Hospital, Shanghai First Medical University, Shanghai

Chen, 48, male, Han nationality, married, cadre. Date of first consultation: December 22, 1981.

CHIEF COMPLAINT: Dizziness, abdominal distention, anuria, anorexia, lassitude, dry mouth, constipation and occasional fever for more than three months.

HISTORY OF PRESENT ILLNESS: Enlargement of the liver and frequent right hypochondriac pain were first noticed in 1976. Because of occurrence of jaundice (icteric index, 39 u and GPT, 400 u), he was treated in January 1978, as an icteric hepatitis patient, and recovered after two months. At the beginning of September 1981, following the occurrence of persistent high fever and stabbing pain in the hypochondriac region, the patient had ascites with an abdominal circumference of more than

110 cm, and was treated in Lanzhou, Gansu Province, with no effect. He was subsequently transferred to our hospital for further treatment.

On admission, the patient was emaciated, spoke with a soft voice and had a brown and yellowish complexion. He complained of abdominal pain with sensation of fullness and abdominal distention (abdominal circumference 118 cm). Some vascular spiders on the chest and neck were noted. Accompanying signs and symptoms were congested eyes, dry lips, constipation and scanty urine, about 200 ml per day.

PERTINENT PHYSICAL EXAMINATION & LABORATORY FINDINGS: Liver function tests: thymol turbidity, 18 u; zinc turbidity, 22 u; icteric index, 10 u. Protein electrophoresis revealed albumin, 40.1%; α-globulin, 12.9%; α, 29.5%; ß, 12.7%; γ, 34.8%.

INSPECTION OF TONGUE: Dry and white fur.

PULSE CONDITION: Rapid, wiry and fine.

MODERN MEDICINE DIAGNOSIS: Cirrhosis of the Liver with Ascites.

TRADITIONAL CHINESE MEDICINE DIAGNOSIS: Accumulation of Heat and Blood Stasis; Retention of Water and Dampness; Insufficiency of Middle Jiao Qi.

THERAPEUTIC PRINCIPLES: Benefit the Qi and strengthen the Spleen, activate Blood circulation to eliminate Blood stasis, clear up Heat and dispel Water.

Prescription: Radix astragali, 30 gm; Rhizoma atractylodis macrocephalae, 60 gm; Radix codonopsis pilosulae, 15 gm; Radix et rhizoma rhei, 9 gm; Eupolyphaga seu steleophaga, 9 gm; Semen perdicar, 9 gm; Fructus gardeniae, 9 gm; Squama manitis, 9 gm; Fructus forsythiae, 9 gm; Carapax trionycis, 15 gm; Semen and pericarpium arecae, 9 gm each; Caulis akebiae, 9 gm; Pericarpium Poria, 15 gm, Fructus Auranti immaturus, 12 gm; and Rhizoma imperatae, 30 gm. Decoct for oral ingestion. In addition, Mirabilitum, 60 gm, was used for external application.

FOLLOW-UP/COURSE OF TREATMENT:

Second consultation: After taking 14 doses of this prescription, fever was lowered and the patient was noted to have thin and white tongue fur and wiry, fine pulse. Constipation was relieved and amount of urine increased to about 1,200 ml per day. Abdominal distention and pain alleviated and he was able to take some food. These indicated that Heat had been cleared away, but Dampness remained severe, with Blood stasis and deficiency of Vital Energy. At this stage, the prescription was modified by adding medicinal herbs which are effective in dispelling Dampness. Prescription: Radix astragali, 60 gm; Rhizoma atractylodis macrocephalae, 15 gm; Semen persicae, 9 gm; Semen and pericarpium arecae, 9 gm each; Carapax trionycis, 9 gm; Squama manitis, 9 gm; Caulis akebiae, 6 gm; Rhizoma tinperatae, 30 gm; and black soybean, 30 gm. Seven doses.

Third consultation: In order to relieve the constipation, Radix et rhizoma rhei, 9 gm, was added to the last prescription. Seven doses.

Fourth consultation: Constipation was relieved but amount of urine still scanty (about 1,200 ml per day). Appetite was normal, coating of tongue thin and white. The pulse was wiry, fine and feeble. Prescription: Radix astragali, 30 gm; Rhizoma atractylodis macrocephalae, 60 gm; Radix et rhizoma rhei, 9 gm; Eupolyphaga seu steleophaga, 9 gm; Semen persicae, 9 gm; Poria, 15 gm; Caulis akebiae, 9 gm; Rhizoma tiperatae, 30 gm; Pericarpium lagenariae cerariae, 15 gm; and Moth-eaten bamboo shoot, 30 gm. Fourteen doses.

Fifth consultation: The patient's condition was much better with gradually improving appetite. Emaciated appearance was gone and his abdominal pain and distention relieved. He had two bowel movements every day and an increased amount of urine (2,500 ml per day). His abdominal circumference had been reduced to 95 cm. Still present were signs of congested eyes, dry lips, sleep disturbance, reddish tongue with white fur, fine and wiry pulse. Additional ingredients for clearing away the Heat-Evil and nourishing the Yin were applied, i.e., Rhizoma coptidis, 15 gm; Colla corii asini, 9 gm; and Caulis lonicerae, 15 gm. These were added to the last prescription.

Sixth consultation: The patient's mentality and appearance had improved significantly. Symptoms had subsided completely. Vascular spider absent from abdominal wall and abdominal circumference was 87 cm. Liver function test: thymol turbidity, 8 u; zinc turbidity, 12 u; icteric index, 6 u. Protein electrophoresis: albumin, 58.4%; α-globulin, 2.4%; α, 4.6; ß, 12.3%; γ, 22.3%. There was general improvement of the patient's condition, but he still had dreamful sleep. Semen jujubae, 12 gm, was added to the previous prescription. After 14 doses of this modified prescription, the patient recovered fully. He went back to Gansu Province and continued to take the prescription, which was discontinued when he had consumed all of the preparations he brought back with him. Liver function tests and protein electrophoresis results were normal.

DISCUSSION: In this case, abdominal distention was due to Jaundice, Blood stasis and accumulation of stagnant Heat-Evil in the Liver as well as retention of Wetness caused by blockade of the water passages. With the passing of time, body's Primordial Energy was damaged and Spleen-asthenia resulted. Based on clinical experience of the author and in accordance with the teaching of *Nei Jing (Canon of Internal Medicine)* that obstruction-syndrome should be treated by bonics in cases with severe ascites due to liver cirrhosis and insufficiency of the Middle Jiao Qi, a large dosage of Radix rehmanniae and Rhizoma atractylodis macrocephalae was used to prevent hepatic coma and to eliminate Blood stasis. For cases of Blood stasis complicated with Heat, Fructus gardeniae, Fructus forsythiae and black soybean are added to clear away Heat, cool the Yin and decrease the hemorrhagic tendency and clinical sign of vascular spider. Rhizoma imperatae and black soybean have the effect of increasing the albumin level and regulating the ratio of albumin and globulin which are crucial to the recovery of hepatic metabolic functions. Moth-eaten bamboo shoot, Poria and Caulis akebiae can speed up diuresis to remove ascitic fluid. For Yin deficiency, hyperactivity of Fire and mental disorder, Rhizoma coptidis and Colla corii asini are applied.

Application of effective TCM treatment not only leads to remission of abdominal distention but also reverses the abnormal laboratory findings.

3.15 LIVER CIRRHOSIS WITH ASCITES
(LIVER STAGNATION WITH SPLEEN DEFICIENCY)

Li Congfu
Hunan Academy of Traditional Chinese Medicine and Materia Medica, Changsha

Hu, 45, male, Han nationality, married, cadre. Date of first consultation: April 15, 1962.

CHIEF COMPLAINT: Abdominal fullness, loss of weight and general weakness of two years duration; appearance of greenish vessels on the abdominal wall for six months.

HISTORY OF PRESENT ILLNESS: In the summer of 1956, the patient suffered from jaundice with xanthochromic sclera and skin. Accompanying signs and symptoms were fatigue, weakness, nausea and aversion to fatty food, poor appetite and xanthochromic urine. He was then diagnosed as having acute icteric hepatitis. After treatment, jaundice and symptoms were relieved (the patient could not recall the names of drugs used). He went back to work full-time and started to experience vague distending pain in the right hypochondrium as well as distending pain under the xiphoid process, which was tender when pressed. He also complained of general fatigue, lassitude and lack of vigour. These signs and symptoms occurred at irregular intervals. In the past two years, his condition took a turn for the worse. He complained of xanthochromic sclera and skin, rapid deterioration of appetite, aversion to fatty food, nausea, dizziness, palpitation, loose stool and oliguria. Condition of the patient continued to deteriorate progressively. Symptoms and signs experienced by the patient recently, in addition to those mentioned above, were strain and distending pain of abdominal wall and appearance of nevus araneus on the shoulders and neck. Therapeutic attempts using modern medications (the patient could not recall the names of drugs used) failed to afford any relief from the condition. The patient subsequently came to our clinic for further treatment.

PERTINENT PHYSICAL EXAMINATION & LABORATORY FINDINGS: Dull complexion, emaciated, abdominal fullness, visible greenish vessels on abdominal wall, ascites, nevus araneus on the neck. Liver function test: icteric index, 9 u; thymol turbidity, 10 u; zinc sulfate turbidity test, 27 u; cephalin cholesterol flocculation test (CCFT) positive; Takata-Ara test positive. General serum protein, 4.95 gm/l; serum albumin, 1.64 gm/l; seroglobulin, 3.31 gm/l; A/GM ratio inversion.

INSPECTION OF TONGUE: Greenish edges of tongue substance with yellowish and greasy fur.

PULSE CONDITION: String-like and rapid.

MODERN MEDICINE DIAGNOSIS: Hepatocirrhosis with Ascites.

TRADITIONAL CHINESE MEDICINE DIAGNOSIS: Tympanitic Disease (Depression of Liver Energy and Asthenia of the Spleen).

THERAPEUTIC PRINCIPLES: Disperse the depressed Liver energy and rectify the Spleen; promote Vital Energy and Blood circulation.

PRESCRIPTION: Liver Soothing Decoction, to be modified according to different stages of the illness. Carapax trionycis, 16 gm; Poria, 13 gm; Radix angelicae, 10 gm; Radix paeoniae alba, 10 gm; Rhizoma atractylodis macrocephalae, 10 gm; Radix salviae, 13 gm; Rhizoma alismatis, 10 gm; Radix glycyrrhizae praeparatae, 3 gm; Radix aucklandiae, 5 gm; Fructus aurantii, 7 gm; Radix curcumae, 9 gm; and Pericarpium citri reticulatae et viride, 6 gm. One dose per day.

FOLLOW-UP/COURSE OF TREATMENT:

Second consultation: After administration of 40 doses of this prescription, dull and somber complexion lightened up with gradual appearance of ruddy complexion. Greenish edges of the tongue also got lighter and tongue coating changed from yellowish and greasy to a thin one. Pulse mild and even. Abdomen was very much relaxed now. The patient felt well generally. His sense of taste had returned and the amount of urine increased. Modified the original prescription by adding herbs effective in invigorating the Spleen and promoting digestion. Carapax trionycis, 13 gm; Radix salviae, 13 gm; Radix paeoniae alba, 10 gm; Rhizoma atractylodis macrocephalae, 10 gm; Radix codonopsis, 10 gm; Poria, 10 gm; Radix angelicae, 10 gm; Pericarpium citri reticulatae et viride, 10 gm; Radix curcumae, 6 gm; Fructus aurantii, 6 gm; Fructus hordei germinatus, 10 gm; Radix glycyrrhizae praeparatae, 3 gm; and stir-fried Liuqu, 10 gm.

Third consultation: After taking 40 doses of the second prescription, the patient's complexion was lustrous now and his appetite improved day by day. The patient was feeling much better. Applied the therapeutic principle of coordinating the functions of the Liver and Spleen. Prescription: Radix salviae, 13 gm; Radix codonopsis, 10 gm; Radix angelicae, 10 gm; Poria, 10 gm; Rhizoma atractylodis macrocephalae, 10 gm; Radix paeoniae alba, 10 gm; Fructus hordei germinatus, 10 gm; Pericarpium citri reticulatae, 6 gm; Radix glycyrrhizae praeparatae, 3 gm; fructus oryzae germinatus, 10 gm; and Endothelium corneum gigeriae galli, 5 gm.

The patient's health was completely restored after taking this prescription for a long period of time.

DISCUSSION: Hepatic cirrhosis with ascites is part of the tympanitic disease due to parasitic infection according to traditional Chinese medicine. This is a serious case of "state of evil domination and asthenia of health energy" produced by development of "asthenia of both the Liver and Spleen." Shen Jinao of the Qing Dynasty states that "tympanitic disease due to parasitic infection, which manifests with only abdominal distention without swelling of the limbs and face, is also known as spider tympanitis due to parasitic infection." Varicosis of the abdominal wall is a characteristic sign of the disease. Pathogenesis of this disease is internal impairment caused by over-straining, resulting in depressed Vital Energy. Liver energy, which regulates the activity of the Vital Energy, is likewise depressed. The sequence of events following this will be obstruction of Blood circulation leading to Blood stasis and impairment of the transport and conversion functions of the Spleen leading to Spleen asthenia. As such, the Spleen is not able to transport and convert the pathologic Wetness. Retention of Wetness leads to abdominal distention. The ability to convert demonstrates the interdependent relationship of the Vital Energy-Blood-Water process. The principal clinical manifestation of this case was severe Spleen deficiency and disintegration of the Visceral Energy. Taking this into consideration, the main thrust of treatment in this case was aimed at obtaining a "strong Spleen" state. Consequently, Wu Wei Yi Gong San (Composition of Herbs of Five Flavours) was employed to replenish the Spleen energy. Radix aucklandiae, Fructus aurantii, Pericarpium citri reticulatae and Fructus hordei germinatus were used to promote the function of the Spleen; Radix salviae, Radix angelicae and Radix paeoniae alba to regulate the functional relation between Liver-energy and Blood and Carapax trionycis; and Pericarpium citri reticulatae et viride and Radix curcumae to dissipate Liver stasis. "The Vital Energy is in Blood, Blood houses the Vital Energy. Stagnation of the Vital Energy produces Blood stasis." Therefore the therapeutic principles for this case were to supplement the Spleen energy, regulate the Vital Energy, regulate the functional relation between the Liver and Blood, dissipate Blood stasis and alleviate mental depression, resulting in simultaneous elimination of evil factors and restoration of a healthy Vital Energy.

As modern medicine sees it, this is a case of cirrhosis of the liver, the diagnosis being established based on the signs and symptoms as well as a positive history of hepatitis. In addition to the apparent compensatory-period signs and symptoms, the patient also had varicosis of the abdominal wall, which reflects presence of portal hypertension. He also had severely impaired liver functions. Jaundice and ascites were also present, making surgical procedures contraindicated in this case. Splenectomy, whose therapeutic efficacy probably would be minimal, could be considered after a reasonably healthy condition was sustained by medical treatment. Our clinic resorts to the alternate route of treating the patient by TCM with all therapeutic measures based on the science of symptom-complex differentiation. This therapeutic effect is very significant.

3.16 ASCITES DUE TO PORTAL CIRRHOSIS (BLOODY ABDOMINAL DISTENTION)

Kang Liangshi
Xiamen Traditional Chinese Medicine Hospital, Xiamen

Chi, 33, male, Han nationality, married, technician. Medical record number: 831027. Date of first consultation: November 27, 1983.
CHIEF COMPLAINT: Hematemesis and bloody stool for 17 days.
HISTORY OF PRESENT ILLNESS: During the period from January to October of this year, the patient had three episodes of massive upper gastrointestinal tract hemorrhage. Blood transfusion, fluid infusion and hemostatic administration were the main modes of treatment. Later on the patient noticed melena, epistaxis and petechiae on the lower extremities. On the morning of consultation, he experienced nausea, distress and distention of the abdomen, vertigo and irritability. He spat blood and

noticed passage of bloody stool. There was an accompanying fever of 39.0°C. He also complained of thirst and scanty amount of dark urine.

PAST HISTORY: The patient had infectious hepatitis at age nine. Presence of hepatomegaly and splenomegaly as well as abnormal liver function tests findings since then. Esophagogram revealed presence of esophageal varix.

PERTINENT PHYSICAL EXAMINATION & LABORATORY FINDINGS: Pale, emaciated; fatigue with general weakness. Blood pressure, 80/50 mmHg. Dull sallow colour of the cheeks and forehead, yellowish conjunctivae and skin. Dilated epigastric veins visible on the chest and lower abdomen; moist skin; and pale nail beds. Edema of the lower extremities; scaly skin with presence of petechiae. Hemoglobin, 5 gm%; RBC, 1.74M/mm^3; total protein, 4.8 gm; albumin, 2.3 gm; globulin, 2.5 gm. TFT, (+++); TTT, 12 u; ZnTT, 15 gm.

INSPECTION OF TONGUE: Pale, swollen and delicate tongue substance with fissures and bristles; no coating.

PULSE CONDITION: Rapid pulse, weak when pressed; pulse rate 104/min.

MODERN MEDICINE DIAGNOSIS: Ascites Secondary to Portal Cirrhosis accompanied by Upper Gastrointestinal Tract Hemorrhage.

TRADITIONAL CHINESE MEDICINE DIAGNOSIS: Bloody Abdominal Distention; Liver Fire Affecting the Stomach due to Internal Accumulation of Dampness and Heat.

Symptom-complex differentiation: When the jaundice had disappeared, a mass was noted in the hypochondrium. This was caused by the existence of pathogens and stagnation of the Vital Energy in the Blood. The patient was pale and emaciated and complained of abdominal distention, hypochondriac pain, bitter taste in the mouth and dark and hot urine. These are signs of accumulation of Fire in the Liver affecting the Stomach, Dampness and Heat impairing the Liver and Spleen. Zhu Danxi describes it as "combination of Dampness and Heat, mixture of the Clear and Turbid, obstruction of the Channels causing distention" and "internal accumulation of Dampness and Heat leading to yellowish skin." When the Liver does not store the Blood, hematemesis, epistaxis and bloody stool result. Liver is concerned with the coagulation process, and this prolonged stasis of Wood and Fire disseminates a vigorous Fire to other organs resulting in hemorrhagic tendencies, i.e., hematemesis, epistaxis and bloody stool. *Ling Shu (Miraculous Pivot)*, a medical classic on acupuncture, states that "if a patient has irregular diet and daily habits of life, his Luo-Mai (the collateral Channels) may be damaged." Injury of Yang Channels causes external bleeding, so epistaxis occurs. Likewise, injury of Yin Channels causes internal bleeding that leads to melena. Due to the large amount of blood lost, the patient fell into a stuporous state quickly with pallor, sweat and thirst, rapid pusle and general weakness, swollen and delicate tongue with fissures. His pulse was barely palpable. All these indicated the patient's Vital Energy and Blood had been damaged seriously. So emergency measures were instituted for resuscitation.

THERAPEUTIC PRINCIPLES: Based on the teaching "to treat the Biao for emergency first," apply the principles of tonifying the Vital Energy and reducing body fluid to bring about hemostasis and sustain the patient from collapse, eliminating Heat and detoxifying and eliminating the stagnant Blood and activating Blood circulation.

PRESCRIPTION: Folium Callicarpae Pedunculatae Decoction for slow oral ingestion. Callicarpae pedunculatae pulverized, Radix notoginseng, 8 gm; and Natural bezoar, 1.5 gm. Ground ingredients into powder and divided into eight shares. One share for two hours. Cut Radix panacis quinquefolii (American ginseng) into 1 gm slices. Sucked frequently, not to be swallowed.

FOLLOW-UP/COURSE OF TREATMENT:

Second consultation on November 22, 1983: Hematemesis and melena had been stopped. The patient passed grass-green stool, loose to dry, once a day. Nasal mucus with blood streaks. Occasional ecchymotic spots on the tongue. Abdominal and hypochondriac pain alleviated. The patient still complained of thirst and sweating, fever in the afternoon (37.8°C), abdominal distention, frequent borborygmus and flatulence, scanty dark urine and dysuria, frequent dreams.

The patient's mental state had improved very much. He was calm though still lethargic. Jaundiced; fissured lips and oral ulcer; pale tongue without coating; rapid pulse; blood pressure elevated; borborygmus present; petechiae on skin and edema of lower extremities.

These signs and symptoms indicated that the damaged Luo-Mai (collateral Channels) had recovered from danger and internal stagnation had been partially dissipated. Jaundice, fissured lips and oral ulcer, scanty dark urine and dysuria reflected internal stasis of Dampness and Heat. At this stage, the patient had deficiency of the Vital Energy with stagnation of Dampness and Heat. The appropriate treatment was now to clear away Dampness and Heat in order to eliminate jaundice and distention.

Therapeutic principles: to excrete the Dampness by tasteless herbs; to harmonize the relationship between the Liver and Spleen.

Prescription: Herba artemisiae, 30 gm; Talcum, 24 gm; Extract poriae, 24 gm; Polyporus umbellatus, 10 gm; Rhizoma alismatis, 10 gm; Pericarpium arecae, 10 gm; Medulla tetrapanacis, 3 gm; Semen coicis, 15 gm; Fructus gardeniae, 10 gm; Fructus citri, 10 gm; Radix notoginseng, 3 gm; Radix curcumae, 5 gm; and Pericarpium citri reticulatae et viride, 5 gm.

After taking this prescription for a week, the patient reported an increased appetite, normal urine and bowel movement. There was no dysuria and he passed a large amount of clear urine. Jaundice started to subside. Abdominal distention and edema of lower extremities gradually diminishing. There was still a little blood in the nasal mucus and the petechiae persisted. The patient had taken Equus asinus once which resulted in increase of the petechiae, borborygmus and frequent passing of gas, fullness of the chest and bitter taste with tidal fever of 37.8°C. In the last four weeks, there were three bouts of high fever. When this fever occurred, the patient had aversion to cold first and then fever. Headache, general malaise and profuse sweating when the fever was brought down. After each of these bouts of fever, his appetite decreased a little bit and the amount of urine was scanty.

History and physical examination revealed that the patient had light red tongue substance, rapid pulse, dry throat, cracked lips and oral ulcer, muscle pains on the extremities, and difficulty in falling asleep before dawn because of restlessness. These signs and symptoms indicated stasis of the Liver and Gallbladder, hemorrhagic shock and deficiency of Yin, accumulation of pathogens in the Yin and internal stagnation of the "Primordial Fire."

Therapeutic principles: clear the Liver channels, dispel the Primordial Fire, and eliminate stasis.

Prescription: Radix stellariae, 3 gm; Herba artemisiae, 3 gm; Carapax trionycis, 6 gm; Urina hominis, 20 ml; Radix scutellariae, 3 gm; Rhizoma coptidis, 3 gm; Radix angelicae, 3 gm; Radix glycyrrhizae, 2 gm; Radix paeoniae alba, 6 gm; Cortex lycii radicis, 10 gm; Radix gentianae, 6 gm; Rhizoma anemarrhenae, 5 gm; Cortex moutan radicis, 5 gm; and Radix panacis quinquefolii, 3 gm.

Fourth consultation on January 6, 1984: Tidal fever had been relieved. The patient reported increased appetite. He did not experience vertigo when getting out of bed. There were still complaints of thirst and lassitude, recurrence of epistaxis because of taking dried human placenta and inability to fall asleep at night because of restlessness. Light red tongue substance; petechiae on the skin of the chest and back; and slow pulse. These signs showed that the stasis had been dissipated partially and pathogens eliminated gradually. Adopting the same therapeutic principles of the last visit, prescribed medicinal herbs effective in nourishing the Yin and the Liver.

Prescription: Replace Herba artemisiae, Rhizoma anemarrhenae and Radix glycyrrhizae of the last prescription with Herba dendrobii rhizoma, 10 gm; Rhizoma alismatis plantago-aquatica, 10 gm; and Concha haliodis, 24 gm.

Fifth consultation on January 18, 1984: Symptoms of thirst and bitter taste in the mouth had been eliminated. There was occasional fullness of the chest, slight restlessness with change of climate since he left extremities exposed during sleep. He complained of sensation of heat in the orbits, nostrils and centre of palms.

Improved mental state; light red and enlarged tongue with white and thin coating. Adopted the same treatment as the last one, adding Plastrum testudinis, 10 gm, and Radix scrophulariae, 10 gm, to tonify and replenish the Yin in order to nourish the Wood.

Sixth consultation on February 3, 1984: The patient made up a prescription by adding Cuscuta chinensis, 10 gm, into Yiguan Jian. After seven doses, scanty amount of urine was noted and other symptoms were aggravated. This was because the harmful Fire had not been eliminated completely. It would not be appropriate to give just tonics. Thus, 10 gm of Radix scrophulariae were added to the previous prescription.

Seventh consultation on February 23, 1984: The patient could fall asleep at night now and did not leave his extremities exposed during sleep. He did not feel restless with climate change. There was no warm sensation in the orbits, nostrils and centre of palms. No vertigo nor coldness of feet when getting out of bed. No epistaxis. Increased appetite. Normal urine and bowel movement. Laboratory tests: hemoglobin, 5 gm%; RBC, 4.48M/mm^3; total protein, 8 gm; albumin, 3.3 gm; globulin, 4.7 gm; TFT, 13 u. It would be appropriate now to tonify the Spleen and Kidney.

Prescription: Fructus lycii, 10 gm; Radix rehmanniae, 10 gm; Poria, 10 gm; Euryale ferox, 10 gm; Semen nelumbinis, 10 gm; Rhizoma alismatis, 10 gm; Radix ophiopogonis, 10 gm; Radix adenophorae, 6 gm; Fructus meliae toosenden, 6 gm; and

Radix angelicae, 5 gm.

DISCUSSION: According to the TCM teaching of "treating the Biao first for emergency," Folium Callicarpa Pedunculatae Decoction was administered initially to stop the hemorrhage. Callicarpa pedunculatae is known to be a hemostatic agent through clinical experience. It has been confirmed through animal tests that Callicarpa pedunculatae can contrict blood vessels, including intestinal blood vessels, and produces a series of hemostatic factors as well. But this effect can only last for three minutes. It was thus necessary to administer it by a small powder dose and a large liquid dose alternately. When this is given together with medicinal herbs effective in tonifying the Vital Energy and producing Blood, dissipating the Heat and detoxifying, such as Radix panacis quinquefolii and Radix notoginseng, a more pronounced therapeutic effect could be obtained.

When hemostasis was achieved, relief of jaundice and ascites became the priority. The patient's condition at this stage was one of hemorrhagic shock, deficiency of the Vital Energy complicated by accumulation of Dampness and Heat. The therapeutic principle would naturally be to eliminate Dampness and Heat, clear the Liver and regulate the Spleen. Accordingly, on the second visit, in addition to the use of Citri curcumae and notoginseng to sustain the Vital Energy, to activate the Blood and to regulate the Spleen, other medicinal herbs were also used to dispel the Dampness and Heat.

3.17 CIRRHOSIS OF THE LIVER
(DEFICIENCY OF BOTH QI AND YIN, DEPRESSION OF THE LIVER DUE TO BLOOD STASIS)

Jiang Chunhua

Zhongshan Hospital, Shanghai First Medical University, Shanghai

Yang, 42, male, Han nationality, married, teacher. Date of first consultation: December 31, 1981.

CHIEF COMPLAINT: Stomachache, tarry stool, edema, pain in the liver region, lassitude and emaciation.

HISTORY OF PRESENT ILLNESS: The patient was admitted to the hospital because of acute perforation of gastro-duodenal ulcer and acute peritonitis on December 13, 1981. Surgical repair of the perforation was done and diffuse nodular liver cirrhosis was noted. The patient complained of anorexia, right hypochondriac distention with stabbing pain, stomachache, dry mouth with bleeding gum, dizziness and loss of weight.

PAST HISTORY: The patient had hepatitis in 1969; suffered from liver cirrhosis for one year.

PERTINENT PHYSICAL EXAMINATION & LABORATORY FINDINGS: Lusterless and dark complexion; crimson lips; vascular spiders on abdomen. Liver palpable 3 cm below right costal margin, hard in consistency. Laboratory findings normal except ZnTT, 16 u.

INSPECTION OF TONGUE: Tongue substance red.

PULSE CONDITION: Wiry pulse.

MODERN MEDICINE DIAGNOSIS: Diffuse Nodular Cirrhosis of the Liver.

TRADITIONAL CHINESE MEDICINE DIAGNOSIS: Deficiency of Both Qi and Yin; Depression of the Liver due to Blood Stasis.

THERAPEUTIC PRINCIPLES: Replenish the Qi and nourish the Yin, activate Blood circulation to soften the mass.

PRESCRIPTION: Radix codonopsis pilosulae, 9 gm; Radix astragali, 15 gm; Radix rehmanniae, 9 gm; Semen persicae, 12 gm; Radix salviae miltiorrhizae, 9 gm; Carapax trionycis, 12 gm; Herba agrimoniae, 15 gm; Eupolyphaga seu steleophaga phaga, 9 gm; Radix et rhizoma rhei, 3 gm; and Concha arecae, 15 gm. Fourteen doses.

FOLLOW-UP/COURSE OF TREATMENT:

Second consultation: Because of right hypochondriac distending pain, Olibanum, 9 gm, was added to the above prescription.

Third consultation: The symptoms of bitter taste in the mouth, dry mouth, yellow fur of the tongue, red-brown urine, and right hypochondriac pain were remitting. Cortex moutan radicis, 9 gm, and Fructus forsythiae, 9 gm, were added to the original prescription. Fourteen doses were prescribed.

Fourth consultation: Deficiency of both Spleen and Stomach Qi and disorder in food digestion and fluid transportation were manifested as distending pain of the stomach. Anorexia, bowel movements two to three times per day, yellow urine, reddish tongue with white, thick and greasy fur. For treatment, charred Fructus crataegi medicated leaven, 9 gm; fried membrane of chicken's gizzard-skin, 9 gm; and husked sorghum, 15 gm, were added. Seven doses.

Fifth consultation: To treat symptoms of stomachache and poor appetite, frequent bowel movements, mild edema of the feet, unsound sleep, thin and greasy fur of the tongue and soft pulse, Concha arecae was replaced in the original prescription with Rhizoma atractylodis macrocephalae, 30 gm; black soybean, 30 gm; and Caulis lonicerae, 15 gm. Twenty-eight doses were given.

After this treatment, symptoms gradually disappeared. Facial colour and appetite returned to normal. Hypochondriac pain was alleviated and no vascular spider was found. ZnTT level normal. Taking the advice of the surgeon, the patient underwent subtotal gastrectomy and gastrojejunostomy on April 3, 1982. During the operation, instead of the original diffuse nodular cirrhosis of the liver, nodules on the right lobe of the liver had disappeared but some nodules still remained on its left lobe.

DISCUSSION: It is rare to have a case of cirrhosis of the liver concomitant with two abdominal operations for gastric disorders, whereby the condition of the liver can actually be visualized. During the first operation, diffuse nodular cirrhosis of the liver was found, while in the second, i.e., after three months of TCM treatment, the nodules on the right lobe of the liver had completely disappeared. This indicates that for the liver cirrhosis patient, the therapeutic principle of replenishing the Qi, strengthening the Spleen and activating Blood circulation to eliminate Blood stasis not only could improve the signs but also might have the capability to reverse the parenchymatous pathology of liver cirrhosis.

3.18 PRIMARY LIVER CANCER
(LIVER MASS)

Yu Rencun

Department of Oncology, Beijing Traditional Chinese Medicine Hospital, Beijing

Li, 50, male, Han nationality, married, cadre. Medical record number: 97642. Date of first consultation: January, 1971.

CHIEF COMPLAINT: Nausea, poor appetite and liver ache for more than a year.

HISTORY OF PRESENT ILLNESS: It has been a year since the patient had poor appetite, nausea and pains in the right hypochondriac region. In 1971, he had liver function tests in a hospital with a GPT value between 120 and 200 units. His case was diagnosed as chronic hepatitis. After six months of treatment, the symptoms persisted and a hard nodule could be felt at the upper part of the abdomen. Ultrasound examination was performed in one of the hospitals in Beijing revealing the lower border of the liver extending 6 cm below the right costal margin. In December of the same year, the patient had isotope scan of the liver which showed a space-occupying lesion in the liver. Meanwhile, he also had an AFP test and was finally diagnosed as having liver cancer with extensive pathological changes. Chemotherapy consisting of 5-Fu, 10 gm and TSPA, 600 mg was instituted instead of surgical treatment. It was discontinued when WBC count decreased to $3,000/mm^3$ and platelet count to $20,000-70,000/mm^3$. From then on, the patient complained of pain in the liver region with visible abdominal distention, vomiting, dizziness, unhealthy pulse condition, weakness, difficulty in locomotion and weight loss of over 10 kg. He subsequently came to our clinic for consultation.

PAST HISTORY: The patient denies previous history of hepatitis and tuberculosis.

PERTINENT PHYSICAL EXAMINATION & LABORATORY FINDINGS: Chronic disease facies, emaciated. Abdomen flat with swelling on the epigastric region which extended 8 cm below the right costal margin. Hard, tender and fixed. Varicose veins visible on the abdominal wall. FP test, (++); SGPT, 186u; TTT, (-). Isotope scanning findings: close microwave and vertical microwave noted. The liver extended 8 cm under the right hypochondrium. Space-occupying pathological changes, probable liver cancer; isotope scanning indicated abnormality of the liver, imbalance of absorption of isotope 198 and space-occupying pathological changes. WBC count, $3,100/mm^3$; platelet count $54,000/mm^3$.

INSPECTION OF TONGUE: Tongue proper deep red with yellowish, thin and sticky coating.

PULSE CONDITION: Thready and rapid.

MODERN MEDICINE DIAGNOSIS: Primary Liver Cancer.

TRADITIONAL CHINESE MEDICINE DIAGNOSIS: Liver Mass.

THERAPEUTIC PRINCIPLES: Regulate the function of the Liver and Vital Energy, disperse Blood stasis and stop pain, eliminate Heat and clear away harmful factors, and promote Vital Energy.

FOLLOW-UP/COURSE OF TREATMENT:

First course of treatment (January 1971 to February 1973): The patient's major symptoms were pain in the liver region, prominent abdominal distention, vomiting, light-headedness, lack of strength, difficulty in walking, swelling in the abdomen, low peripheral blood counts, deep red tongue, yellowish, sticky tongue coating and thready, rapid pulse. Medications were prescribed to regulate the function of the Liver and Vital Energy, soften the hardness and dispel the nodules, replenish the Spleen and Stomach, and promote Vital Energy and Blood.

PRESCRIPTION: Radix bupleuri, 6 gm; Herba artemisiae scopariae, 30 gm; Rhizoma pinelliae, 9 gm; Herba lysimachiae, 15 gm; Radix aucklandiae, 6 gm; Fructus meliae tousendan, 9 gm; Colla corii asini, 15 gm; Radix angelicae, 9 gm; Radix paeoniae alba and rubra, 9 gm each; Carapax trionycis, 30 gm; Cortex magnoliae officinalis, 9 gm; Rhizoma zedoariae, 6 gm; Radix astragali, 15 gm; Radix polygoni multiflori, 30 gm; Radix isatidis, 15 gm; Caulis spatholobi, 30 gm; Spica prunellae, 15 gm; Fructus polygoni orientalis, 30 gm; Bungei decne, 30 gm; Prunella vulgaris, 15 gm; and Polygonum orie orientale, 30 gm. One dose a day. Decocted twice and taken separately.

Other management: (1) Bie Jiajian Pill, one in the morning and one in the evening; and (2) Royal Jelly, 5 ml, once or twice a day.

The patient took this regimen for a period of two years. During this time, the symptoms, to varying extents, were alleviated. He was on the mend with normal peripheral blood counts (Hemoglobin, 13.6 gm%, WBC, 8,200/mm^3; platelet, 150,000/mm^3). There were signs of remission of abdominal swelling.

Second course of treatment (February 1973 to May 1977): To consolidate the therapeutic effects of the first treatment course, the following medications were used along with the original prescription: (1) Ping Gan Shu Luo Pill, one pill every other day; (2) Bie Jiajian Pill, one in the morning and one in the evening, every other day; and (3) Oliminate Atumour Pill, one in the evening, every other day.

After two courses of treatment, though still with pain in the liver region, the patient reported improvement of appetite and lessening of the nauseating feeling. He had gained weight, from 56 kg to 70 kg. On the whole, he was getting better and was working half-time. The swelling in his abdomen had turned smaller and softer and less painful. Isotope scanning indicated the absorption of isotope 198 and visible reduction of the blank area. AFP examination was negative on two occasions; SGPT, 63; hemoglobin, 12.6 gm%; WBC count, 7,700/mm^3 and platelet count, 130,000/mm^3.

DISCUSSION: *Canon of Internal Medicine*, one of the most ancient books of traditional Chinese medicine, records the cause, signs and symptoms of a disease very much like those of what we know today as liver cancer. Its pathogenesis is considered to be damage of the main and collateral Channels by anorexia, chills and fever, fatigue and unhappiness. Mass is caused by deficiency of Vital Energy, damage of the Liver and Spleen, stagnation of the Vital Energy and Blood stasis and internal invasion by Blood stasis. Symptoms manifested are retention of toxic materials in the Liver, hypochondriac pain, loss of appetite and abdominal distention, nausea, fatigue and dizziness. Accumulation and retention of toxins internally gradually damage the Vital Energy and Blood and lead to deficiency of the Vital Energy and Yin deficiency of the Liver and Kidney. Application of traditional prescriptions in this case is aimed at relaxing the Liver and regulating the function of the Vital Energy, clearing away Heat and softening the mass, nourishing the Blood, clearing away harmful pathogens and nourishing the Liver and Kidney. The key part of the treatment is to control the neoplastic process, alleviate the symptoms and improve the well-being of the patient.

In China, primary liver cancer carries a high mortality rate and a low curative rate. The course of disease usually develops rapidly and is generally difficult to treat, which has earned it the sobriquet "king of cancers." It is estimated that the natural survival period of those who suffer from liver cancer with no medical treatment averages about 4.9 years and the median survival period is between 2.6 and 3.8 months. With the more comprehensive therapeutic regimens of recent years, the one-year survival rate has risen slightly. Chemotherapy is of reasonable effectiveness as a treatment for liver cancer. Generally, the chemical agents used are TSPA and 5-Fu. It has been reported that 5-Fu and TSPA, together with supplementary traditional Chinese medicine, can maintain an average survival rate of 28% with the highest being 34%. The patient in this particular case had been consulting us for six to seven years. After being treated by the combination of both traditional Chinese and modern medicine, his symptoms were alleviated remarkably. He is in apparent good health and is able to attend to light work duties. This case is a fine illustration of the advantage of a combined therapeutic regimen using both traditional Chinese and modern medicine.

3.19 ACUTE HEMORRHAGIC NECROTIC ENTERITIS (VISCERAL INTOXICATION)

Hong Yongshen and Chen Jianyong
Hangzhou Red Cross Hospital, Hangzhou

Yu Huigeng, 24, male, Han nationality, single, farmer. Medical record number: 13836. Admitted on May 29, 1982.

HISTORY OF PRESENT ILLNESS: The patient felt dull pain around the umbilical region after eating pork and two pieces of raw cucumber two days ago. The pain was tolerable initially but became persistent later on with intermittent intensification of severity. There was no radiation to other parts of the body. He had three bowel movements and the stool was noted to be soft, yellow in colour and with a small amount of mucus. There was no blood or pus noted and he did not experience tenesmus. Persistent pain and intermittent colics were experienced after each bowel movement. He vomited "coffee-coloured," liquid gastric contents twice. He sought medical advice that night at a local clinic. Anagelsics and anitihelmintics were administered which did not afford any relief. He visited another local hospital where fluid administration and gentamycin injection likewise did not relieve the symptoms. The next day, he passed jam-like, loose stools. Tenesmus was not present but he had abdominal fullness and bitter taste. He was low in spirits. Stool examination was done in the Yuhang First Hospital showing jam-like stool, WBC (+), RBC (++++), pus cells minimal, occult blood (++++). He was diagnosed as having "hemorrhagic necrotic enteritis" and was subsequently transferred to our hospital.

On admission, the patient had a slight fever without chill, poor appetite and lack of sleep. No jaundice noted.

PAST HISTORY: Non-contributory.

PERTINENT PHYSICAL EXAMINATION & LABORATORY FINDINGS: Temperature, 37°C; pulse rate, 86/min; respiratory rate, 16/min; blood pressure, 106/56 mmHg. Conscious, acute and drawn facies. Head and EENT, normal. Heart and lung findings negative. No tenderness or percussion on the kidney area. Abdomen slightly rigid, marked tenderness around umbilical region with light rebound tenderness. Peristaltic sounds 1-2/min. No mass palpated. Liver and spleen not palpable. Shift dullness negative. No edema on lower extremities and no pathological reflexes elicited. WBC, 12,800/mm^3; neutrophils, 92%. Hemoglobin, 10.5 gm%; platelet, 95,000/mm^3. Stool examination showed a jam-like appearance; WBC, (+); RBC, (++++); pus cells, few; occult blood (++++).

INSPECTION OF TONGUE: Red Tongue substance with thick, greasy and yellowish coating.

PULSE CONDITION: Weak, floating and rapid.

MODERN MEDICINE DIAGNOSIS: Acute Hemorrhagic Necrotic Enteritis.

TRADITIONAL CHINESE MEDICINE DIAGNOSIS: Visceral Intoxication (Retention of Wetness and Heat Evil).

THERAPEUTIC PRINCIPLES: Clear away the Wetness-Heat Evil, cool the Blood and remove the toxins.

PRESCRIPTION: Decoction for Clearing Intestine and Expelling Intoxication (author's preparation). Radix pulsatillae, 30 gm; Herba portulacae, 30 gm; Herba euphorbiae humifusae, 15 gm; Radix sanguisorbae, 15 gm; Flos sophorae, 12 gm; Rhizoma coptidis, 10 gm; and Radix et rhizoma rhei, 6 gm. Three doses. One dose per day. Boil the ingredients in 600 ml of water with proper intensity of heat for an hour to obtain 200 ml of decoction. Add 6 gm of Raw Rhubarb and boil for two more minutes. Divide decoction into two equal parts, to be taken orally twice a day.

Other treatment: Nothing per orem. IV glucose and normal saline infusion with vitamins, kalium chloride, etc. The patient received 2,500 ml of infusion every day in order to correct dehydration and acid-base imbalance.

FOLLOW-UP/COURSE OF TREATMENT:

Second consultation: Abdominal pain and diarrhea were relieved three days after the management. The amount of bloody stool was not as much as before. Body temperature 37.2°C. WBC, 10,200/mm^3; neutrophils, 80%. Stool: WBC, (++) and occult blood, slightly positive. Red Tongue with thin and yellowish coating. Weak, floating and rapid pulse. Continued the previous prescription and replaced Herba portulacae, Flos sophorae and Radix et rhizoma rhei with Radix paeoniae rubra, Fructus aurantii and Poria to enhance the effect of cooling the Blood, promoting Blood circulation, removing stasis and relieving pain. Five doses.

Third consultation: Abdominal pain and diarrhea were relieved progressively. Passage of bloody stool ceased and body temperature was normal. The patient complained only of poor appetite. The treatment of invigorating the Spleen and dredging the Stomach was adopted at this stage. Radix pulsatillae, 15 gm; Radix paeoniae rubra, 15 gm; Radix paeoniae alba, 15 gm; Rhizoma dioscoreae, 15 gm; Radix glycyrrhizae, 6 gm; Poria, 12 gm; Radix aucklandiae, 6 gm; Semen coicis, 15 gm; and Pericarpium citri reticulatae, 6 gm. Seven doses.

All symptoms disappeared after the treatment. The patient's appetite returned. Blood and stool examinations revealed no abnormality. The patient recovered completely and was discharged from hospital.

DISCUSSION:

This case has these clinical features:

1) History of eating raw food;

2) Abdominal pain, diarrhea, jam-like stool with offensive smell; and

3) Red tongue substance with thick, greasy and yellowish coating; weak, floating and rapid pulse.

This is a common disease in children and the young. Bloody stool and toxemia are the main clinical manifestations. The stool is blood-streaked with presence of clots and offensive smell. Disturbance of microcirculation may occur in severe cases.

According to traditional Chinese medicine, this disorder belongs to the category of "visceral intoxication." Appearance of the characteristic stool was first described in the classic *Yan Yonghe (Recipes for Saving Lives)* as "the stool with fresh blood means viceral intoxication." The etiology of this disease is intake of greasy and raw cold food which causes retention of Wetness-Heat Evil and intoxication in the body when the pathogens invade the intestines. These pathogens damage the Yin-Channels and obstruct the Qi and Blood circulation resulting in symptoms of abdominal pain, diarrhea and bloody stool with offensive smell. In accordance with TCM therapeutic principles, the Heat-syndrome is to be treated with "cooling management." In the initial stage of treatment of this disease, emphasis was placed on purgation and clearing away the Evils out of the body and in so doing satisfactory results were obtained. Radix pulsatillae and Radix et rhizoma rhei were the chief therapeutic herbs in the first prescription. Theormer has the function of clearing away the Heat, expelling Evils and cooling the Blood which have been recorded in the classic text of traditional Chinese medicine *Collected Notes to the Canon of Materia Medica*. It is also the chief therapeutic ingredient in treating dysentery. The latter not only has the capability to purge but also the properties of cooling the Blood and expelling stagnation. When combined with Radix pulsatillae, it is able to rectify the Qi and Blood disturbance and to expel the Evils from viscera. Herba euphorbiae humifusae has the nature of controlling bleeding without causing Blood stasis and promoting Blood circulation. Radix sanguisorbae enhances the hemostatic effect, while Rhizoma coptidis and Herba portulacae have the function of clearing away the Evil, cooling the Blood and controlling bleeding. Prescription containing these herbs clears away Heat Evil, promotes the Qi circulation, cools Blood and eliminates stasis. This prescription must be applied in the early stage of the disease. Radix paeoniae rubra is effective in cooling the Blood, promoting Blood circulation and removing Blood stasis. It was employed in a large dosage in the second prescription to treat abdominal distension and pain as well. Modern medicine holds that toxemia can be cured by improvement of microcirculation. Rhizoma dioscoreae, Poria, Radix aucklandiae, Pericarpium citri reticulatae, Semen coicis and Radix glycyr-rhizae were effective in invigorating the Spleen and facilitating the patient's recovery.

4. URINARY DISEASES

4.1 ACUTE PYELONEPHRITIS (DAMP-HEAT STRANGURIA)

Chen Kechong and Zhang Jidong
Shandong Medical University Hospital, Jinan

Wang Manli, 27, female, Han nationality, married, teacher. Medical record number: 266258. Date of first consultation: February 6, 1982.

CHIEF COMPLAINT: Urgent, frequent and painful urination for three days, exacerbated over the last half day.

HISTORY OF PRESENT ILLNESS: The patient complained of urgent, frequent and painful urination with red-colour urine for three days accompanied by lumbago, fatigue, fever, thirst and dry stools. She was admitted to hospital for treatment.

PAST HISTORY: Non-contributory.

PERTINENT PHYSICAL EXAMINATION & LABORATORY FINDINGS: Acute facies. Body temperature, 38°C. Routine urinalysis: protein, (++); puric B.C., (+++); RBC, (+++).

INSPECTION OF TONGUE: Red tongue tip with thick, yellowish fur.

PULSE CONDITION: Slippery and rapid pulse.

MODERN MEDICINE DIAGNOSIS: Acute Pyelonephritis.

TRADITIONAL CHINESE MEDICINE DIAGNOSIS: Damp-Heat Stranguria.

THERAPEUTIC PRINCIPLES: Remove Heat, eliminate Dampness through diuresis and treat stranguria.

PRESCRIPTION: Modified Bazheng Powder. Semen plantaginis, 12 gm; Herba polygoni avicularis, 12 gm; Radix et rhizoma rhei, 9 gm; Cortex moutan radicis, 12 gm; Rhizoma rehmanniae, 12 gm; Cortex phellodendri, 9 gm; Fructus forsythiae, 12 gm; Flos loniscerae, 10 gm; Folium pyrrosiae, 30 gm; and Herba ecliptae, 12 gm. Six to One Powder, 12 gm. Decoct for oral ingestion. Three doses, one dose per day.

FOLLOW-UP/COURSE OF TREATMENT:

Second consultation on February 8, 1982: The patient's menstruation began the previous day. The flow was profuse with clots accompanied by abdominal pain and lumbago. Bacillus proleus was found in urine culture. Her tongue was red with thin, yellowish fur and her pulse fine and rapid. Continued the prescription minus Six to One Powder, Radix rehmanniae and Cortex phellodendri. Added Radix angelicae, 9 gm, and Herba loniscerae, 15 gm. Three doses.

Third consultation on February 11, 1982: Symptoms such as urgent and painful urination noticeably alleviated, but there was still thirst and palpitation. The tongue was pink and the pulse fine and rapid. Added Rhizoma anemarrhae, 12 gm, to the prescription. Four doses.

Fourth consultation on February 15, 1982: The patient felt well. Took another four doses of the above prescription.

Fifth consultation on February 18, 1982: Three routine urinalyses were performed consecutively and no abnormality found. The patient was discharged from the hospital along with six doses of the previous prescription.

DISCUSSION: Acute pyelonephritis belongs to Heat and Excess syndrome of traditional Chinese medicine. The disease results from attack by pathogens leading to accumulation of Dampness and Heat which are transferred downward to the urinary bladder. The general clinical manifestation is urgency, frequency and dysuria. This disturbance in urine excretion and internal accumulation of Damp-Heat would certainly fumigate and steam the Kidney and cause visceral and bowel diseases. It may also induce symptoms, such as lumbago, to appear. In this case, the patient had symptoms of urinary irritation, constipation, slippery and rapid pulse as well as red tongue with thick, yellowish coating. According to the TCM principle of "knowing the cause of the disease and treating the symptoms accordingly," the treatment would naturally be to dispel the invading pathogenic factors by means of removing evil Heat and excreting Dampness. Modified Bazheng Powder was prescribed for attaining these objectives. Dahuang chosen in the recipe not only to relieve constipation, expel evil Heat and stop bleeding but also to control inflammatory process and growth of bacteria. Animal experiments have been performed using these herbs in removing Heat and Dampness. The results demonstrate that they are very potent in facilitating urine excretion. Meanwhile, they improve the function of the Kidney and rectify the inflammatory process. Experimental results also show that herbs which are effective in removing Heat and Dampness, such as Semen plantaginis, Folium pyrrofiiae, Herba polygoni avicularis, etc., also possess, to various extents, an inhibitory function on some pathogens. Clinically, chronic pyelonephritis is characterized by presence of deficiency syndrome. The main manifestations are deficiency of the Spleen and Kidney Qi or deficiency of Spleen-Yin. Since Heat and Dampness are present in both cases, i.e., acute infection or chronic state, it's imperative for the therapeutic regimen to contain medicinal herbs effective in dissipating Heat, detoxifying stranguria and eliminating Dampness through diuresis.

A similar case was seen in an adult female patient suffering from the same disease. She was given many kinds of antibiotics as well as herbs effective in removing Heat and Dampness. Little improvement of her condition was obtained. She still had pain and weakness in the lumbar region and knees, poor appetite and bacteriuria. Based on TCM symptom-complex differentiation, the case was diagnosed as deficiency of both the Spleen and Kidney. The following recipe was prescribed: Rhizoma atractylodis macrocephalae, 12 gm; Poria, 15 gm; Rhizoma anemarrhae, 9 gm; Cortex phellodendri, 9 gm; Fructus corni, 9 gm; Folium pyrrofiiae, 20 gm; Rhizoma dioscoreae hypoglaucae, 15 gm; and Fructus crataegi, 20 gm. The patient was treated using this prescription for a month or so. Her symptoms took a favourable turn and bacteriuria was negative. This case demonstrates that in order to simultaneously strengthen the body resistance and to eliminate the pathogenic factors, it is important to obtain an equilibrium between Yin and Yang of the body so as to bring about the necesssary defense mechanism against invading pathogens. It must be noted that such an equilibrium can only be achieved if one is to approach the therapy bearing in mind the relationship between the Part and the Whole. This is one of the significant ways to improve the therapeutic effects of acute pyelonephritis.

4.2 CHRONIC PYELONEPHRITIS (URINATION DISTURBANCE SECONDARY TO OVERSTRAIN)

Chen Keji

Xiyuan Hospital, China Academy of Traditional Chinese Medicine, Beijing

Zheng, 30, female, Han nationality, married, cadre. First seen in the outpatient department on December 10, 1960.

CHIEF COMPLAINT: Frequent facial puffiness, back pain, urinary frequency, dysuria, positive urinary culture for E. coli for the past two years.

HISTORY OF PRESENT ILLNESS: In March 1957, without any apparent cause, the patient experienced urinary frequency, about 14 times a day accompanied by burning pain of the urethra and minimal gross hematuria at the end of micturition. Her case was diagnosed as "acute cystitis" and was subsequently cured. Since then the patient had similar episodes about twice a year. The episode in February 1960 was more severe. Aside from hematuria, frequency of micturition and dysuria, the patient also had fever, facial puffiness and back pain. Urinary bacterial culture revealed a positivity for E. coli and she was diagnosed as having "pyelonephritis." Symptoms remitted after the patient was treated with a regimen of combined modern and traditional medications. Thereafter, symptoms of urinary frequency, dysuria, back pain and facial puffiness recurred occasionally. Other associated symptoms reported by the patient were headache and insomnia.

PAST HISTORY: The patient underwent partial hysterectomy in 1956 because of uterine myoma. Menstrual cycles after surgery were normal but there was occasional dull pain on the left lower quadrant of the abdomen.

PERTINENT PHYSICAL EXAMINATION & LABORATORY FINDINGS: Facial colour dull; blood pressure 108/68 mmHg; heart and lungs negative; liver, spleen and kidneys not palpable; no tenderness on the area of urinary bladder; urinary culture positive for E. coli; and routine urinalysis indicative of trace protein and occasional WBC.

INSPECTION OF TONGUE: Tongue substance pale and tongue fur absent.

PULSE CONDITION: Slippery and rapid.

MODERN MEDICINE DIAGNOSIS: Chronic Urinary Tract Infection (Pyelonephritis and Cystitis).

TRADITIONAL CHINESE MEDICINE DIAGNOSIS: Urinary Disturbance Secondary to Overstrain.

THERAPEUTIC PRINCIPLES: Simultaneous clearing and replenishing of the System.

PRESCRIPTION: Radix rehmanniae, 12 gm; Radix astragali, 12 gm; Rhizoma smilacis glabrae, 10 gm; Rhizoma alismatis, 10 gm; Polyporus umbellatus, 10 gm; Fructus lycii, 12 gm; Semen plantaginis, 12 gm; Radix achyranthis bidentatae, 10 gm; Flos chrysanthemi, 10 gm; Pericarpium citri reticulatae, 5 gm; and Radix glycyrrhizae, 10 gm.

FOLLOW-UP/COURSE OF TREATMENT: After taking this prescription for about a month, there was significant remission of the symptoms. Cystoscopy and ureteral catheterization were performed on January 13, 1961. Bladder content turbid, cystic and ureteral mucosa intact, no ulcers nor locus of bleeding; urinary trigone moderately hyperemic; right ureteral meatus edematous; urine flow relatively sluggish. Examination of urine collected separately from the calyces showed presence of red blood cells on both sides at 20/hpf and occasional WBC and epithelial cells. Phenolsulfonphthalein excretion test: time of detection for the right side was five to seven minutes (density + to ++++), and for the left, two minutes (density + to ++++); routine bacterial culture negative. At this juncture the occurrence of urinary frequency and dysuria had been reduced significantly but there was still dull pain on the left lower abdominal quadrant. Based on these physical signs, a working diagnosis had been reached that the patient still suffered from the general syndrome of Stasis. Hence, she was given Danggui San (Chinese Angelica Powder) with Guizhi Fuling Pill in order to improve the flow of Qi-Blood. After taking successively more than 10 decoctions, the dull pain totally disappeared, but signs and symptoms of general malaise, back pain, urinary spotting, slippery and rapid pulse persisted. These signs served as indications for administration of a prescription based on Shengji Decoction in order to replenish the deficiencies, remove stasis, clear away Heat and dispel Dampness. The modified prescription was composed of raw Radix astragali, 12 gm; Radix salviae miltiorrhizae, 10 gm; Resina myrrhae, 10 gm; Talcum, 12 gm; Caulis clematidis armandii, 3 gm; Fructus gardeniae, 3 gm; and Radix glycyrrhizae, 10 gm. Successive taking of this prescription for more than six months led to disappearance of the symptoms of urinary frequency and dysuria; results of routine urinalysis were reverted to normal. Urinary culture also showed a negative growth. The patient was later given Xiangsha Yangwei Wan (Stomach Pills with Cyperus and Amomum) for her complaints of general malaise and lack of appetite. For the past year, except for occasional bouts of common cold and mild back pain, there was no recurrence of the previous symptoms and her condition was rendered stable. Last urinary culture done in September 1962, also showed no growth and a first-hour 55% excretion for the phenolsulfonphthalein test. Serum non-protein nitrogen 38.7 mg%, general health condition improving steadily.

DISCUSSION: The treatment of this particular case was successful by applying simultaneously the principles of clearing and replenishing the System. The clearing aspect of this case, including application of febrifugal and diuretic medications, which are effective in removing the Heat and eliminating Dampness, and other herbs effective in eradicating Blood stasis, probably helped in facilitating the destruction and passage of bacteria from the urinary tract and thus nipped the whole pathological process in the bud. As to the injured urinary tract tissue, application of Qi-replenishing and granulation-promoting prescriptions had a reparative effect.

4.3 CHRONIC PYELONEPHRITIS, UREMIC STAGE (GUANGE)

Kang Ziqi

Department of Medicine, Peking Union Medical College Hospital, Beijing

Huang, 38, female, cadre. Medical record number: C-207027.

CHIEF COMPLAINT: Recurrent urinary tract infection for more than 10 years. Nausea and vomiting for one month.

HISTORY OF PRESENT ILLNESS: For more than 10 years prior to admission the patient had recurrent urinary tract irritation symptoms (frequency, urgency and urodynia) associated with lumbago and edema. She also experienced nausea and vomiting with epistaxis, itching, dry mouth, dry stool and oliguria for the past one month. There was no fever.

PERTINENT PHYSICAL EXAMINATION & LABORATORY FINDINGS: Anemic in appearance with uremic breath. Blood pressure, 160/100 mmHg. Pericardial rub and murmurs appreciated. Liver palpable 2.5 cm below the right costal margin. Edema of both lower extremities. Chest X-ray showed lung edema. BUN, 186 mg%; SCr 15.0 mg%; CCr, 3.8 ml/min; CO_2Cp, 24 vol%; hemoglobin, 6.8 gm%.

INSPECTION OF TONGUE: Tongue proper pale with thin, yellowish and greasy fur.

PULSE CONDITION: Taut but slightly slippery.

MODERN MEDICINE DIAGNOSIS: Chronic Pyelonephritis, Uremic Stage.

TRADITIONAL CHINESE MEDICINE DIAGNOSIS: Guange (Vomiting, Simultaneous Retention of Urine and Stool).

Symptom-complex differentiation: Internal retention of Dampness and Turbidity; accumulation of Damp-Heat.

THERAPEUTIC PRINCIPLES: Discharge Turbidity by catharsis.

PRESCRIPTION: Radix et rhizoma rhei, 10 gm (to be put in separately); Herba taraxaci, 20 gm; Concha ostreae, 30 gm (boil first). Decoct the ingredients in 500-600 ml of water.

Other management: Hypotensive drugs and vitamins.

FOLLOW-UP/COURSE OF TREATMENT:

Second consultation: One week after administration of the prescription, nausea and vomiting disappeared. Two weeks later, X-ray showed disappearance of pulmonary edema. Four weeks later, cutaneous pruritus and sensation of numbness disappeared. There was no marked change in SCr. BUN, 75 mg%; hemoglobin, 7.5 gm%.

DISCUSSION: This is a case of uremia due to retention of Dampness and Turbidity in the Middle Jiao causing nausea, vomiting and intolerance to food. Loss of appetite resulted from accumulation of Water in the Large Intestine impeding the proper descent of Stomach-Qi. Accumulation of Dampness-Heat in the Large Intestine and stasis of Qi led to disturbance of the Qi in Sanjiao. This condition was probably also due to failure of the Turbid Yin to descend. Subsequent upward attack of Turbid Dampness resulted in a series of symptoms. Radix et rhizoma rhei has the properties of an antiphlogitstics, eliminating stagnation and activating Blood, regaining appetite and discharging bile and lowering blood pressure by diuresis. It is valuable to uremic patients because it prevents infection, controls bleeding and promotes appetite as well as lowers the blood pressure. Herba taraxici is effective in dissipating Heat and detoxifying as well as in promoting peristalsis of the large intestine. Combined with Radix et rhizoma rhei, they strengthen the function of downward transport.

4.4 RENAL INSUFFICIENCY IN CHRONIC PYELONEPHRITIS (INTERNAL ACCUMULATION OF DAMP-HEAT)

Xie Zhufan

Department of Traditional Chinese Medicine, First Teaching Hospital, Beijing Medical University, Beijing

A woman, 47, was admitted to the urology ward of this hospital on June 1, 1978, for kidney transplantation and transferred to the ward of traditional Chinese medicine on June 19 for herbal medication owing to temporary lack of appropriate transplant.

HISTORY OF PRESENT ILLNESS: The patient first contracted urinary infection in 1974. Though controlled by antibiotics, it recurred three to five times every year. Four months prior to admission, after an acute attack, she began to suffer from epigastric discomfort, nausea and vomiting. There was also marked nocturia. Her general condition became worse and worse with manifest emaciation. After admission to the urology ward, alkali infusion was given to treat acidosis, and there was slight amelioration of the gastric symptoms. Because no appropriate transplant kidney could be obtained at that time, the patient was subsequently transferred to this ward for further treatment.

PERTINENT PHYSICAL EXAMINATION & LABORATORY FINDINGS: Pale and listless. Severe anemia with a blood hemoglobin level of 6.1 gm% and seriously impaired kidney function, the blood urea nitrogen being 37.8 mg/dl, creatinine clearance rate 19.5 ml/min, and PSP excretion 0 in two hours. There was marked acidosis, CO_2 Combining Power being 33.5 vol/dl. Radioisotope renography also revealed serious impairment of bilateral renal function with disappearance of ß phase. Urinalysis showed albuminuria (+), glucosuria (++) and microscopically, scanty white and red cells. Gastroscopic examination revealed superficial inflammation in the antral region; no abnormality was found on barium meal examination of the upper gastrointestinal tract.

INSPECTION OF TONGUE: Darkened in colour with tooth prints at its borders and yellow and greasy coating.

PULSE CONDITION: Thready.

MODERN MEDICINE DIAGNOSIS: Chronic Pyelonephritis with Renal Insufficiency; Acidosis and Renal Glucosuria.

TRADITIONAL CHINESE MEDICINE DIAGNOSIS: Internal Accumulation of Damp-Heat with Dysfunction of the Stomach; Deficiency of the Spleen and Kidney.

THERAPEUTIC PRINCIPLES: Remove Damp-Heat and regulate Stomach function.

PRESCRIPTION: Modified Erchen Tang plus Ermiao San. Pericarpium citri reticulatae, 10 gm; Rhizoma pinelliae, 10 gm; Endothelium corneum gigeriae galli, 10 gm; Poria, 15 gm; Cortex phellodendri, 10 gm; Rhizoma atractylodis, 12 gm; Radix glycyrrhizae, 6 gm; Caulis bambusae in taeniam, 10 gm; and Semen amomi cardamomi, 6 gm. Make into decoction as a daily dose for oral administration. In addition, put 3 gm of powdered ingredients at the root of the tongue in several divided doses to be swallowed gradually for arresting nausea and vomiting.

FOLLOW-UP/COURSE OF TREATMENT: After ten days of treatment, the patient's condition improved and appetite became better. There was no more vomiting. After 20 days there was marked increase of food intake, disappearance of nausea and improvement of vigour. Her condition steadily improved during her five-month stay in the hospital. She was discharged on November 16, 1978. On discharge, laboratory findings showed blood urea nitrogen, 26.5 mg/dl; creatinine clearance rate, 35.1 ml/min; PSP excretion, 20% in two hours; blood hemoglobin, 13 gm/%; and erythrocyte sedimentation rate lowered from 50 mm/hr to 8 mm/hr. After the discharge she received follow-up treatment in the outpatient department, and the prescription of modified Erchen Tang plus Ermiao San was continued with gradual deduction of the Heat-removing ingredients as the Heat manifestations faded away but the Dampness symptoms persisted. The course of this treatment lasted for 440 days. Re-examination of renal functions in June 1979 (i.e., after one year of herbal medication administration) showed the following results: blood urea nitrogen, 16.4 mg/dl; creatinine clearance rate, 71 ml/min and PSP excretion 50% in two hours. Doctors checked her progress periodically for the next three years, and her health was well maintained. Radioisotope renogram also showed marked improvement of the bilateral renal function in 1981.

DISCUSSION: The gastric symptoms were so prominent in this case that a stomach disease was first suspected on admission. However, the patient had no past history of gastric troubles, and her renal function was seriously damaged after repeated episodes of pyelonephritis. The superficial antral gastritis discovered by endoscopy could be attributed to azotemia and acidosis.

There are various views on the relationship between renal and gastric symptoms in renal failure cases. In general, renal insufficiency is usually taken as the primary derangement, and gastric troubles are considered curable only when the renal function has improved or the metabolic disorders have been corrected. However, it is also reasonable that persistent gastric troubles may aggravate renal insufficiency and metabolic disorders. Different views result in different therapeutic approaches. TCM concepts, which hold the Spleen and Stomach as the organs responsible for providing the material basis for the acquired constitution, agree more with the latter view. Prolonged Stomach dysfunction consumes Qi and Yin and inevitably makes the patient's condition worse. That is why regulation of the Stomach function is stressed as one of the major objectives of treatment. In this case, removal of Damp-Heat was necessary because Stomach dysfunction was caused by internal accumulation of pathogens. This is true in other cases of renal insufficiency, and the case we presented here is by no means the only one that has been satisfactorily treated by such an approach in our clinic. One of the reasons for selecting this case as illustration of this concept is the simplicity of the prescriptions which were only slightly modified during the prolonged course of treatment.

It is worth mentioning that during the follow-up period, there were no more episodes of pyelonephritis. Apparently, herbal medication is also helpful for long-term control and prevention of infection in this case.

4.5 ACUTE NEPHRITIS WITH RENAL FAILURE (YANG WATER)

Hong Yongshen and Tao Xiaojue
Hangzhou Red Cross Hospital, Hangzhou

Wang Xiaoling, 17, female, Han nationality, single, student. Medical record number: 27510. Date of admission: January 25, 1985.

CHIEF COMPLAINT: Puffiness, oliguria with dizziness, nausea and vomiting for 10 days.

HISTORY OF PRESENT ILLNESS: Twenty-five days prior to admission, the patient experienced sore throat without chill, fever, headache and cough. She did not receive any treatment. Two weeks later, puffiness of the eyelids and swelling of the face appeared. Swelling was also noted on the back and lower extremities. In the past 10 days, the amount of urine had decreased. The patient experienced nausea, dizziness and headache. Other accompanying symptoms were lumbago, general weakness and loss of agility. In the past two days, she had had frequent episodes of nausea and vomiting, failed to take any food and passed black tea-like urine. The amount of urine was only 150 ml daily. She had no frequency, urgency nor burning sensation upon urination. Routine urinalysis showed: protein, (++++); RBC, (++++) and granular cast, (++). She was admitted as a case of acute nephritis.

PAST HISTORY: Non-contributory.

PERTINENT PHYSICAL EXAMINATION & LABORATORY FINDINGS: Temperature, 37.6°C; pulse rate, 86/min; respiratory rate, 20/min; blood pressure, 160/100 mmHg. Conscious but in low spirits. No skull deformity but with apparent puffy face. Silkworm-like eyes. Edematous bulbar conjunctivae. Non-icteric sclera. Isocoric with normal light reflex. Throat: enlarged and congested tonsils with edema of the uvula. No enlargement of superficial lymph nodes. Heart and lungs negative. Abdomen smooth and soft. No tenderness, no mass. Liver and spleen not palpable. Shifting dullness (?). Pitting edema on the back and lower extremities. No pathological reflexes elicited. hemoglobin, 13 gm%; WBC count, 10,200/mm^3; neutrophils, 80%; creatinine, 4.6%; BUN, 89 mg%; CO_2CP, 40 vol/%; Blood C3, 40.3 mg%; cholesterol, 20 mg%; A/GM = 3.4/2.6; Ccr, 23 ml/min. Urine: protein, (++++); RBC, (++++); WBC, (+) and granular cast, (++).

INSPECTION OF TONGUE: Red, flabby and tender tongue body with purple spots, yellow, thick and sticky tongue coating.

PULSE CONDITION: Rapid.

MODERN MEDICINE DIAGNOSIS: Acute Nephritis; Acute Renal Failure.

TRADITIONAL CHINESE MEDICINE DIAGNOSIS: Yang Water; Retention of Water and Dampness; Accumulation of Heat with Blood Stasis.

THERAPEUTIC PRINCIPLES: Clear away the Evil Factors, cool the Blood and promote Blood circulation.

PRESCRIPTION: Yi Shen He Ji (Mixture for Tonifying the Kidney, author's own preparation). Herba scutellariae barbatae, 15 gm; Herba lobeliae radicantis, 15 gm; Radix rubiae, 12 gm; Herba leonuri, 20 gm; Pollen typhae, 12 gm; Radix salviae, 10 gm; and Radix et rhizoma rhei, 15 gm. Three doses. One dose daily. Place ingredients in 500 ml of water, boil to obtain 150 ml of decoction. Add fresh rhubarb and boil for one more minute. Divide decoction into two parts. One part, twice a day.

Other management: Complete bed rest. Low-protein diet without salt. Water intake limited to about 1,000ml daily.Anti-hypertensives for controlling the blood pressure and penicillin for concurrent infections. Five hundred ml Dextran with 80 mg Ligustiqing Injection and 40 gm Lasix, IV, once daily.

FOLLOW-UP/COURSE OF TREATMENT:

Second consultation: Puffiness was reduced a little after treatment. The amount of stool was about 500 ml daily. Symptoms of nausea and vomiting were relieved. She was able to take semi-liquid food. Blood pressure, 150/90 mmHg, manifestation of pulse and tongue coating remained unchanged. Continued the same prescription for three more days.

Third consultation: Amount of urine increased to 1,400 ml a day. Puffiness of the face had disappeared. Mild pitting edema on the back and lower extremities. The patient felt much better. There were no nausea and vomiting. Blood pressure, 130/90 mmHg. She could take some low-salt food. Instead of dextran, 500 ml of 10% glucose and Ligustiqing, 80 mg, were administered, IV, once a day. Tongue substance red with purple spots on the edges, tongue fur yellow. Pulse floating. Radix et rhizoma rhei of the prescription replaced by Rhizoma atractylodis macrocephalae, 15 gm; Poria, 15 gm; and Rhizoma imperatae, 30 gm. Seven doses.

Fourth consultation: All the symptoms were relieved. Urinalysis showed protein, (++) and RBC, (+). Blood creatinine: 1.8 mg% and BUN, 24 mg%. Blood pressure, 120/80 mmHg. Red tongue body with thin coating. Ligustiqing injection was discontinued. Last prescription added 15 gm of Radix astragali for fifteen days as well as Yi Shen Chong Ji (Granule Mixture for Tonifying the Kidney), one package, three times a day.

Fifth consultation: Yi Shen Chong Ji (Granule Mixture for Tonifying the Kidney) had been taken for more than half a year at the dosage of one package three times a day. All symptoms were relieved. Proteinuria negative for three months, no RBC nor cylindruria. Blood pressure normal. Blood creatinine, 1.2 mg%; BUN, 17 mg%; Ccr, 73 ml/min. Hemoglobin, 13 mg%, WBC, 9,000/mm^3 and blood C3, 90 mg%.

DISCUSSION: In modern medicine, acute nephritis is a common disease causing puffiness, transient elevation of blood pressure, proteinuria and hematuria. Its clinical symptoms are similar to those of Yang Water in traditional Chinese medicine. The six Evil Factors attack the body resulting in dysfunction of the Lung, Spleen and Kidney, disturbance of Vital Energy and retention of turbid Dampness and Heat toxin. These pathological changes lead to functional failure of the Kidney, retention of Water and Dampness and Heat accumulation throughout the course of the disease.

This case had the following clinical features:

1) The patient had sore throat without treatment three weeks before developing kidney problems.

2) Two weeks later, puffiness appeared and the patient's condition worsened.

3) The patient had symptoms of black tea-like urine, oliguria, nausea, vomiting, headache, general malaise and low spirits.

4) Red, flabby and tender tongue body with purple spots on the edges and yellow, thick and sticky tongue coating. Rapid pulse.

It is not difficult to establish that the patient was affected by exogenous Evil Factors which caused the pathological changes of Water retention, accumulation of Dampness and Heat toxin with Blood stasis. All these belong to excess type of pathology. Therefore, the principle of treatment should be to expel and clear away the Evils, cool the Blood and promote Blood circulation. Measures to tonify could not be employed at the early stage. The prescription was based on Yi Shen Chong Ji. Herba scutellariae barbatae and Herba lobeliae radicantis are the main ingredients; they are effective in clearing away Heat, expelling the Evils, promoting diuresis and eliminating edema. Radix rubiae, Pollen typhae and Radix salviae have the functions of cooling Blood, promoting Blood circulation and removing Blood stasis. Radix et rhizoma rhei was used to move up the turbid Qi and discharge it from the urine and stool. With this application, edema and fever were relieved rapidly. IV injection of Ligustiqing was used to strengthen the effect of removal of Blood stasis. All the Evils like Dampness, Heat and stasis could then be removed as well as most of the symptoms. However, if a purgation regimen is used for a prolonged period of time, it may damage the healthy energy and cause an imbalance between Yin and Yang. This is a principle of treatment in traditional Chinese medicine. So on the third visit Radix et rhizoma rhei was omitted. Rhizoma atractylodis macrocephalae and Poria were added to invigorate the Spleen and Rhizoma imperatae to promote diuresis. On the fourth visit, Radix astragali was added to tonify Qi. These herbs were used together to obtain the effects of clearing away the Heat and Dampness and promoting Qi and Blood circulation. The symptoms were alleviated progressively. The Granule Mixture was made of these herbs and its dosage was three packages every day. The patient adapted to this form of administration easily because of its convenience. The Granule Mixture was used in treating 162 cases of acute nephritis and complete cures were obtained in 109 cases or 67.3%. In animal studies, these herbs are effective in dilating vessels, inhibiting aggregation of RBC, improving microcirculation and increasing survival rate. These findings were confirmed by experimental studies in rats where acute disturbance of renal microcirculation was induced by injecting deactivated bacillus typhosus. In comparison with the control group, the experimental group showed significant alleviation of kidney problems.

4.6 CHRONIC NEPHRITIS
(EDEMA OR INJURY OF THE KIDNEY)

Zhou Zhongying
Nanjing College of Traditional Chinese Medicine, Nanjing

Fan Yongfang, 25, female, Han nationality, single, accountant. Medical record number: 801136. Date of first consultation: July 4, 1980.

CHIEF COMPLAINT: Recurrent attacks of lower extremities, edema for nine years.

HISTORY OF PRESENT ILLNESS: Nine years prior to consultation, the patient noted that she was affected by edema over the whole body with scanty amount of urine. She was hospitalized in Nanjing and was diagnosed as having acute nephritis. Having been treated for six months, the edema subsided and she was discharged from the hospital. However, edema of the lower extremities recurred frequently whenever she caught a cold or became tired after physical exertion. Routine urinalysis often demonstrated presence of protein and red blood cells. She was diagnosed then as having chronic nephritis in a hospital where she was treated with corticosteroids and Radix tripteryqii wilfordii without significant results. Recently, when affected by a common cold, she had edema of the lower extremities, sore throat, dry mouth, lumbar soreness and burning sensation on urination.

PAST HISTORY: Non-contributory.

PERSONAL AND FAMILY HISTORY: Non-contributory.

PERTINENT PHYSICAL EXAMINATION & LABORATORY FINDINGS: Throat reddish and right tonsil enlarged (Grade I hypertrophy) with dispersed small ulcers on the surface the size of rice grains. Heart and lung findings negative. Abdomen soft; liver and spleen not palpable. Slight tenderness by percussion on both renal areas.

Slight pitting edema on the lower extremities. Urinalysis showed protein, (++); RBC, (+) and WBC, trace. BUN, 19 mg% and creatinine, 1.5 mg%.

INSPECTION OF TONGUE: Tongue substance red and with thin and yellow tongue fur.

MODERN MEDICINE DIAGNOSIS: Chronic Glomerulonephritis.

TRADITIONAL CHINESE MEDICINE DIAGNOSIS: Edema; Injury of the Kidney.

THERAPEUTIC PRINCIPLES: Remove Evil Heat from the Lung, nourish the Kidney, invigorate the Vital Energy and replenish the Vital Essence.

PRESCRIPTION: Sha Shen Mai Men Dong Tang and Modified Bolus of Rhizoma anemarrhenae, Cortex phellodendri and Rhizoma rehmanniae.

Ingredients: Radix adenophorae strictae, 12 gm; Radix glehniae, 12 gm; Radix ophiopogonis, 12 gm; Radix trichosanthis, 12 gm; Radix scrophulariae, 12 gm; Radix pseudostellariae, 12 gm; Radix astragali seu hedysari (stir-bake with adjuvants), 12 gm; Rhizoma dioscoreae, 12 gm; Radix rehmanniae, 12 gm; Rhizoma anemarrhenae, 9 gm; Rhizoma smilacis glabrae, 15 gm; Herba pyrolae, 15 gm; Achyranthes bidentata BI, 15 gm; and Serissae, 15 gm.

Decoct for oral ingestion, one prescription divided in two doses per day.

The patient was asked to avoid over exertion, spicy and fried food, seafood such as crabs and prawns and to eat a low-salt diet. She was encouraged to eat foods such as white gourd, Job's seed, water chestnut, red bean, lean meat, crucian carp and old duck.

FOLLOW-UP/COURSE OF TREATMENT:

Second consultation on July 18, 1980: By clearing the Lung and nourishing the Kidney, edema of the lower extremities apparently disappeared. Sore throat was relieved, too. Symptoms such as headache, sensation of heat in the palms and soles, lumbar soreness, dry mouth, foamy and dark-coloured urine still remained. These symptoms indicated Yin deficiency of both the Lung and Kidney and retention of Dampness and Heat. It was then appropriate to apply the principles of nourishing the Lung and Kidney and expelling the evil Heat and Dampness.

Prescription: Folium mahoniae, 10 gm; Radix scrophulariae, 10 gm; Rhizoma anemarrhenae, 10 gm; Cortex moutan radicis, 10 gm; Cyclea hypoglauca (Schau.), 10 gm; Radix rehmanniae, 12 gm; Radix ophiopogonis, 12 gm; Poria, 12 gm; Cortex phellodendri (baked and stirred), 8 gm; Herba commelinae, 15 gm; Rhizoma dioscoreae hypoglaucae, 15 gm; and Sambucus williamsii hance, 15 gm. Ten doses.

Third consultation: Urinalysis findings were getting better. No edema; lumbar soreness and sensation of heat in the palms and soles were experienced. The patient still had recurrent attacks of heat sensation of the body and headache. She had sore throat due to common cold a few days before. Tongue fur yellow and sticky, pulse thready. Continued to apply the principles of clearing the Lung and nourishing the Kidney.

Prescription: Radix glehniae, 12 gm; Radix rehmanniae, 12 gm; Herba pyrolae, 12 gm; Rhizoma dioscoreae, 12 gm; Radix ophiopogonis, 10 gm; Radix scrophulariae, 10 gm; Cortex phellodendri (baked and stirred), 6 gm; Rhizoma anemarrhenae, 6 gm;

Plastrum testudinis (stir-baked with adjuvants), 20 gm; Herba solidaginis, 20 gm; Rhizoma smilacis glabrae, 20 gm; Achyranthes bidentata Bl, 20 gm; and Rhizoma imperatae, 20 gm. Ten doses.

Fourth consultation on August 15, 1980: Urinalysis findings better. Protein and WBC trace and no RBC seen. Lumbar soreness had disappeared. The patient still complained of symptoms such as sensation of heat in the palms and soles, dry mouth, dark-coloured urine and occasional watery stools. Thin and yellowish tongue fur, pulse thready. Continued to apply the same therapeutic principles.

Prescription: Radix glehniae, 12 gm; Radix rehmanniae, 12 gm; Rhizoma dioscoreae, 12 gm; Poria, 12 gm; Herba pyrolae, 12 gm; Radix astragali seu hedysari, 10 gm; Cortex phellodendri (backed and stirred), 5 gm; Rhizoma anemarrhenae, 6 gm; Radix ophiopogonis, 10 gm; Plastrum testudinis (stir-baked with adjuvants), 20 gm; Rhizoma polygoni cuspidati, 15 gm; and Herba solidaginis, 15 gm. Twenty doses.

Fifth consultation on November 5, 1980: Urinalysis findings: protein trace, WBC and RBC negative. The patient complained of headache which could be relieved by cold pack and there was no lumbar soreness experienced. She caught colds easily. Stool was dry. Tongue substance red with thin fur, pulse thready. This syndrome was due to deficiency of the Kidney and weakness of the Lung which made her vulnerable to evil factors. To treat this, the Lung and Kidney were reinforced.

Prescription: Radix adenophorae strictae, 12 gm; Radix ophiopogonis, 12 gm; Rhizoma dioscoreae, 12 gm; Cortex eucommiae (baked and stirred), 12 gm; Radix rehmanniae, 12 gm; Radix astragali seu hedysari, 15 gm; Rhizoma polygonati odorati (baked and stirred), 10 gm; Cortex moutan radicis, 10 gm; Rhizoma alismatis, 10 gm; Pills for Nourishing Kidney-Yin, 10 gm; and Periostracum cicadae, 3 gm. Ten doses.

Sixth consultation on February 18, 1981: Lately the patient had common cold and urine protein was (+). She still complained of symptoms such as nasal stuffiness, sore throat with itchy sensation, dry mouth, mild watery stools, thin tongue coating and red tongue substance. The underlying pathology was deficiency of the Kidney and weakness of the Lung which rendered her vulnerable to invading pathogens. Therapeutic measures instituted were to clear and ventilate the Upper Burner followed by reinforcement of the Kidney.

Prescription: Herba solidaginis, 15 gm; Herba taraxaci, 15 gm; Herba pyrolae, 15 gm; Rhizoma polygoni cuspidati, 15 gm; Herba serissae, 15 gm; Periostracum cicadae, 3 gm; Radix platycodi, 3 gm; Physalis alkekengi L. var. franchetii (Mast.) Mak, 3 gm; Radix glycyrrhizae, 3 gm; Radix adenophorae strictae, 12 gm; Radix scrophulariae, 10 gm; and Rhizoma imperatae, 20 gm.

Seventh consultation on March 4, 1981: Because of the chronic nature of nephritis, the patient was weak in constitution and was vulnerable to infiltration by external evil factors because of her Kidney and Lung deficiencies. Kidney deficiency in particular prevented her from retaining the Essence which flows downward and away easily. This explained the positive finding of proteinuria. She also had dry mouth, red tongue substance with thin tongue fur, thready and rapid pulse and other symptoms of internal accumulation of Heat. Therefore, therapeutic principles to follow would be to nourish the Yin, reinforce the Lung and Kidney and restore the retaining power.

Prescription: Radix adenophorae strictae, 10 gm; Radix glehniae, 10 gm; Rhizoma anemarrhenae, 10 gm; Cortex moutan radicis, 10 gm; Radix scrophulariae, 10 gm; Colla corii asini (baked and stirred), 10 gm; Radix ophiopogonis, 12 gm; Rhizoma dioscoreae, 12 gm; Herba pyrolae, 12 gm; Glycine max (L.) Merr., 12 gm; Radix rehmanniae, 15 gm; Radix astragali seu hedysari, 15 gm; Plastrum testudinis (stir-baked with adjuvants), 20 gm; Cortex phellodendri (baked and stirred), 3 gm; and Bombyx bombycis, 7 gm. Sixty doses.

Eighth consultation on August 12, 1981: By continuous administration of large dosages of herbs effective in reinforcing the Lung and Kidney and restoring the retaining power, findings of repeated urinalysis were better; only a trace of protein was found even when the patient had attacks of common colds. She still had, occasionally, dry mouth, dry nose, dark-coloured urine and lumbar soreness. These symptoms were likely caused by Kidney Yin deficiency and retention of Dampness and Heat. Principles of treatment were to nourish the Kidney Yin and to clear the Lower Burner.

Prescription: Radix rehmanniae, 12 gm; Radix ophiopogonis, 12 gm; Rhizoma alismatis, 12 gm; Rhizoma dioscoreae, 12 gm; Radix scrophulariae, 10 gm; Cortex moutan radicis, 10 gm; Fructus ligustri lucidi (stir-baked with adjuvants), 10 gm; Herba ecliptae, 10 gm. Radix dipsaci, 10 gm; Concha ostreae, 30 gm; Cortex phello-dendri, 8 gm; Rhizoma anemarrhenae, 8 gm; and Rhizoma smilacis glabrae, 15 gm. Zhi Bai Di Huang Wan, 5 gm. B.i.d.

The patient was asked to take this prescription for a period of 10 months. During this period, the prescription was modified according to the patient's condition. Herba solidaginis, Radix platycodi, Physalis alkekengi L. Var. franchetii (Mast.) Mak, and Radix glycyrrhizae were added to treat the colds and sore throat; if dark-coloured urine appeared, Herba salviae plebeiae, Rhizoma imperatae, Herba pyrolae, Herba serissae and Rhizoma polygoni cuspidati were added; Radix patrimiae heterohyllae and White cockscomb flower were added for leukorrhea; Radix astragali seu hedysari, Poria and Semen coicis were added for deficiency of Lung and Spleen Qi; and Semen cuscutae, Cortex eucommiae, Radix dipsaci and Fructus corni were added for lumbago.

Ninth consultation on June 22, 1983: In the last two months, findings of urinalysis were normal. Symptoms remaining were slightly coloured and turbid urine which was somewhat hot and foul in smell, dry mouth and feverish sensation. Signs of red tongue substance and thin tongue fur and thready pulse remained unchanged. Continued to apply the principles of reinforcing the Lung and nourishing the Kidney.

Prescription: Radix adenophorae strictae, 12 gm; Radix glehniae, 12 gm; Radix ophiopogonis, 12 gm; Rhizoma alismatis, 12 gm; Poria (with the outer cover intact), 12 gm; Radix rehmanniae, 15 gm; Rhizoma smilacis glabrae, 15 gm; Rhizoma dioscoreae, 10 gm; Cortex moutan radicis, 10 gm; Cortex phellodendri, 10 gm; Rhizoma anemarrhenae, 10 gm; Radix scrophulariae, 10 gm; Fructus corni, 6 gm; and Rhizoma imperatae, 20 gm. Zhi Bai Di Huang Wan, 5 gm. B.i.d.

Tenth consultation on September 17, 1983: Having taken the last prescription (with minor modifications from time to time) for almost three months, the patient's condition got much better. Urinalysis was negative. She complained only of mild symptoms such as sensation of heat in her body, mild dry mouth, slightly dry stools, slightly coloured and turbid urine, minimal tongue coating and reddish tongue proper and rapid pulse. These symptoms, however mild, were still due to retention of Dampness and Heat, deficiency of Yin and flaring-up of the Fire. Therefore, the same therapeutic principles and prescriptions identified during the last consultation were applied for another period of time.

Repeated urinalysis during the one year follow-up showed negative results. This indicated that, after this long course of treatment, the disease was now in remission.

DISCUSSION: It is known that protracted chronic nephritis often has a poor prognosis because of recurrent attacks. Only when this vicious cycle is stopped can the patient really get into a long and uneventful remission. The patient in this case had a history of chronic nephritis for eight years. Though this case did not involve renal failure, repeated urinalysis were all abnormal; the prognosis would have been more than evident if the case had been left untended.

4.7 CHRONIC RENAL FAILURE
(ANURIA)

Hu Longcai

Department of Traditional Chinese Medicine, First Affiliated Hospital, Suzhou Medical College, Suzhou

Zhao Shanjin, 67, female, Han nationality, married, pensioner. Medical record number: 170326. Date of admission: July 20, 1981.

CHIEF COMPLAINT: Recurrent anasarca for 12 years, exacerbated for the past one month.

HISTORY OF PRESENT ILLNESS: In July 1966, the patient had generalized edema and malaise. She was examined in a local clinic and diagnosed as having acute nephritis. Both modern and traditional Chinese medications were given and the symptoms were relieved after two months of treatment. However, in August 1968, the patient suddenly had severe headache and high blood pressure (180/100 mmHg) with abnormal urinalysis findings. She was diagnosed as having renal hypertension and traditional Chinese medications were administered. The symptoms were relieved after several months but routine urinalysis still revealed proteinuria. In May 1979, edema appeared on her face and lower limbs which was subsequently put under control after a long period of treatment with traditional Chinese medications. Recently, the edema aggravated and the patient felt heaviness of the head with pounding sensation and pain in her shoulders and toes. She was diagnosed as having chronic nephritis, renal insufficiency and skin infections of the dorsum of the left foot and was admitted to hospital. Her symptoms persisted after treatment with antibiotics, diuretics, anti-hypertensives, etc. For more than a month, her urine output gradually decreased. On August 18, anuria appeared and it did not respond to intravenous injection of hydragogue. The patient was transferred to traditional Chinese medicine department.

PAST HISTORY: Positive history of typhoid fever and malaria when the patient was a child.

PERTINENT PHYSICAL EXAMINATION & LABORATORY FINDINGS: Temperature, 37.3°C; pulse rate, 84/min; blood pressure, 190/88 mmHg. Conscious but appeared tired and drowsy. Neck supple and thyroid not enlarged. Chest symmetrical and not deformed. Breath sounds harsh, moist rales appreciated over both lung bases. Heart rate 84/min with regular rhythm. No pathological murmur appreciated. Abdominal circumference 107.5 cm. Liver and spleen not palpable. Blisters, redness, edema and tenderness present on the dorsolateral part of the left foot. Pitting edema of the lower extremities positive. Neurological examination negative. Hemoglobin, 5.5 gm%; WBC, 9,200/mm³; neutrophils, 88%; lymphocytes, 12%. Routine urinalysis: protein, (++); RBC and WBC, trace. BUN, 53 mg%; Cr, 4.8 mg%; CO_2CP, 24.4 vol/%. Blood K^+, 21.7 mg%. Renogram: Function of both kidneys severely damaged.

INSPECTION OF TONGUE: Tongue substance light in colour, with a midline fissure. Tongue fur yellowish and greasy.

PULSE CONDITION: Taut and fine.

MODERN MEDICINE DIAGNOSIS: Chronic Nephritis; Chronic Renal Failure.

TRADITIONAL CHINESE MEDICINE DIAGNOSIS: Anuria; Edema.

THERAPEUTIC PRINCIPLES: Clear away Heat and Wetness, promote Blood circulation and eliminate Blood stasis, reinforce the Spleen and nourish the Qi.

PRESCRIPTION: Modified Zhibai Dihuang Tang. Rhizoma anemarrhena, 10 gm; Cortex phellodendri, 10 gm; Radix paeoniae rubra, 10 gm; Radix paeoniae alba, 10 gm; Rhizoma ligustici Chuanxiong, 3 gm; Radix angelica, 10 gm; Rhizoma rehmanniae, 10 gm; Herba leonuri, 30 gm; Flos carthami, 10 gm; Radix astragali, 10 gm; Rhizoma atractylodis, 10 gm; Rhizoma dioscoreae, 30 gm; Herba hedyotis diffusae, 30 gm; Semen plantaginis, 10 gm; and Radix glycyrrhizae, 3 gm. Two doses.

FOLLOW-UP/COURSE OF TREATMENT:

Second consultation on August 20: The patient began to pass urine after taking the first dose of the prescription. After taking the second dose, she passed as much as 1,700 ml of urine per day (without taking any diuretics). Lower extremities edema diminished markedly and dyspnea alleviated. Since the medication prescribed was effective, the patient was instructed to continue the treament. Six doses.

Blood examination on September 7 showed Cr, 3.1 mg%. Daily urine output was around 1,500 ml. Dyspnea had disappeared. Lower extremities edema had disappeared. The patient was discharged with condition much improved.

DISCUSSION: Anuria, or renal shutdown, in cases of asthenia syndrome, is usually caused by accumulation of Wetness-Heat evil, obstruction to the passage of fluid or by asthenia of both the Spleen and Kidney accompanied by abnormal ascending and descending movement of Qi. Our case involved a senile and weak patient suffering from the illness for a long time. The accumulation of Wetness-Heat evil and obstruction to the passage of fluid caused anuria. Accordingly, the therapeutic principle adopted in this case was to clear away the evil Heat and Wetness, invigorate blood circulation, eliminate Blood stasis and remove obstruction to the passage of fluid. Li

Dongyuan (A.D. 1180-1251) indicated that "diseases of the Spleen render the Nine Orifices out of order." In this case, our patient was deficient in Qi. Once the Qi of the Middle Burner rises properly, it benefits the functions of both the Middle and Lower Burners. As a result, the Qi of the Middle and Lower Burners help each other. Since the prescription was appropriate, the curative effect was immediate and satisfactory.

4.8 CHRONIC NEPHRITIS, RENAL HYPERTENSION, RENAL ANEMIA OR UREMIA (ASTHENIA OF THE KIDNEY)

Zhang Jingren

Shanghai First People's Hospital, Shanghai

Chen, 62, male, Han nationality, married, cadre. Medical record number: 422878. Date of first consultation: January 31, 1980.

CHIEF COMPLAINT: Dizziness with edema of the lower extremities for one month.

HISTORY OF PRESENT ILLNESS: In the past four years prior to consultation, the patient noticed that his urine volume had increased with frequent urination, especially obvious at night, but he was still able to work and did not pay much attention to it. Since April 1978, he experienced dizziness, so he went to see a doctor and was diagnosed as having hypertension. After taking some medications (the patient could not recall the names), the symptoms were relieved. He also noticed increased pallor and experienced lumbago. In the first months of 1980, symptoms aggravated due to over fatigue. A mild edema was found on the lower extremities, so he came to our outpatient department (OPD) for medical consultation. Routine urinalysis and renal function tests were done which showed poor renal functions, and he was admitted to our hospital. Shortly after admission, symptoms such as lethargy, nausea, vomiting, etc., developed and the renal functions continued to deteriorate. The patient refused to undertake dialysis therapy, so conservative treatment with traditional Chinese medicine was to be the mainstay of his treatment. At the time of first consultation, the patient was pale and somnolent with nausea, vomiting, halitosis, dizziness, lumbago, weakness, palpitation and shortness of breath after exertion.

PERTINENT PHYSICAL EXAMINATION & LABORATORY FINDINGS: Blood pressure, 200/96 mmHg; urinary protein, (+); hemoglobin, 4.5 gm%; urea nitrogen, 70-140 mg%; creatinine, 8.6-11.2 mg%.

INSPECTION OF TONGUE: Pale tongue with thin, yellow and dry coating.

CONDITION OF PULSE: Wiry and weak.

MODERN MEDICINE DIAGNOSIS: Chronic Nephritis; Renal Hypertension; Renal Anemia and Uremia.

TRADITIONAL CHINESE MEDICINE DIAGNOSIS: Asthenia of the Spleen and Kidney; Consumption of Vital Energy and Blood; Abnormal Flaring-Up of

Liver-Yang; Disorder of the Stomach; Inability of the Energy to Descend; Retention of Dampness Depressing the Mental Activity.

THERAPEUTIC PRINCIPLES: Invigorate the Spleen to eliminate Dampness, replenish the Kidney to purge Dempness Evil, regulate Stomach functions to clear away Heat.

PRESCRIPTION: Rhizoma atractylodis macrocephalae, 9 gm; Radix salviae, 9 gm; Black soybean, 3 gm; Rhizoma coptidis, 3 gm; Radix pinelliae praeparatae, 5 gm; Pericarpium citri reticulatae, 5 gm; Caulis bambusae in taeniam, 5 gm; Fructus aurantii, 5 gm; Semen coicis, 30 gm; Faeces bombycis, 9 gm; Folium apocyni veneti, 15 gm; Herba serissae, 30 gm; Radix cynanchi paniculi, 15 gm; and Fructus oryzae germinatus, 12 gm. Decoct for oral ingestion; seven doses.

FOLLOW-UP/COURSE OF TREATMENT:

Second consultation on February 7, 1980: Signs and symptoms of nausea, drowsiness, halitosis, feeble and wiry pulse, and pale tongue with dry, yellow coating were somewhat alleviated. This indicated insufficiency of nutrients and Blood, deficiency of both Vital Energy and Yin and retention of Dampness in the Middle Burner. As a result, the Lucid Yang failed to spread. So herbs effective in perking up the patient from drowsiness by eliminating Phlegm were added to the last prescription.

Prescription: In addition to the herbs in the last prescription, added Radix ginseng, 9 gm, decocted separately then mixed with other herbs; Rhizoma acori gramine, 6 gm; Radix polygalae, 3 gm; and Radix curcumae, 9 gm. Seven doses.

Following the treatment with traditional Chinese medications for more than one month, the patient was discharged from the hospital on March 6, 1980, with slight improvement of renal functions and symptoms. He was followed up in OPD and treated with the same therapeutic principles with occasional minor modifications of the prescription. Radix ginseng was replaced by Shen Shai Shen (sun-dried ginseng). Retention enema was employed which included Radix rhei, 9 gm; Radix cynanchi paniculati, 15 gm; Herba serissae, 30 gm; Concha ostreae, 30 gm; and Semen gleditsiae, 9 gm. These herbs were decocted in water and concentrated to 200 ml for retention enema; once daily.

Follow-up laboratory examinations were done on November 11, 1980, which showed hemoglobin, 5.7 gm%; urea nitrogen, 85 mg% and creatinine, 7.7 mg%. The patient could take care of himself, had a good appetite and slept soundly. He continued the TCM treatment and his condition was stable until the end of 1981 when he got an uncontrollable lung infection and passed away.

DISCUSSION: This was a case of chronic progressive renal insufficiency. From traditional Chinese medicine's point of view, this case was characterized by retention of Dampness and Heat secondary to dysfunction of the Three Burners in the transformation of Qi. As a consequence, food could not be digested into refined substances; it turned to Dampness and Evil instead. Because of asthenia in both the Spleen and Kidney which leads to disturbance in the ascending and descending forces, failure to control the Vital Energy was evident. Under these conditions, turbid substance fails to be absorbed and secreted out and Water Evil instead of being drained is retained. As a result, the flow of Turbid-Yin is obstructed and moves upward. The impairment of visceral functions and accumulation of stagnant Turbid Evil are cause and effect in relation and form a vicious cycle. This condition was evidently a crisis manifesting a prevalence of pathogenic factors and a weakened body resistance. The TCM principle of treatment at this stage emphasizes the Spleen and Kidney and handling properly the relationship between expelling the Turbid Evil and supporting the healthy energy. Expelling Turbid Evil should not injure the healthy energy, while supporting the healthy energy does not mean to over-nourish and over-invigorate. To replenish both the Vital Energy and Yin, Radix ginseng is suitable; Radix angelicae or Radix salviae regulate the nutrients and Blood; Huang Lian Wen Dan Tang (Coptis Root Decoction for Warming the Gallbladder) eliminates the Dampness Evil and expels Turbid Evil; Radix cynanchi and Herba serissa for detoxication clear away the Heat Evil; black soybean is used for diuresis by invigorating the Kidney; Faeces bombycis dispels Turbid Evil; Rhizoma acori graminei, Radix polygalae and Radix curcumae resuscitate by eliminating Phlegm. During the later stage of the treatment, retention enema using Radix rhei, etc., is to be used. Potent herbs which excrete the Turbid Yin should be used carefully. Under proper treatment, the symptoms are often relieved and the life of the patient prolonged.

It has been reported in medical literature that the average survival period of 112 cases with blood creatinine of more than 10 mg% is 210 days. In this case, our patient has a creatinine level higher than 10 mg% and after TCM treatment, his symptoms were relieved and he survived for two years, which was much longer than the average survival period reported. This case illustrates that TCM treatment is effective in delaying the progressive deterioration of renal functions. Mechanisms of action by which traditional Chinese medications correct the Kidney asthenia may be explained as follows:

1) By regulating the metabolism of the body, the amount of harmful material generated from abnormal metabolism due to Kidney insufficiency may be reduced;

2) By regulating body metabolism, the production of toxic wastes can also be reduced, so the burden of the kidneys is lightened; and

3) By paying attention to reinforcement of body resistance, the causative processes which aggravate the condition can be prevented and controlled, so as to protect the residual healthy nephrons from damage and prevent further deterioration of the patient's condition.

4.9 NEPHROTIC SYNDROME (INSUFFICIENCY OF SPLEEN AND KIDNEY YANG, DERANGEMENT OF THE KIDNEY QI)

Wang Chenbai

Department of Traditional Chinese and Western Medicine, No. 302 Hospital of the People's Liberation Army, Beijing

Hao Jingyi, 48, male, Han nationality, married, cadre. Medical record number: 86073. Date of admission: October 31, 1978.
CHIEF COMPLAINT: General dropsy and proteinuria for six months.

HISTORY OF PRESENT ILLNESS: General dropsy was first noted in May 1978. Urinalysis performed then showed large quantity of protein. He was admitted to hospital with a diagnosis of "nephritis." Treatment using cyclophosphamide, prednisone and traditional Chinese medications relieved the symptoms, but symptoms exacerbated once the prednisone was withdrawn. Recently, he came to Beijing for medical consultation when he noted that edema and proteinuria could not be controlled by prednisone any more. He was admitted to our hospital because of acute bacillary dysentery which was cured within a week. A consultation was made on his request for his edema and proteinuria. At the time of first consultation, the patient complained of shortness of breath, cold extremities, abdominal distention, large amount of clear urine and frequent nocturia (five to six times). Urine output 200 ml a day.

PAST HISTORY: Toxic bacillary dysentery in July 1978.

PERTINENT PHYSICAL EXAMINATION & LABORATORY FINDINGS: Body weight, 78 kg. Blood pressure, 130/90 mmHg, pulse rate and temperature normal. Edema of the eyelids, bulbar conjunctivae and face. Heart and lung findings negative. Abdominal girth 94.5 cm, positive sign of ascites; liver and spleen palpable. Pitting edema of the lower extremities. Blood non-protein nitrogen, 35 mg%; carbon dioxide combining power, 40.08 vol/L. Blood potassium, sodium and chloride, 4.7 mEq/L, 149.5 mEq/L and 84 mEq/L, respectively. Total cholesterol, 350 mg%; plasma albumin/globulin, 2.21/1.96 gm%. Urinary protein, (+++) to (++++).

INSPECTION OF TONGUE: Light-coloured tongue proper with yellowish greasy fur.

PULSE CONDITION: Deep and thready.

MODERN MEDICINE DIAGNOSIS: Nephrotic Syndrome.

TRADITIONAL CHINESE MEDICINE DIAGNOSIS: Insufficiency of Spleen and Kidney Yang; Deficiency of Kidney Qi.

THERAPEUTIC PRINCIPLES: Warm the Yang to promote diuresis, replenish the Qi and reinforce the Kidney.

PRESCRIPTION: Decoction for Strengthening the Spleen Yang and Modified Powder of Ginseng, Poria and Atractylodis. Radix aconiti praeparatae, 10 gm; Poria, 30 gm; Radix astragali, 30 gm; Rhizoma cimicifugae, 6 gm; Rhizoma dioscoreae, 30 gm; Radix scutellariae, 15 gm; Rhizoma ligustici, 15 gm; Radix angelicae, 15 gm; Cortex cinnamomi, 3 gm; and Semen euryale, 20 gm.

The patient continued to take prednisone (40 mg a day) after he was admitted to our hospital. Its dosage was reduced to 30 mg per day since November 15, 1978, and to 20 mg per day from November 20, 1978, onward when Chinese herbs were given.

FOLLOW-UP/COURSE OF TREATMENT:

Second consultation on November 14, 1978: Having taken five doses of the prescription, the patient had progressive increase of urine output (3,600-4,900 ml a day) with noticeable relief of edema. He lost 7 kg in body weight and his abdominal girth was reduced to 88.5 cm from 94.5 cm. He had a moderate appetite and slept much better than before. The sensation of cold extremities was also alleviated. His tongue tip remained red and pulse deep and thready. Modified the prescription by increasing the dosage of Radix aconite praeparatae to 12 gm and that of Cortex cinnamomi to 6 gm.

Examinations done on November 20, 1978, showed plasma albumin/globulin, 3.22/1.60 gm% and urine protein, trace. Body weight 70 kg.

Third consultation on November 22, 1978: The patient was noted to be in high spirits. Symptoms of shortness of breath and lower extremities edema had been relieved, and general dropsy had disappeared. He still complained of sensation of heaviness of the head and body. Frequency of nocturia had decreased to one to two times, its volume being about 300 ml. Urinary protein negative. Tongue proper dark-red with white greasy fur. Pulse condition normal. Modified the prescription to contain: Radix aconiti praeparatae, 15 gm; Cortex cinnamomi, 6 gm; Poria, 30 gm; Radix astragali, 30 gm; Rhizoma dioscoreae, 30 gm; Semen euryale, 20 gm; Rhizoma ligustici, 10 gm; Radix angelicae, 15 gm; Radix scutellariae, 18 gm; Flos carthami, 9 gm; Semen persicae, 9 gm; and Fructus crataegi, 30 gm.

Fourth consultation on December 6, 1978: Though the patient was found to be in good spirits, he had not been able to sleep well and complained of bitter taste with a decrease in the amount of urine as well as mild edema of the lower extremities. Tip of tongue red with thick and greasy fur; pulse taut. Urinary protein (+++) to (++++). Modified the prescription to contain: Radix aconiti praeparatae, 15 gm; Ramulus cinnamomi, 15 gm; Poria, 30 gm; Stamen nelumbinis, 15 gm; Rhizoma alismatis, 15 gm; Rhizoma dioscoreae, 30 gm; Radix astragali, 30 gm; Radix angelicae, 15 gm; Radix scutellariae, 18 gm; and Rhizoma ligustici, 10 gm.

Fifth consultation on December 26, 1978: The patient felt quite well. Condition of tongue and pulse same as previous visit. Plasma albumin/globulin was 4.11/2.60 gm% and urinary protein negative. Continued the same prescription with dosage of Radix aconiti praeparatae changed to 20 gm. When the patient was discharged from hospital against medical advice, he was instructed to reduce the dosage of prednisone gradually and to continue the administration of traditional Chinese medications. The patient was contacted by mail and we were informed that he had stopped taking prednisone one year after discharge from our hospital and that he was in good health and urinary protein had been negative. There was no recurrence of edema at the end of the third year when we lost contact of him.

DISCUSSION:

1) Diagnosis and treatment of modern medicine: At present, the etiology and pathogenesis of nephrotic syndrome remains undetermined. Diagnosis could be established by these findings: large amount of protein lost in urine, hypoproteinemia, general dropsy and its complication of hydrothorax and ascites, hypercholesterolemia which is often higher than 300 mg% and lipiduria. Among these findings, large quantity of proteinuria and hypoproteinemia is regarded as pathognomic. The diagnosis of this case was established because the urinary protein was (+++) to (++++), plasma albumin/globulin ratio 2.21/1.96 gm% with severe general dropsy and ascites, body weight being 8 kg more than before and his serum cholesterol level 350 mg%. The patient was treated with common traditional Chinese and modern medicine treatment as well as long-term application of prednisone which failed to effect a cure.

2) Diagnosis and treatment of traditional Chinese medicine: This is a case of edema

according to traditional Chinese medicine's point of view. It is pointed out in *Prescriptions with Specially Good Effects* that "onset of edema might result from diseases of the Heart and Kidney." It was stated in *Complete Works of Jing-Yue: Swelling* that "syndrome of edema is a disease due to discordance of the Lung, Spleen and Kidney. Fluid is extreme of Yin and is derived from the Kidney." If fluid due to insufficiency of the Spleen could not be removed, accumulation of excessive fluid would certainly lead to injury of Spleen Yang which would aggravate the Spleen deficiency and result in insufficiency of Kidney Yang. Transformation of Qi and distribution of fluid in the body is accomplished principally by promoting Kidney-Yang. Qi transformation of fluid in the body is accomplished principally by promoting Kidney-Yang. Qi transformation of fluid would be disturbed and general dropsy occur if Kidney-Yang is suffering from insufficiency.

Kidney-Yang insufficiency is manifested as general dropsy, weakness of the knees, intolerance of cold, difficulty in micturition, frequent nocturia, whitish tongue proper and weak cubit pulse. This kind of edema is classified as "Yin edema." Such is the situation we saw in our case.

Zhang Zhongjing laid stress on reinforcing the Spleen and Kidney in the treatment of edema. He pointed out in *Complete Works of Jing-Yue: Swelling* that "edema syndrome should be treated by reinforcing the Spleen and Kidney because it is an insufficiency syndrome due to transformation of Essence and Blood into fluid." The prescription commonly used for treatment is Jin Kui Qi and Decoction for Strengthening the Spleen-Yang.

Instead of drawing indiscriminately from the experiences of our forefathers, the author concluded that the lowered plasma protein was due to severe edema. Hypoproteinemia was the result of a vast amount of protein lost in the urine, while visible components lost in the urine were due to disintegration of Kidney-Qi. Based on the diagnosis of Yang insufficiency of the Spleen and Kidney, Radix aconiti praeparatae and Cortex cinnamomi were used to remove edema by warming the Yang and transforming the Qi, while Stamen nelumbinis and Rhizoma dioscoreae were used to enrich the Blood and invigorate Blood circulation so that the fluid would be set in motion when Blood circulation was invigorated. Large doses (30-60 gm) of Radix astragali were effective in inducing diuresis, reducing edema and eliminating proteinuria. Its efficacy would be much greater if Poria was added. It is documented in *Good Prescriptions Based on Experiences* that the "Radix astragali (25 gm) and Poria (50 gm) are effective in removing Dampness and supplementing the Qi." If they are used in combination with Rhizoma cimicifugae, they will not only elevate the Spleen Qi but also accelerate the removal of edema of the lower extremities.

After administration of the prescription based on these principles, the patient's daily amount of urine excretion was increased to 4,900 ml and he lost 8 kg of body weight within 12 days, while his plasma albumin increased to 3.22 gm% from 2.21 gm% with no or trace urinary protein being found.

Very satisfactory therapeutic effects were obtained in this treatment course by reducing the dose of steroids on the one hand and by increasing the dose of Chinese herbs to warm the Kidney on the other. The patient's condition worsened when steroids were about to be withdrawn, therefore steroid had to be used, but its dosage gradually reduced to maintain its long-term therapeutic effect. We could draw a lesson from *On Inquiring into the Properties of Matters: Abdominal Distention* which states that "since this disease is deeply ingrained and severe, one would bring disaster to himself if he is too anxious for quick therapeutic effects."

4.10 CHRÒNIC NEPHROPATHIC NEPHRITIS (DROPSY, DEFICIENCY OF THE SPLEEN AND ACCUMULATION OF HEAT IN THE LUNG)

Gao Chiyan and Du Jinhai

Xiamen Traditional Chinese Medicine Hospital, Xiamen

Cheng Qinghai, 25, male, Han nationality, single, worker. Medical record number: 17764. Date of first consultation: December 8, 1982.

CHIEF COMPLAINT: Puffy face and gradual swelling of the body for two months.

HISTORY OF PRESENT ILLNESS: Two months prior to consultation, the patient had one episode of sore throat accompanied by fever of three days duration. After taking traditional Chinese medications, his temperature came down gradually. He felt listless and weak but did not take it seriously and still went to work. One week later, he suffered from edema of the eyelids for several days. The condition worsened progressively and general edema appeared, with accompanying symptoms of dizziness, sore throat, loss of appetite, numbness of lower limbs with heaviness, oliguria and panting even on slight physical activities. Routine urinalysis then showed urine protein, (++++); RBC, (+) and granular cast, 1-4/hpf. He was diagnosed as having chronic nephropathic nephritis and was treated by penicillin, hydrochlorothiazide, triamterene and traditional Chinese medicine. Urine output increased slightly but the edema remained and symptoms stayed unchanged. He was then transferred to our hospital.

PAST HISTORY: The patient had chronic epigastric pain and was diagnosed by barium meal examination as having chronic gastritis. No history of arthritis. He had acute tonsillitis two years ago and came to our hospital for treatment because of edema of the eyelids several days later. His illness was diagnosed as acute nephritis. After taking traditional Chinese medications for two weeks, the edema disappeared and results of urine tests were normal. Further treatment was given, but the edema recurred occasionally thereafter. No further treatment was given.

PERTINENT PHYSICAL EXAMINATION & LABORATORY FINDINGS: Temperature, 37°C; pulse rate, 88/min; and blood pressure, 130/88 mmHg. Conscious and ambulant, pale, marked puffy eyelids. Non-icteric sclera, no palpable superficial lymph nodes, midline trachea, no secretion from the ears, throat congested with proliferation of lymph follicles, swollen tonsils. Symmetrical thorax; heart normal in size; heart rate, 88/min; regular rhythm; no pathological murmur appreciated; P2>A2.

Lungs clear. Abdomen soft, no ascites, liver and spleen not palpable. Pitting edema on the lower extremities, especially at the ankles. Routine urinalysis: specific gravity, 1.008; protein, (++++); RBC, 2-3/hpf; WBC, 2-4/hpf; granular cast, 1-3/hpf. Routine blood test: hemoglobin, 8.5 gm%; WBC, 9,800/mm³; neutrophils, 70%; lymphocytes, 28%; eosinophils, 2%. Cholesterol, 400 mg%; total protein, 3.21 gm; albumin, 1.8 gm; globulin, 1.41 gm; non-protein nitrogen, 62 mg; creatinine, 1.24 mg; CO_2CP, 42.8 vol%. Antinuclear antibody, (+). Liver function tests normal. HBsAg, (-). Chest X-ray: heart and lungs normal. ECG examination: normal. Fundoscopy findings: pale with little exudate.

INSPECTION OF TONGUE: Light-red tongue swollen with dental indentation, light-red tongue with slightly yellowish coating.

PULSE CONDITION: Deep, small and rapid.

MODERN MEDICINE DIAGNOSIS: Chronic Nephropathic Nephritis.

TRADITIONAL CHINESE MEDICINE DIAGNOSIS: Dropsy (Deficiency of the Spleen and Accumulation of Heat in the Lung).

THERAPEUTIC PRINCIPLES: Purge and clear the Lung Heat, strengthen the Spleen and induce diuresis.

PRESCRIPTION: Modified Pu Yu Mixture and Si Jun Zi Tang. Herba taraxaci, 18 gm; Rhizoma imperatae, 30 gm; Rhizoma atractylodis macrocephalae, 9 gm; Herba houttuyniae, 18 gm; Semen armeniacae amarum, 6 gm; Radix glycyrrhizae, 3 gm; Radix astragali seu hedysari, 15 gm; Radix isatidis, 18 gm; Radix platycodi, 9 gm; Poria, 15 gm; Fructus forsythiae and Flos lonicerae, 9 gm each. One dose a day.

FOLLOW-UP/COURSE OF TREATMENT:

Second consultation on December 22, 1982: Edema of the face and lower extremities relieved slightly but the patient still suffered from dizziness, lassitude and sore throat. Slight increase in urine output (about 1,300 ml a day). Lustreless complexion, throat congested, light-red tongue with slightly yellowish fur and small, slightly rapid pulse. Although the edema was relieved a little, Heat in the Lung had not been purged completely and Spleen-Qi not yet recovered. Continued the same therapeutic principles. Modified the last prescription by adding plantago seed to facilitate diuresis.

Prescription: Herba taraxaci, 18 gm; Rhizoma imperatae, 30 gm; Rhizoma atractylodis macrocephalae, 9 gm; herba Houttuyniae, 18 gm; Semen armeniacae amarum, 9 gm; Radix glycyrrhizae, 3 gm; Radix astragali seu hedysari, 15 gm; Radix isatidis, 18 gm; Radix platycodi, 9 gm; Semen plantaginis, 15 gm; Fructus forsythiae and Flos lonicerae, 9 gm each. One dose a day.

Third consultation on January 8, 1983: Large amounts of clear urine (about 2,000 ml a day) excreted, edema of the face and lower limbs markedly decreased, sore throat alleviated, appetite slightly improved but lassitude remained. Routine urinalysis: protein, (++); WBC, 0-1/hpf; RBC, 0-2/hpf. Routine blood test: hemoglobin, 10 gm%; WBC, 8,100/mm³; neutrophils, 70%; lymphocytes, 30%. Light-red tongue with slightly yellowish and glossy fur. Small, slightly rapid pulse. At this stage, urinary output was normal with edema essentially absent. The patient still complained of sore throat and listlessness. These signs and symptoms indicated that Heat in the Lung had not been purged completely, though Spleen-Qi showed signs of gradual recovery. Since diuresis consumes the Qi and impairs the Yin, therapeutic principles would be to strengthen the Spleen, tonify the Qi and Yin while purging and clearing the Heat.

Prescription: Radix codonopsis pilosulae, 18 gm; Poria, 18 gm; Semen armeniacae, 9 gm; Herba taraxaci, 18 gm; Radix astragali hedysari, 18 gm; Radix scrophulariae, 9 gm; Radix polycodi, 9 gm; Herba houttuyniae, 18 gm; Rhizoma atractylodis macrocephalae, 9 gm; Radix rehmanniae, 9 gm; and Radix glycyrrhizae, 3 gm. One dose a day.

Fourth consultation on January 15, 1983: The edema had disappeared completely and large amounts of clear urine (2,000-2,500 ml per day) excreted. All clinical symptoms had faded away essentially by this time. Routine urinalysis: protein, trace; dregs, (-); specific gravity, 1.012-1.016. Routine blood test: N.P.N, 51.6 mg; CO_2CP, 65 vol%. Red tongue substance with white fur, slow pulse. Biao (superficial manifestations) had been cured and now the treatment must proceed to the aspect of Gu Ben (to consolidate the foundation), in which the principles of tonifying the Spleen and Qi were adopted.

Prescription: Radix codonopsis pilosulae, 18 gm; Poria, 18 gm; Semen nelumbinis, 18 gm; Radix astragali seu hedysari, 18 gm; Rhizoma dioscoreae, 18 gm; Radix glycyrrhizae, 3 gm; Rhizoma atractylodis macrocephalae, 9 gm; and Semen euryales, 18 gm. One dose daily.

From then on the patient was treated by following the principles of strengthening the Spleen and tonifying the Qi. After one month of treatment, the clinical symptoms disappeared and several tests for presence of protein in urine were all negative. N.P.N., 40 mg and CO_2CP 52 vol%. The patient's condition was stable, so he was discharged from the hospital on February 15, 1983. He resumed his work duties. When checked one year later, urine test was normal and symptoms had not recurred.

DISCUSSION: The main symptoms of this case were edema, severe albuminuria, low plasma albumin and high blood cholesterol; all of these are manifestations of nephrotic syndrome. The cause of the illness was probably streptococcus infection, resulting in nephritis. Infection by hepatitis virus B can be ruled out on account of the negative HBsAg test. The patient was treated by modern medicines in other hospitals for a long time without satisfactory results, so he turned to our hospital for TCM treatment.

In traditional Chinese medicine, "nephritis" as a clinical entity is known as "dropsy." This patient manifested generalized edema, scanty amount of urine, dizziness, lassitude, sore throat, indigestion and loss of appetite; light-red tongue with slightly yellowish fur; and deep, small and rapid pulse when he was admitted to our hospital. Taking into consideration the past history of epigastric symptoms, acute nephritis two years ago, sore throat and fever one week prior to admission, it can be concluded that, based on the Four Methods of Diagnosis, the main pathology lay in the Spleen and Lung. The spleen, as interpreted by traditional Chinese medicine, is one of the Five Solid Organs and its physiological functions are concerned mainly with transmission and digestion, tonification of Qi and control of Blood. *Jin Kui Yao Lue (Synopsis of the Golden Chamber)* states that "pathogens do not invade the body as long as the Spleen function is strong." In his classic *Pi Wei Lun (On the Spleen and Stomach)*, Li Dongyuan points out that "all diseases are caused by deficiency of the Spleen and Stomach." The patient had epigastric pain for a long time, causing Spleen and Stomach deficiencies along with deficiency of Yuan Qi (Primordial Energy), Jing (Essence) and Blood, resulting in, internally, an inadequacy in nourishing the Five Solid Organs, the Six Hollow Organs and the four extremities and, externally, a low body resistance vulnerable to attacks by exogenous pathogens. Thus, the patient was asthenic and susceptible to disease invasion. The Lung is one of the Five Solid Organs and according to *Su Wen: Lu Jie Zang Xiang Pian,* it is "the foundation of Qi." It communicates through its external openings, the nose, throat and larynx, and through the skin and hair. *Su Wen: Lu Jie Zang Xiang Pian* also states that "from the Lung, the second most important organ, comes the regulatory functions." It is thus evident that the Lung can put in order and regulate the activities of Qi in the body which in turn is also dependent on the digestion and transformation of nutrients governed by the Spleen. This patient was deficient in the Spleen with weakness of its transformation function and also deficient in Lung Qi. In the event of invasion by exogenous pathogens, the Lung would be the first to be attacked. So his illness began from the Lung with a sore throat and fever, and then with edema on the eyelids to the whole body. As for dropsy, classical teachings dictate that "the root is in the Kidney, the manifestation in the Lungs while the control rests in the Spleen." Clinically, because of an imbalance of Lung and Spleen functions, exogenous pathogens were able to invade the Lung, leading to accumulation of Lung Heat and stagnation of Qi. This pathology was due to external blockade of the sweat glands, whereby water and moisture in the body could not change into sweat to be excreted by the sweat glands. Lung Qi thus lost its normal functions to purify and to descend. With its regulatory functions lost, unusual activities of Qi resulted in the San Jiao (Three Burners). This lost regulatory function of the flow of fluids led to the manifestation of a scanty amount of urine. As a result, water and moisture spread unchecked throughout the body, causing edema. Since the Spleen controls digestion and transformation, it is closely related to the transportation and disposition of water. *Su Wen: Lu Jie Zang Xiang Pian* states that "the Spleen controls the Stomach to transport fluid" and "the Spleen pertains to Earth and is the sole parenchymatous viscera transmitting nutrients to other organs." This shows that water in the Stomach depends on Spleen Qi to be absorbed and be transported to the Five Solid Organs and the Six Hollow Organs. In addition, the flow of water and moisture also depends on the descending action of the Lung Qi to reach the bladder. The patient in our case was deficient in the Spleen and his condition was made worse by a concomitant invasion of the Lung by Evil Heat, resulting in a progressive decline in the digesting and transporting ability of the Spleen. Consequently, water accumulated in the body and edema worsened. It is evident at this point that edema resulted from deficiency of the Spleen and Qi, complicated with invasion by external pathogens. At the time of his admission, the patient had both the Ben (the root, primary) and the Biao (the superficial, secondary) syndromes present. As his condition progressed, Lung Heat was more serious than Spleen deficiency. The treatment was then focused mainly on purging and clearing the Heat first followed by strengthening the Spleen with diuresis. By following closely the TCM principles of symptom-complex differentiation, a satisfactory outcome was realized in this case.

4.11 CHRONIC GLOMERULAR NEPHRITIS (EDEMA DUE TO QI DEFICIENCY AND BLOOD STASIS)

Liu Yuzhao

Shandong Institute of Traditional Chinese Medicine and
Materia Medica, Jinan

Wang Guilan, 42, female, Han nationality, married, nursery governess. Date of first consultation: April 14, 1977.

CHIEF COMPLAINT: Edema and proteinuria for eight years.

HISTORY OF PRESENT ILLNESS: The patient has had edema and proteinuria since 1960. She was admitted to hospital on February 14, 1970, because of exacerbation of the two ailments. The diagnosis was chronic glomerular nephritis. She was discharged on August 1, 1970, but the symptoms recurred frequently. Her blood pressure was high and fluctuating, sometimes reaching 200/110 mmHg. Prednisone and other medications as well as Chinese herbs were given. The principles of treatment were invigorating the Spleen, warming the Kidney and promoting diuresis, but they were not able to afford relief from the symptoms. Her edema could only be relieved temporarily when diuretics were used. The symptoms became worse since last October, with proteinuria (+) to (+++). Headache, dizziness, soreness of the loins and lumbago appeared with anorexia and fatigue. She also had frequent urination at night and susceptibility to common cold.

PAST HISTORY: History of dermapruritus for two years.

PERTINENT PHYSICAL EXAMINATION & LABORATORY FINDINGS: Conscious, medium build and poorly nourished. Pitting edema on the face and lower extremities. HEENT, heart, lung and abdomen findings were normal. No pathological reflex elicited. Hemoglobin, 9.5 gm%; RBC, 3.8M/mm³. Total serum protein, 4.5 gm%; albumin, 2.3 gm%; globulin, 2.2 gm%; ESR, 20 mm/h; N.P.N., 30 mg%. Urine protein, (++), RBC, 1-3/hpf and WBC, trace. Total urinary protein, 5.8 gm/24h.

INSPECTION OF TONGUE: Tongue substance pink, with whitish and greasy fur.

PULSE CONDITION: Wiry and thin.

MODERN MEDICINE DIAGNOSIS: Chronic Glomerular Nephritis (CGN); Nephrotic Type.

TRADITIONAL CHINESE MEDICINE DIAGNOSIS: Edema due to Deficiency of Vital Energy and Blood Stasis.

THERAPEUTIC PRINCIPLES: Reinforce the Vital Energy, activate Blood circulation to eliminate stasis and promote diuresis.

PRESCRIPTION: Radix astragali seu hedysari, 24 gm; Radix salviae miltiorrhizae, 24 gm; Radix angelicae sinensis, 12 gm; Radix paeoniae alba, 12 gm; Rhizoma ligustisi chuanxiong, 9 gm; Flos carthami, 9 gm; Herba leonuri, 24 gm; Poria, 15 gm; Rhizoma imperatae, 30 gm; Semen phasiole, 24 gm; Radix cynanchi paniculati, 15 gm; Ramulus loranthi, 12 gm; and Herba cistanchis, 12 gm. Preparation: mix the ingredients in an adequate amount of water and boil for two periods of time after infusing, about 20 minutes each time. Remove the dregs from the liquid (about 250 ml should remain). To be taken orally, 125 ml, b.i.d. Thirty doses.

FOLLOW-UP/COURSE OF TREATMENT:

Second consultation on April 28, 1977: A week ago, after taking the prescription, the patient's urinary output increased and edema of the face and lower extremities reduced. But in the last few days, she experienced headache, pharyngoxerosis and sore throat. Her urinary output had decreased and was accompanied by irritability. Tongue substance red, fur thin and yellowish. Wiry pulse, smooth and rapid.

Principle of Treatment: Activate Blood circulation to eliminate stasis, clear away Heat and remove toxic materials.

Prescription: Modified the last prescription by adding Flos lonicerae, 18 gm; Fructus forsythiae, 15 gm; Folium isatidis, 15 gm; and Radix platycodi, 9 gm. Twelve doses.

Third consultation on May 9, 1977: The patient's urinary output had increased and the edema reduced after taking the decoctions. Symptoms of headache and sore throat had disappeared, but she complained of anorexia and fatigue. Urine protein (++). Tongue appearance similar to that during the first consultation. Pulse wiry and smooth.

Prescription: Removed Lianqiao and Daqingye and added Pericarpium citri reticulatae, 9 gm, Herba lophatheri, 9 gm, and Semen plantaginis, 15 gm (wrapped in gauze), to the last prescription. Twenty-four doses.

Fourth consultation on July 7, 1977: The patient's edema had subsided. Her appetite was quite good. Blood pressure was normal, too. She slept well but still complained of fatigue. Urine protein negative. Hemoglobin, 11 gm%; RBC, 3.8M/mm^3. Urine protein, (-).

Prescription: Radix astragali seu hedysari, 24 gm; Radix codonopsis pilosulae, 15 gm; Radix salviae miltiorrhizae, 24 gm; Radix paeoniae rubra, 12 gm; Rhizoma ligustisi chuanxiong, 9 gm; Herba leonuri, 24 gm; Radix cynanchi paniculati, 15 gm; Herba cistanchis, 24 gm; Semen cuscutae, 24 gm; Rhizoma rehmanniae praeparatae, 15 gm; and Cortex moutan radicis, 12 gm. Method of preparation: same as above. Twelve doses.

Fifth consultation on June 20, 1977: The patient did not complain of fatigue any more. No other symptoms experienced. Both appetite and sleep were good. Tongue substance red, fur whitish and thin. Pulse tardy. Urine protein, (-).

Principle of treatment: Reinforce the Vital Energy, invigorate Spleen functions, activate Blood circulation to eliminate stasis, clear away Heat and remove toxic materials.

Prescription:

1) Same as last decoction. Twelve doses.

2) Patent Pills, 9 gm, t.i.d. Composition: Radix astragali seu hedysari, 120 gm; Rhizoma atractylodis macrocephalae, 60 gm; Radix salviae miltiorrhizae, 12 gm; Radix angelicae sinensis, 45 gm; Cortex moutan radicis, 12 gm; Radix paeoniae rubra, 45 gm; Herba leonuri, 120 gm; Radix cynanchi paniculati, 90 gm; Flos lonicerae, 90 gm; Fructus forsythiae, 60 gm; Folium isatidis, 60 gm; Fried hirudo, 15 gm; Pericarpium citri reticulatae, 45 gm; Semen amomi cardamomi, 45 gm; and Placenta hominis, 150 gm. Method of preparation: Grind the ingredients into powder, mix with water and adjuvants, then make into small pills.

Sixth consultation on August 3, 1977: The patient's condition was good and her symptoms were all gone. She had a good appetite and gained 3 kg in weight. Repeated laboratory examinations showed normal findings in blood and urine. Tongue and pulse essentially same as last consultation. Urine protein, (-) 24 hr urinary protein undetected. Total serum protein, 6.7 gm%; albumin, 3.7 gm%; globulin, 3.0 gm%.

Prescription: Continued taking the Patent Pills. Removed Pericarpium citri and Placenta hominis and added Radix astragali, 45 gm, to the recipe.

Follow-up on July 23, 1988: The patient's CGN was cured after taking the pills. Her health condition was satisfactory, and she seldom catches a cold. Blood and urine tests remained normal.

DISCUSSION: Traditional Chinese medicine interprets this disease as edema due to Yang-deficiency of the Spleen and Kidney and inefficiency in distribution of Wetness. The therapeutic principles of invigorating the Spleen, warming the Kidney, promoting Blood circulation and eliminating Blood stasis proved to be effective.

It has been reported that Radix astragali can exert its actions on the immune system and is effective in enhancing the generation of antibodies, the phagocytic function of the macrophages and the function of T-lymphocytes. In experimental studies, its effects in promoting Blood circulation to eliminate stasis and clearing away Heat to remove toxic materials have proven significant in reducing allergic inflammation, improving rehabilitation of nephropathy, restoring blood supply of the kidney and increasing the excretory functions of renal tubules.

In this case, the course of disease would be quite long and the disease unresponsive to treatment initially. The patient's clinical manifestations were secondary to retention of fluid in the body due to deficiency of both the Spleen and Kidney. On account of long course of the disease, the stagnation of the Blood and obstruction of the Collaterals by stasis, and aggravation of the symptoms due to fever and sore throat, the appropriate therapeutic principles adopted in the first stage of the treatment were to reinforce the Vital Energy, activate Blood circulation to eliminate stasis and promote diuresis. The second stage emphasized activating Blood circulation to eliminate stasis, clearing away Heat and removing toxic materials. The last stage of the treatment was to continue implementing the principles used in the second stage together with those of reinforcing the Vital Energy and invigorating the Spleen.

The author has adopted these therapeutic principles in treating various cases of CGN. The results have been most satisfactory.

4.12 CHRONIC NEPHRITIS WITH ACUTE EPISODES (IMPAIRMENT OF BOTH THE SPLEEN AND KIDNEY)

Li Congfu

Hunan Academy of Traditional Chinese Medicine and Materia Medica, Changsha

Li, 52, male, Han nationality, married, cadre.

CHIEF COMPLAINT: Lumbago, puffiness of the face and edema of the lower extremities of four years duration, exacerbation of symptoms in the past six months.

HISTORY OF PRESENT ILLNESS: During the past four years, the patient suffered frequently from pitting edema accompanied by soreness in the mid-section of the body, lumbago, lassitude, oliguria and cough. After undertaking medical treatment, the symptoms were relieved, but the patient could not recall the names of the medications he took. He went back to work without paying much attention to his condition. At the beginning of this year, as a result of exposure to cold, he was sick again, this time with sudden chills and fever, nausea, anorexia, cough, abdominal flatulence, general anasarca and oliguria. He was consequently admitted to hospital with a diagnosis of acute episodes of chronic nephritis and impairment of renal functions. Condition worsened during his several months of hospitalization. Especially pronounced was generalized edema with extreme distention of the abdomen and swelling of the lower extremities extending to the scrotum. The patient was subsequently referred to our clinic.

At the time of first consultation, the patient complained of dry mouth without sensation of thirst, hypochondriac pain, abdominal pain associated with flatulence, indigestion of food, fatigue, somnolence and inability to lie flat.

PAST HISTORY: Positive history of nephritis and hepatitis.

PERTINENT PHYSICAL EXAMINATION & LABORATORY FINDINGS: Conscious, emaciated, pale and acute sickness facies. Pitting edema evident on the face, abdomen and extremities had a translucent appearance of the skin. Tachypnic, blood pressure, 150/98 mmHg. Blood examination: hemoglobin, 8.5 gm%; CO_2CP, 46 vol%; cholesterol, 293 mg%; urea nitrogen, 48 mg%. Urinalysis: protein, (++++); RBC, 1-4/hpf; WBC, 3-5/hpf; granular cast, (+).

INSPECTION OF TONGUE: Maroon-coloured tongue substance, yellowish and greasy fur.

PULSE CONDITION: Floating, bowstring-like and rapid.

MODERN MEDICINE DIAGNOSIS: Acute Exacerbation of Chronic Nephritis; Impairment of Renal Functions.

TRADITIONAL CHINESE MEDICINE DIAGNOSIS: Edema (Impairment of Both the Spleen and Kidney).

THERAPEUTIC PRINCIPLES: Invigorate and activate the Spleen, control and treat the renal edema.

PRESCRIPTION: Modified Decoction of Radix Astragali and Radix Stephaniae

Tetrandrae; Powder of Five Drugs containing Poria and Five Peels Decoction. Radix astragali, 15 gm; Rhizoma alismatis, 10 gm; Radix stephaniae tetrandrae, 10 gm; Radix achyrantheis, 10 gm; Pericarpium citri reticulatae, 8 gm; Poria, 15 gm; Cortex acanthopanacis radicis, 10 gm; Pericarpium arecae, 10 gm; Semen coicis, 12 gm; Rhizoma atractylodis macrocephalae, 10 gm; Polypporus umbellatus, 10 gm; and Semen phasedi, 12 gm. To be decocted and taken one dose per day.

FOLLOW-UP/COURSE OF TREATMENT:

Second consultation: After taking more than 50 doses of the prescription, the patient's condition improved. Amount of urine output increased, tongue had thin coating. General anasarca alleviated. Pulse empty and wiry. The patient still experienced chills. His condition was described as Yin-edema, a type of edema caused by insufficiency of Yang-Qi, manifested as deficiency and cold syndrome, and Yang against external pathogenic factors becoming empty and hollow. Continued the previous prescription with minor modifications.

Modification: Removed Semen coicis and Semen phasedi from the prescription and added Ramulus cinnamomi, 5 gm; Semen plantaginis, 9 gm; and Radix salviae, 10 gm (stir-fry in wine). One dose per day.

Third consultation: Having taken more than 50 doses of this prescription, the edema was eliminated. The patient still had abdominal distention, flabby muscles, emaciation and general debility. His skin was rough, dry, brownish, hyperkeratotic and scaly, and he was severely emaciated. Pulse feeble, slow and deep. He complained of heaviness of the loins and placidity of the feet. It was evident that Kidney Qi had been impaired. Prescriptions to treat the Spleen and Lung were not appropriate for the patient's present condition. It was essential now that the Kidney be treated.

Prescription: Radix astragali, 15 gm; Rhizoma dioscoreae, 10 gm; Fructus corni, 5 gm; Ramulus cinnamomi, 5 gm; Radix tetrandrae, 10 gm; Poria, 15 gm; Rhizoma alismatis, 10 gm; Cortex moutan radicis, 5 gm; Rhizoma atractylodis macrocephalae, 10 gm; Radix achyranthis, 9 gm; Rhizoma rehmanniae praeparatae, 10 gm; Pericarpium citri reticulatae, 8 gm; Semen plantaginis, 7 gm; Radix aconiti praeparatae, 5 gm; and Radix angelicae, 10 gm. One dose per day. Put Pilose asiabell root in the decoction and stir before oral ingestion.

After taking more than 60 doses of this prescription, the patient's condition recovered gradually. The symptoms were relieved and he was energetic. Abdomen soft and appetite improved. Pulse broad, slow and even. Laboratory findings were all within normal limits. The patient looked healthy.

DISCUSSION: It is difficult to treat chronic nephritis when it is characterized by multiple acute episodes, presence of severe edema and impairment of renal functions.

In the early stage, this case manifested excess of evil and deficiency of healthy energy. Fluid retention, which spread both internally and externally, was the main pathology.

Pathogenesis (the mechanism of a disease including its etiology, site of lesion, manifestations and change of the vicera, Vital Energy and Blood) of this case was due to the failure of the Spleen to transport and convert and impairment of the regulatory function of the Lung (Lung is responsible for the coordination of viceral activities).

Therapeutic principles used in this case were to invigorate the Spleen, protect the Lung and drain the stagnant Water. When the edema was eliminated from the body, emphasis of the treatment was then focused on treating the Kidney instead of the Spleen.

In the prescriptions, eight kinds of Pill for Invigorating Kidney Energy were used to warm the Kidney-Yang and to dissipate the Fire from the Gate of Life to activate Kidney Energy, thus regulating the opening and closing of the renal hilus. Radix achyranthis and Semen plantaginis were used to alleviate Water retention and support the eight kinds of ingredients to regulate Yin and Yang. In order to avoid more sweat and stagnation, Rhizoma zingiberis and Fructus ziziphi jujubae were removed from the Decoction of Radix Stephaniae Tetrandrae and Radix Astragali seu Hedysari, and Radix glycyrrhizae from the Decoction of Radix Stephaniae Tetrandrae, Poria and Radix Angelicae, while Radix astragali was added to tonify the Blood. Pericarpium citri reticulatae assists Rhizoma atractylodis macrocephalae in regulating the Vital Energy. Application of Radix codonopsis pilosulae was to treat both the Spleen and Stomach and to balance the Yin and Yang. Therefore the functional activities of the Spleen and Kidney Energy (referring to the functional activities of the Kidney) could recover.

This was a case of chronic nephritis by modern medicine diagnosis, and this diagnosis can be established based on clinical findings such as edema, protein cast and cholesterol. The disease had transformed from renal disease into a secondary syndrome of renal failure. The patient's condition tended to deteriorate progressively as evidenced by the presence of anemia, impairment of renal functions, puffiness of the face and elevated blood pressure. It is difficult to control these aggravated symptoms by modern medicine. At present, adrenocortical hormones are often used to treat renal diseases. With this treatment, the condition of the patient may be stable for a period of time but its side effects are serious.

When treated by Chinese medicinal herbs, which are selected based on the principles of symptom-complex differentiation, instead of adrenocortical hormones, the patient's condition could be improved significantly and recovery obtained progressively.

4.13 GLOMERULONEPHRITIS-IGA
(URINE WITH BLOOD)

Kang Ziqi
Department of Medicine, Peking Union Medical College Hospital, Beijing

Wang, 17, male, student. Medical record number: C21168.
CHIEF COMPLAINT: Gross hematuria without pain for almost three years.
HISTORY OF PRESENT ILLNESS: Two years prior to consultation, the

patient had infection and pus formation of the gum which was cured by incision and drainage and antiphlogistic treatment. Two months later, he had gross hematuria. There was no lumbago or edema. Temperature and blood pressure were normal. He complained of thirst and took a large quantity of water every day. Skin of the face was reported to be tightened. He also experienced constipation with bowel movement every several days. Urine stream was short and colour of urine red. The patient was treated by both traditional Chinese and modern medicine but with no significant effects.

PAST HISTORY: Thrombocytopenic purpura at six months of age.

PERTINENT PHYSICAL EXAMINATION & LABORATORY FINDINGS: Eczematoid changes on the skin of both upper extremities and neck. Routine urinalysis: protein, negative; RBC, full field; WBC, 0-2/hpf. No tuberculous bacteria or tumour cells found in urine samples taken on several occasions. Urine culture negative. Phase-contrast microscopic examination of the urine revealed a large number of abnormal red cells. Findings of plain film of the abdomen, intravenous pyelography, retrograde pyelography and radioisotope renogram were all normal.

INSPECTION OF TONGUE: Tongue proper slightly red in colour with thin, yellow and mild greasy fur.

PULSE CONDITION: Wiry and rolling.

MODERN MEDICINE DIAGNOSIS: IgA-Glomerulonephritis.

TRADITIONAL CHINESE MEDICINE DIAGNOSIS: Urine with Blood.

Symptom-complex differentiation: Internal retention (stasis) of Damp-Heat, Extravasation of disturbed Blood.

THERAPEUTIC PRINCIPLES: Dissipate excessive stagnation, clear away Heat and expel Dampness, cool the Blood and remove the Evil Wind.

PRESCRIPTION: Dioscorea tokoro, 12 gm; Herba polygoni avicularis, 12 gm; Radix scutellariae, 12 gm; Rhubarb, 10 gm; Semen plantaginis, 15 gm; Fructus forsythiae, 12 gm; Semen phaseioli, 30 gm; Radix rehmanniae, 30 gm; Rhizoma imperatae, 30 gm; Herba artemisiae scopariae, 30 gm; Herba ephedrae, 10 gm; and Herba schizonepetae, 10 gm. One dose a day.

FOLLOW-UP/COURSE OF TREATMENT:

Second consultation: Three days after treatment, urine became clear and bowel movement was normal. Urinalysis after one week showed RBC, 0-3/hpf.

Third consultation: Treatment was continued for another 17 days. The patient felt better with normal urine and bowel movement. No RBC seen in urine examination.

The patient was checked for the next six months; there was no recurrence of symptoms, and eczematoid lesions of the skin were also cured.

DISCUSSION: There are several causes for bleeding according to traditional Chinese medicine:

1) Loss of control of the Blood due to deficiency of Qi. Insufficiency of Spleen-Qi is the cause of various kinds of chronic hemorrhage. Spleen Qi controls the Blood.

2) Abnormal flow of the Blood due to excessive Heat.

3) Bleeding due to stagnation of the Blood.

This case had no signs of deficiency of Qi or weakness or insufficiency of

Spleen-Qi. In light of the pulse condition and clinical manifestations, the diagnosis was established to be internal stasis of Dampness and abnormal flow of the Blood. Internal stasis of Dampness and Heat caused the Fire to be wrapped by Cold, which is the result of prolonged administration of herbs bitter and cold in property. Fire in such a condition is difficult to scatter and disperse and pathogenic factors of Dampness and Heat and accumulation of Heat cannot be easily dissipated; it is hard for the herbs to get to the site of pathology. Based on TCM principles of dissipating excessive stagnation, Ephedra vulgaris and Nepeta japonica, which are warm and pungent in nature, were used for their dissipating effects. This method of treatment was supplemented by the principles of clearing the Heat and excreting the Dampness, cooling the Blood and eliminating the stagnant Blood by activation.

4.14 URETEROLITHIASIS (UROLITHIASIS)

Chen Kezhong and Zhang Jidong
Shandong Medical University Hospital, Jinan

Gao Baichun, 23, female, Han nationality, single, worker. Medical record number: 260081. Date of first consultation: June 22, 1981.

CHIEF COMPLAINT: Paroxysmal pain of two years duration in the right lower abdomen, exacerbated in the past two weeks.

HISTORY OF PRESENT ILLNESS: For two years prior to admission, the patient had suffered frequently from paroxysmal pain in the right lower abdomen. About two weeks ago, she had an episode of colicky pain in the same area accompanied by lumbago, sweating and dizziness. At the same time, she experienced painful and disturbed urination as well as dry stools. The patient subsequently came to the emergency room of our hospital where a diagnosis of lithiasis of the right lower ureter was given, and was admitted for treatment.

PAST HISTORY: Non-contributory.

INSPECTION OF TONGUE: Tongue substance pink with thin, yellow fur.

PULSE CONDITION: Taut and rapid.

PHYSICAL EXAMINATION & LABORATORY FINDINGS: Marked tenderness in the right lower abdomen. Plain film of the abdomen showed a bean-sized translucent area. Routine urinalysis: RBC, (++); WBC, 0-1/hpf.

MODERN MEDICINE DIAGNOSIS: Lithiasis of the Right Lower Ureter.

TRADITIONAL CHINESE MEDICINE DIAGNOSIS: Urolithiasis.

THERAPEUTIC PRINCIPLES: Clear up the Heat and relieve the Dampness, eliminate the stone and remove the stranguria.

PRESCRIPTION: Modified San Jin Pai Shi Tang (Sustained Decoction of Three Jin Drugs to Remove Stone). Herba lysimachiae, 30 gm; Spora lygodii, 15 gm; Radix curcumae, 15 gm; Radix achyranthis bidentatae, 15 gm; Radix salviac miltiorrhizae,

30 gm; Radix paeoniae rubra, 15 gm; Endothelium corneum, 9 gm; Cortex moutan radicis, 9 gm; Herba polygoni avicularis, 15 gm; Semen plantaginis (in packages), 12 gm; Talcum, 15 gm; Rhubarb, 6 gm; Succinum Powder, 3 gm (divided into two doses); and Radix glycyrrhizae, 6 gm. Four doses, one dose per day.

FOLLOW-UP/COURSE OF TREATMENT:

Second consultation on June 25, 1981: The paroxysmal pain was still present and radiated to symphysis pubis. Urinary stream short and urine bloody. The tongue was pink with thin, white fur. Pulse taut and rapid. Rhizoma alismatis was added to the previous prescription. Four doses.

Third consultation on June 29, 1981: Absence of abdominal pain in the past few days. Normal diet, normal bowel movement and urination. Condition of the tongue and pulse remained the same. Another three doses of the same prescription.

Fourth consultation on July 2, 1981: Since this morning, the patient had attacks of paroxysmal pain in the right lumbar area and the pain radiated along the course of the ureter. The pain was caused by downward movement of the stone. Urinary stream was intermittent and stool was dry. Tongue substance pink with white fur. Pulse sinking, taut and strong. Added Folium pyrrosiae, 20 gm, Rhizoma alismatis, 30 gm, and Rhizoma zedoariae, 15 gm, to the previous prescription. Dosage of Rhubarb changed from 15 gm to 9 gm. Four doses.

Fifth consultation on July 6, 1981: The patient experienced "bursting" pain in the same area these past few days. Tongue substance was red with thin, white fur. Pulse taut. Took another six doses of the same prescription.

Sixth consultation on July 11, 1981: The pain disappeared yesterday. A stone the size of a bean was discharged in the urine. P-A plain film of the abdomen showed no shadow of the stone. Routine urinalysis was normal. The patient was discharged from hospital and in order to maintain the effect, she was asked to take six more doses of the above prescription at home.

DISCUSSION: In traditional Chinese medicine, ureterolithiasis is grouped under urolithiasis. Its etiology and mechanism are due mainly to everyday dietary habit and partially to factors such as alcoholism, excessive ingestion of pungent, sweet, fatty or acidic food. Such food can encourage Dampness and Heat to accumulate in the Lower Burner, resulting in stone formation. As far as this case is concerned, red tongue, rapid pulse, dry stool and lingering and intermittent urination were all signs of accumulation of Dampness and Heat in the Lower Burner. It was treated accordingly using the principles of clearing up the Heat and Dampness, removing stranguria and eliminating the stone. The recipe of choice San Jin Pai Shi Tang (Sustained Decoction of Three Jin Drugs to Remove Stone) with modifications was used in this case. Succinum was chosen for its effects in removing stranguria and eliminating stasis. All ingredients of the prescription are effective in descending the uretics, clearing Dampness and removing stranguria. When put together, they can exert a concerted and significant effect. In addition, the patient was asked to clap the affected area every day for five minutes and to jump a few dozen times each morning to dislodge the stone and to promote its descent. The patient was also instructed to drink 500-800 ml of water within 5-10 minutes when the stomach was empty to facilitate descent of the stone. Taking into consideration the easy relapse of urolithiasis and to consolidate the therapeutic effect of the present treatment course, she was asked to take two dose of the prescription each week to further clear up the Heat and Dampness and to remove stranguria.

5. GENITAL, ENDOCRINE AND METABOLIC DISEASES

5.1 LOW SPERM SURVIVAL RATE
(*JIN* ESSENCE FAILURE)

Chen Keji

Xiyuan Hospital, China Academy of Traditional Chinese Medicine, Beijing

Lu, 32, male, Han nationality, married, cadre. Medical record number: 21734. Date of first consultation: April 27, 1962.

CHIEF COMPLAINT: Oligospermia.

HISTORY OF PRESENT ILLNESS: The patient had been married for three years at the time of consultation. He claimed to have normal sexual activities, and there were no signs of sexual impotence, premature ejaculation or other sexual disturbances, though the amount of semen was noted to be small. Previous examinations of the semen revealed sperm mortality rate to be as high as 70-80%. The marriage proved to be infertile (spouse examined to be healthy), which prompted the patient to seek medical consultation. Other accompanying signs were insomnia occurring about two or three nights a week, nightmarish sleep, dizziness, easy excitability and frequent lapses of memory. The patient consulted and underwent a course of treatment with an endocrinologist but to no avail.

PAST HISTORY: No serious illness before, no history of prostate gland or testicular pathology.

PERTINENT PHYSICAL EXAMINATION & LABORATORY FINDINGS: Endomorphic, dull facies, general physical examination as well as examination of the testicles, vas deferens and epididymis were all negative. Sperm count and sperm activity assessment: sperm count‹7M/ml, sperm survival rate 30%.

INSPECTION OF TONGUE: Tongue proper plain, tongue fur pale.

PULSE CONDITION: Deep and slow, bilateral cubits weak.

MODERN MEDICINE DIAGNOSIS: Low Sperm Survival Rate.

TRADITIONAL CHINESE MEDICINE DIAGNOSIS: *Jin* Essence Failure, Deficiency of both Kidney-Fire and Kidney-Essence.

THERAPEUTIC PRINCIPLES: Simultaneous tonification of Kidney Yin and Yang.

PRESCRIPTIONS:

1) Zougui Decoction as the basic prescription with additional herbs: Radix reh-

manniae praeparatae, 12 gm; Rhizoma dioscoreae, 12 gm; Fructus lycii, 15 gm; Fructus corni, 10 gm; Radix glycyrrhizae, 10 gm; Poria, 12 gm; and Colla cornu cervi, 10 gm. Dosage: one prescription per day.

2) 10 gm of Ginseng-Nourishing-Essence Pill each morning.

3) 10 gm of Jinkui Shenqi Pill for invigorating the Kidney-Qi at night.

Forty days later (June 8, 1962), re-examination showed improvement of the tongue profile, and pulse had become stronger. Examination showed a 60% survival rate of the sperm cells. The patient reported feeling a great improvement in his general well-being. The same therapeutic regimen was continued. Repeated sperm examinations on the 60th day (August 14, 1962) after start of the treatment course showed sperm survival rate to be 68%.

DISCUSSION: This is a case of low sperm survival rate due to unknown etiology, spontaneous sperm deficiency syndrome, classified as a type of male infertility syndrome. The application of the TCM therapeutic principle of tonifying the Kidney produced a significant rise in sperm survival rate. Unfortunately, a follow-up could not be carried out because the patient was relocated to another city, and no further information could be obtained to determine whether the treatment was effective for a longer period of time. This case is a good illustration of how oligospermia can be treated according to the traditional medical theory which stipulates that "the Kidney masters the reproduction functions."

5.2 OLIGOSPERMIA OR AZOOSPERMIA (STERILITY DUE TO KIDNEY DEFICIENCY)

Xie Renfu

Department of Hematology, Sino-Japanese Friendship Hospital, Beijing

Case 1
Shi Chigen, 30, male, technician. Date of first consultation: July 6, 1983.

CHIEF COMPLAINT: Infertility for three years and diagnosed as having oligospermia for one year.

HISTORY OF PRESENT ILLNESS: The patient got married three years prior to consultation, and the couple has not been able to conceive a baby. Gynecological and other examinations done on his wife did not show any abnormalities. The patient was found to have oligospermia. Sperm count was 11×10^6/ml, 10% mobility and 87% dead or abnormally shaped sperm cells. He had sought medical advice many times, but all treatment had failed to improve his condition. At the time of first consultation, the patient complained of sensation of coldness and wetness on his scrotum, lassitude and tiredness of the loins and legs after sexual activities. To a certain extent, he had impotence and premature ejaculation in the last two years. He was unable to sleep well. Appetite good. Urination and bowel movement were normal.

PAST HISTORY: Habitual masturbation during his youth.

PERTINENT PHYSICAL EXAMINATION & LABORATORY FINDINGS: Dark complexion; heart and lung findings negative. Liver and spleen not palpable. Semen examination: white, thin and viscous, 1.5 ml in volume. Sperm count 12×10^6/ml with 5% mobility and more than 90% of them were dead or abnormal in shape.

INSPECTION OF TONGUE: Tender with thin and white fur.

PULSE CONDITION: Deep and fine, especially at both Chi positions of radial arteries.

MODERN MEDICINE DIAGNOSIS: Oligospermia.

TRADITIONAL CHINESE MEDICINE DIAGNOSIS: Sterility due to Kidney Deficiency.

THERAPEUTIC PRINCIPLES: Nourish the Yin and tonify the Kidney.

PRESCRIPTION: Modified Liuwei Dihuang Tang. Rhizoma rehmanniae, 15 gm; Fructus corni, 10 gm; Fructus lycii, 15 gm; Rhizoma dioscoreae, 15 gm; Poria, 15 gm; Rhizoma alismatis, 10 gm; Ramulus loranthi, 15 gm; and Fructus psoraleae, 15 gm. Served in decoction form, q.i.d. The patient was asked to refrain form sexual activity.

FOLLOW-UP/COURSE OF TREATMENT:

September 20, 1983: The patient had taken more than 30 doses of the prescription. There was no significant improvement in his symptoms. Since in tonifying the Kidney one should pay attention to regulating the Yin and Yang, the herbal decoction was changed to patent pills of Liuwei Dihuang Wan, 10 gm, b.i.d. Another prescription was given. Radix ginseng, 60 gm; Fructus lycii, 30 gm; and Fructus schizandrae, 15 gm. Immerse the ingredients in 500 ml of wine (60% proof) for one week, then take 30 ml, h.s.

November 5, 1983: The patient followed the doctor's order assiduously. Symptoms such as tiredness in loins and lassitude were relieved. Pulse was still sinking and thready. Semen examination showed a sperm count of 21×10^6/ml, 15% mobility and 80% dead or of abnormal shape. Modified Huan Shao Dan was prescribed. Herba cistanchis, 30 gm; Radix morindae, 15 gm; Rhizoma rehmanniae, 15 gm; Fructus lycii, 15 gm; Fructus foeniculi, 10 gm; Radix achyranthis, 15 gm; Radix dipsaci, 30 gm; Poria, 15 gm; Rhizoma acori graminei, 10 gm; Rhizoma polygonati, 30 gm; and Fructus broussonetiae, 10 gm.

December 20, 1983: After taking more than 40 doses of Modified Huan Shao Dan, the patient felt much better, and he also noted improvement in sexual impotence. Tongue had a thin fur and pulse was deep and small. Sperm count was raised to 76×10^6/ml with 50% mobility and a decrease in the number of dead and abnormally shaped sperm cells. Continued to take the prescription.

April 6, 1984: The patient felt good. He did not experience impotence or premature ejaculations any more. He asked to take the prescription for another three months. Sperm count was 85×10^6/ml with 70% mobility. For convenience of administration, the prescription, with minor modifications, was prepared and made into pills. Ingredients: Herba cistanchis, 120 gm; Radix morindae, 15 gm; Rhizoma rehmanniae, 60 gm; Poria, 40 gm; Fructus mori, 60 gm; Fructus broussonetiae, 60 gm; Rhizoma dioscoreae, 60 gm; Fructus foeniculi, 40 gm; Cortex eucommiae, 60 gm; Herba cynomorii, 60 gm; Fructus schisandrae, 60 gm; and Radix polygoni multiflori, 120 gm. Pulverize all ingredients into powder form, mix with honey and make into 10-gm pills. 10 gm, twice a day.

With this home medication, the patient did not come to our clinic for a long period of time. On December 5, 1984, he informed us that his wife was pregnant and a female baby was born on June 6, 1985.

Case 2
Li Zongqiang, 24, male, farmer. Medical record number: 189219. Date of first consultation: March 18, 1987.
CHIEF COMPLAINT: Unable to conceive after 18 months of marriage.

HISTORY OF PRESENT ILLNESS: The patient got married at the end of 1985. Sexual activity had been normal but the couple was not able to conceive a baby. In January of 1987, both of them underwent general examination in a hospital in Shijiazhuang City. No abnormal findings were found during his wife's examinations, while he was told that he had azoospermia. No sperm cells were found in sperm examinations done on five consecutive occasions. Between March and April of 1987, the patient came to Beijing three times to seek medical advice but all the treatment proved to be ineffective. Some doctors told him that the condition was incorrectible. In May 1987, biopsy was done on the testes in the Second Affiliated Hospital of the Hebei Medical University which showed atrophy of seminiferous tubules and absence of sperm production. At the time of first consultation in our clinic, the patient only complained of a little bit of tiredness in the loins and legs after sexual intercourse. Appetite and sleep were good. Urine and bowel movements were normal.

PAST HISTORY: There was one episode of high fever lasting for three days in his early childhood.

PERTINENT PHYSICAL EXAMINATION & LABORATORY FINDINGS: General condition fair. Examination of the heart, lungs and abdomen revealed no abnormal findings. Semen examination: grayish white in colour, thin viscous appearance, 1.2 ml in volume, no sperm cells seen under microscope.

MODERN MEDICINE DIAGNOSIS: Azoospermia.

TRADITIONAL CHINESE MEDICINE DIAGNOSIS: Sterility Secondary to Kidney Deficiency.

THERAPEUTIC PRINCIPLES: Tonify the Kidney.

PRESCRIPTION: Modified Huan Shao San. Semen cuscutae, 15 gm; Herba cistanchis, 30 gm; Radix morindae, 15 gm; Fructus foeniculi, 10 gm; Fructus lycii, 15 gm; Radix achyranthis, 15 gm; Cortex eucommiae, 60 gm; Fructus broussonetiae, 15 gm; Rhizoma rehmanniae, 15 gm; Rhizoma acori graminei, 10 gm; and Fructus corri, 10 gm. Served in decoction form, q.i.d. In addition, the patient was to take Wuji Baifeng Wan, 10 gm, b.i.d. He was asked to refrain from sexual activities.

Since the patient lived far away from Beijing, he did not come back again for follow-up. We received a letter from him on December 6, 1987, which informed us that the patient had been taking the prescription as well as the pills continuously for three months after he went back. His wife was confirmed to be pregnant in September and a semen examination done at the same time showed a sperm count of 51×10^6/ml with 60%

mobility. We were informed later that a male baby was born to them on May 8, 1988.

DISCUSSION: Both of these patients suffered from sterility, the diagnosis being confirmed by seminal fluid findings of oligospermia and azoospermia. Such cases are difficult to treat with modern medicine.

Traditional Chinese medicine holds that the Kidney is functionally the foundation of the human body. It serves as the source of genuine essence of Kidney Yin and original vital force, or Yuan Yang, and is also called the Vital Fire which controls all the human physiological activities. Among its many functions, it promotes the function of the Spleen in absorbing and metabolizing all the nutrients from the diet; it also acts as the source of production of the Essence, Blood and sperm. For a male, the Kidney begins to function fully at the age of sixteen. Therefore, functional and organic impairment of the Kidney will lead to a myriad of problems including oligospermia and azoospermia.

For case 1, this was probably a case of inborn deficiency since the patient had been weak since his childhood. The essence was exhausted further by his habitual masturbation before marriage. This resulted in many symptoms relating to Kidney deficiency including oligospermia.

As for case 2, absence of sperm production and testicular tissue atrophy was already evident when the patient was only 24 years old. This could have been an inborn defect. The essence might have been further impaired by the episode of high fever during his youth.

The primary cause of oligospermia and azoospermia is Kidney deficiency and naturally, the chief therapeutic principle is to tonify the Kidney. Both the Kidney Yin and Kidney Yang must be regulated and replenished. The herbal prescription used for these cases is Huan Shao Dan.

Huan Shao Dan is a well-known recipe; it is recorded in the Chapter on Fertility in *Gujin Tushu Jicheng Yiba Quanji (Complete Collection of Ancient and Modern Books: Medicine)*. It is usually indicated in patients with impotence, premature ejaculation and sterility. It is composed of fourteen herbs: Herba cistanchis, Radix morindae and Fructus foeniculi act on the Kidney to tonify the Vital Energy; Fructus lycii and Rhizoma rehmanniae replenish the Essence; Cortex eucommiae achyranthis strengthens the loins and legs and is also beneficial to the Kidney; Fructus schisandrae supplements the Essence; Fructus corri, Rhizoma acori graminei and Radix polygalae coordinate the physiological relationship between the Heart and Kidney; Poria and Rhizoma dioscoreae dispel Dampness to strengthen the function of Kidney Yang. This original prescription can be modified on a case-by-case basis. Other herbs, such as Rhizoma polygonati, Herba cynomorii, Semen cuscutae, Fructus schisandrae and others which tonify the Kidney and/or the Spleen, can be added or serve as substitutes in the recipe, as we have done in these cases. Wang Ang once said admiringly that "this prescription, warm but not dry in nature, reinforces both Yin and Yang and is a very good recipe for sperm production and fertility."

In case 1, the patient had an inborn defect which was probably accentuated further in youth. Liuwei Dihuang Tang and a herbal medicated liquor were used initially. Later on, Huan Shao Dan was taken for more than a year which was successful in bringing about the desired effect. For case 2, the patient suffered from azoospermia; Huan Shao Dan supplemented by Wuji Baifeng Wan was administered. An excellent response to this regimen was evident in three months time.

Besides the basic principle of tonifying the Kidney in treating infertility, it is very important to keep good personal hygiene and a proper diet. Of particular importance would also be the conservation and storage of Essence and sperm in order to enhance recuperation. Patients in these two cases were asked to refrain from sexual activities during the treatment course. This might have contributed to the favourable outcomes in the two cases.

5.3 HYPERTHYROIDISM
(GOITER)

Liu Cuiyong and Xie Faliang
Hunan Academy of Traditional Chinese Medicine and Materia Medica, Changsha

Chen Zhiping, 22, male, Han nationality, single, Wushu (martial arts) sportsman.
Medical record number: 2030. Date of first consultation: December 26, 1983.

CHIEF COMPLAINT: Palpitation, trembling of hands and enlargement of the neck of one year duration.

HISTORY OF PRESENT ILLNESS: On October 10, 1982, while taking part in a Wushu match, the patient suddenly experienced palpitation and dizziness due to hypertonia. He was immediately sent to hospital for treatment. His condition recovered, though palpitation remained for quite a period of time. In April of 1983, he was diagnosed as having hyperthyroidism in the Hunan Medical College and methylthiouracil was given as treatment. After one month of treatment, palpitation was relieved. But as soon as methylthiouracil was discontinued, symtoms of palpitation and sensation of an enlarging neck recurred. He was treated then in another hospital by a combination of traditional Chinese and modern medicine, but his condition failed to respond.

On December 8, 1983, he came to our hospital for consultation. He complained of palpitation (108/min), feeling of oppression in the chest, polyorexia (250 to 400 gm per meal), irascibility, aversion to heat, profuse sweating, insomnia, dreaminess, urorrhagia and loose stools.

PAST HISTORY: Non-contributory.

PERTINENT PHYSICAL EXAMINATION AND LABORATORY FINDINGS: Temperature, 37°C; pulse rate, 108/min; respiratory rate, 20/min; blood pressure, 120/80 mmHg. Exophthalmic. Thyroid gland: grade II diffusive enlargement, surface smooth, no tenderness. Left and right lobes of the thyroid symmetrical. Cardiac rhythm regular, no palpitation. Tremors of hands, moist palms. WBC, 4,400/mm^3; neutrophils, 77%; lympocytes, 23%; T_3, 2.9 ng/ml; and T4, 21 μgm/dl.

INSPECTION OF TONGUE: Red tongue substance with white fur.

PULSE CONDITION: Thready, wiry and rapid.

MODERN MEDICINE DIAGNOSIS: Primary Hyperthyroidism.

TRADITIONAL CHINESE MEDICINE DIAGNOSIS: Goiter (Ying Bing), Deficiency of Liver and Kidney Yin.

THERAPEUTIC PRINCIPLES: Nourish the Liver and Kidney, soften the hard lumps and dissipate the nodes.

PRESCRIPTION: Jia Kang Ling Tang. Spica prunellae, 15 gm; Herba ecliptae, 15 gm; Radix salviae miltiorrhizae, 15 gm; Rhizoma dioscoreae, 15 gm; Os draconis, 30 gm; and Concha ostreae, 30 gm. Preparation: Immerse all ingredients in 600-700 ml of cold water for 1-2 hours, then boil for 20 minutes over a slow fire. Remove 200 ml from the top of the decoction, add 400 ml of cold water, boil again until 200 ml is obtained. Combine the two portions of decoction, 200 ml of the decoction to be taken, twice a day, by oral administration.

First consultation on December 26, 1983: The patient's condition was due to hypertonia. Initially, he experienced palpitation. Later on, his condition worsened with a host of clinical signs and symptoms such as sensation of neck thickness, profuse sweating accompanied by restlessness, feverish sensation, thirst and polydipsia, polyorexia, listlessness, irritability, trembling of hands, insomnia, urorrhagia, red tongue with dry, thin, white coating and thready, wiry and rapid pulse. All these symptoms resulted from deficiency of Liver and Kidney Yin. Therapeutic principles to apply were to nourish the Liver and Kidney, soften the hard lumps, dissipate the nodes and activate Blood circulation to remove Blood stasis. The patient was given a dose of Jia Kang Ling Tang per day and propranolol, 10 mg, three times a day.

Second consultation on January 12, 1984: Having taken 17 doses of the prescription, the patient's condition improved. Symptoms of irascibility and palpitation eliminated; diet, stools and amount of urine became normal. Tongue with thin, white fur. Pulse thready and weak. Propranolol was discontinued. Continued to take the Chinese herbal prescription.

Third consultation on January 29, 1984: The patient had taken another 17 doses of Jia Kang Ling Tang. All symptoms were eliminated, goiter became small, the values of T_3 and T_4 were reduced to 1.92 ng/ml and 13.81 µgm/dl, respectively. He complained of nocturia and lumbago associated with weak and small pulse. Based on TCM theory, these symptoms may result from Kidney asthenia. The principles of treatment were to nourish and strengthen the Kidney to restore its astringent function. Modified Jia Kang Ling Tang. Rhizoma rehmanniae praeparatae, 15 gm; Radix paeoniae alba, 10 gm; Concha ostreae, 15 gm; Os draconis, 15 gm; Rhizoma dioscoreae, 15 gm; Herba ecliptae, 15 gm; Cortex moutan radicis, 10 gm; Poria, 10 gm; and Radix achyranthis bidentatae, 10 gm. Decoction to be prepared in the same way as before. One dose per day.

Fourth consultation on February 7, 1984: The patient felt much better. Condition marked by relief of lumbago, weakness in the legs and tinnitus. In order to invigorate the Liver and Kidney and strengthen the bones, tendons and muscles, Eucommia Bark,

10 gm, was added to the previous prescription.

Fifth consultation on February 16, 1984: The patient complained of slight lumbago. Diet, stool and urine were normal. He occasionally experienced swelling in the eyes, tremors of the hands, restlessness, insomnia, red tongue and wiry and rapid pulse (96/min). These symptoms indicated deficiency of Yin and hyperactivity of Yang. Added 10 gm each of Radix adenophorae strictae and Semen ziziphi spinosae to Jia Kang Ling Tang to nourish the Yin and tranquilize the mind.

Sixth consultation: Having been treated for two months, palpitation was relieved and goiter eliminated. The patient was able to sleep well, and he had slow and soft pulse (76/min). He continued to take Jia Kang Ling Tang in order to consolidate the therapeutic effects.

Seventh consultation: The patient was in good condition. Findings of laboratory examination showed T_3, 1.24 ng/ml; T_4, 9.52 µgm/dl; WBC, 5,400/mm^3; neutrophils, 73%; and lymphocytes, 27%. These normal values indicated that the patient had been cured clinically.

FOLLOW-UP/COURSE OF TREATMENT: The patient was admitted to a college of physical education in the summer of 1984. He has been studying in the college for four years without recurrence of the symptoms.

DISCUSSION: In traditional Chinese medicine, goiter is classified into three types, namely, the blood goiter, the toxic goiter and the Qi-goiter.

In recent years, hyperthyroidism is considered to be an autoimmune disorder (autoimmune hyperthyroidism). Experimental animal studies have been performed in our laboratory by injecting Jia Kang Ling (JKL) for phagocytosis test of leucocytes in mice. Results indicate that the phagocytic power of leucocytes increased significantly in the JKL group as compared with the control group ($p < 0.05$).

In the case of hyperthyroidism, the values of T_3 (I-triiodothyronine) and T_4 (I-thyroxine) and uptake of radioactive iodide are all higher than normal. Therefore, detemination of serum T_3 and T_4 and radioactive iodine uptake serves as an objective index of the thyroid function status. As for this patient, apart from symptoms and signs, the diagnosis was established on the basis of these laboratory values.

In the past five years, of the 368 cases of hyperthyroidism treated in our clinic, 80% belonged to the Yin Deficiency type which led to hyperactivity of Yang and deficiency of Liver-Yin and Kidney-Yin. Based on the clinical experience in treating these cases, we came up with the JKL prescription which is effective in nourishing the Yin and suppressing the sthenic Yang, dissipating the mass and activating Blood circulation to remove Blood stasis. Patients treated with JKL were all diagnosed definitely; some discontinued original modern medicine treatment because of serious side effects, while others refused thyroidectomy or radioactive iodine therapy. In a series of 234 cases of hyperthyroidism treated by JKL or modified JKL prescriptions, the clinical effective rate was 94-98%. It is concluded that JKL may be considered a safe and effective new herbal medicine for the treatment of goiter (hyperthyroidism).

5.4 DIABETES
(SPLEEN AND KIDNEY DEFICIENCIES AND BLOOD STASIS)

Jean Yu

Santa Barbara College of Oriental Medicine, California, U.S.A.

Cunningham, 32, female, white, single, personnel counselor. Medical record number: 912. Date of first consultation: October 19, 1987.

CHIEF COMPLAINT: Fluctuating blood sugar level due to diabetes and anxiety.

HISTORY OF PRESENT ILLNESS: The patient has been a diagnosed diabetic for 22 years. She is presently receiving laser therapy for the beginning stages of diabetic retinopathy. She suffered from great stress and anxiety at the time. She reported that her blood sugar had been fluctuating in recent weeks. She was suffering from headaches in the region of the eyes and in the sinus area. The patient also suffered from a variation of appetite with upper and lower abdominal pain and slight bloating. Her energy was described as erratic and often as fatigued. She complained of pain in the left eye which was receiving therapy. She usually felt warm and preferred cold drinks but was not overly thirsty. She had occasional constipation. Her menses was regular at 32 days with a light flow of dark blood with clots and cramping. She was currently taking insulin NDH with regular and split dosage.

PAST HISTORY: The patient was diagnosed at age 10 with diabetes (juvenile onset). Five years ago she had sudden hearing loss in the right ear. She had a tubal ligation four years ago.

INSPECTION OF TONGUE: Dark body, red tip, puffy, tooth marks and thin white coating.

PULSE CONDITION: Thin or thready, slippery and rapid (84/min). The first and third positions were deep.

MODERN MEDICINE DIAGNOSIS: Diabetes; Diabetic Retinopathy.

TRADITIONAL CHINESE MEDICINE DIAGNOSIS: Spleen Qi Deficiency and Deficiency of Qi and Yin; Blood Stasis in the Eye Region.

THERAPEUTIC PRINCIPLES: Tonify the Spleen Qi, tonify the Yin and remove Blood stasis.

PRESCRIPTION: Radix codonopsis pilosulae, 9 gm; Radix astragali, 9 gm; Rhizoma polygonati odorati, 9 gm; Fructus corni, 9 gm; Flos chrysanthemi, 12 gm; Folium mori, 9 gm; Herba cistapchis, 9 gm; and Radix salviae miltiorrhizae, 9 gm. Four doses. Patent medicine: Liuwei Dihuang Yan, eight pills, three times a day.

FOLLOW-UP/COURSE OF TREATMENT:

Second consultation on October 26, 1987 (one week): The patient reported a marked decrease in anxiety and sound sleep. She indicated that her recovery time from retinal laser treatments was reduced. She did not suffer from headaches. She had no abdominal bloating and had an increased appetite. She said her energy level was good. From the improvement in condition, it was determined that the formula was having the desired effect of tonifying the Qi and Yin as well as moving the Blood and benefiting the eyes. The prescription was continued and modified to further tonify the Yin and benefit the eyes.

Modification: Rhizoma polygonati odorati increased to 12 gm, Herba dendrobii, 15 gm; and Flos eriocauli, 9 gm. Four doses.

Fifth consultation on November 16, 1987: The patient reported continued and uninterrupted relief from anxiety, insomnia, headache, poor appetite, abdominal pain and tiredness. She reported that her blood sugar levels were remaining stable in the normal range. Her left eye had recovered from laser therapy with some resultant night blindness and photophobia. Her tongue was now a pink colour with glossy sides and tooth marks. Her pulse was slippery and rapid (85/min).

DISCUSSION: The patient's root imbalance was Spleen Qi deficiency and Yin deficiency of the Heart and Kidney. The retinal laser therapy was causing local Blood stagnation in the eye. The herbs Radix salviae miltiorrhizae and Radix astragali were used to tonify the Qi and stabilize the blood sugar. Rhizoma polygonati odorati, Fructus corni and Herba dendrobii were used to tonify the Yin and produce fluids as well as to clear heat. Flos chrysanthemi, Flos buddleiae, Folium mori and Flos eriocauli were prescribed to benefit the eyes, clear the eyes and reduce corneal opacity. In addition, Folium mori was used as an antidiabetic herb. Radix salviae miltiorrhizae was used to increase microcirculation in the arterioles to move stagnant Blood. Herba cistanchis was included as a Kidney tonic and to moisten the stool. Most herbs used in this formula have an antihypertensive effect. In all, the prescription was an effective therapy for this patient's condition.

(Collator: Brock Haines)

5.5 DIABETIC GASTROINTESTINAL AUTONOMIC NEUROPATHY
(XIAO KE DISEASE, DIARRHEA)

Guo Saishan

Department of Traditional Chinese Medicine, Peking Union Medical College Hospital, Beijing

Tian Baoshan, 36, male, married, shop assistant. Medical record number: C-336428. Date of first consultation: January 13, 1987.

CHIEF COMPLAINT: Polydipsia and polyuria for eight years, diarrhea for two years, exacerbated in the last four days.

HISTORY OF PRESENT ILLNESS: Since 1979, the patient had been suffering from polydipsia and polyuria. He was diagnosed as having diabetes mellitus in 1984, with fasting serum glucose level at 280 mg%, urine sugar (+++). He had blindness due to diabetic retinopathy. A year later, he developed diabetic nephropathy and gastrointestinal autonomic neuropathy. After being treated with insulin (50 u per day), fasting serum glucose was decreased to 120 mg%, urine sugar negative or trace. However, he began to complain of increasing frequency of bowel movement ranging from three or four to ten times a day, especially during the nighttime. Frequency of bowel movement was decreased to one or two times a day by taking berberine 0.3 to 0.9 gm a day, but diarrhea recurred whenever he stopped taking berberine. He had his stool examined three times in 1986, the results were all normal. The patient has been taking berberine regularly (0.6-0.9 gm a day) for the last two years. In the past four days, diarrhea aggravated and administration of berberine did not relieve the symptom. He had watery diarrhea up to 10 times a day even to the extent of fecal incontinence. He also had intolerance to cold, especially in the abdomen and lumbar areas. The patient was depressed and anxious.

INSPECTION OF TONGUE: Thin, white fur.

PULSE CONDITION: Slippery.

MODERN MEDICINE DIAGNOSIS: Diabetic Gastrointestinal Autonomic Neuropathy.

TRADITIONAL CHINESE MEDICINE DIAGNOSIS: Xiao Ke Disease; Diarrhea; Deficiency of Both Spleen and Kidney-Yang.

THERAPEUTIC PRINCIPLES: Warm and invigorate the Spleen and Kidney, nourish the Liver and regulate the Spleen-Qi.

PRESCRIPTION: Radix astragali, 30 gm; Ramulus cinnamomi, 10 gm; Radix paeoniae alba, 20 gm; Radix glycyrrhizae, 6 gm; Rhizoma zingiberis, 8 gm; Rhizoma atractylodis macrocephalae, 10 gm; Radix ledebouriellae, 8 gm; Pericarpium citri reticulatae, 10 gm; Semen cuscutae, 15 gm; Fructus psoraleae, 10 gm; Fructus schisandrae, 10 gm; and Margaritifera usta, 30 gm. Twelve doses. Q.i.d.

FOLLOW-UP/COURSE OF TREATMENT:

Second consultation on February 2, 1987: The patient's symptoms were alleviated after taking six decoctions, and he had bowel movement once a day. However, he had nocturnal diarrhea, as many as eight times per night when he stopped taking the decoctions. Over the last couple of days, he had diarrhea two times a day. The dosage of insulin was decreased to 46 u a day, and his urine sugar was trace or negative. Tongue with thin, white fur. Pulse slippery.

Radix astragali, 30 gm; Ramulus cinnamomi, 10 gm; Radix paeoniae alba, 20 gm; Radix glycyrrhizae, 6 gm; Rhizoma zingiberis, 8 gm; Rhizoma atractylodis macrocephalae, 10 gm; Radix ledebouriellae, 8 gm; Pericarpium citri reticulatae, 10 gm; Semen cuscutae, 15 gm; Fructus psoraleae, 10 gm; Fructus schisandrae, 10 gm; Concha margaritifera usta, 30 gm; and Cornu cervi, 15 gm. Twelve doses. Q.i.d.

After being treated with this prescription plus Semen coicis, 30 gm, and Poria, 30 gm, for three months, the patient had bowel movement once a day or once every other day with formed stool. He only complained of sensation of cold in the lumbar area and below the knees. Insulin was decreased to 44 u and fasting serum glucose level was 148 mg%. Urine sugar (examined on four occasions), (±). He continued to take the decoctions for one year until he had normal bowel movement. The symptom of intolerance to cold in the lumbar area, abdomen and lower extremities was relieved. The symptoms did not recur after he stopped taking the decoctions.

DISCUSSION: Diarrhea, nocturnal diarrhea or alternating constipation and diarrhea are the most common symptoms of diabetic gastrointestinal neuropathy. Although the patient's fasting serum glucose level was controlled quite well by insulin (fasting serum glucose, 150 mg%; urine sugar negative), he suffered from intractable diarrhea for two years. The symptom was alleviated for a period of time after taking berberine, which has an anti-acetylcholine effect. However, since the condition was essentially due to deficiency of Spleen- and Kidney-Yang, diarrhea was not well-controlled. Xiao Ke disease itself is weakness of the Kidney, which eventually leads to Yang deficiency. Deficiency of Spleen-Yang disturbs the warm transportation resulting in abdominal cold and diarrhea. Diarrhea occurred at dawn when Yin reaches its higest point and Yang its lowest. Insufficiency of Yang leads to fecal incontinence and failure to warm up the body and to propel Blood circulation normally. This is why the extremities were cold and tongue substance pale. After suffering from this illness for such a prolonged period of time, the patient was depressed and the promoting function of the Liver impaired. Therefore, the therapy was to warm and invigorate the Spleen and Kidney, to inhibit diarrhea and nourish the Liver, and to regulate the Spleen-Qi.

In the prescription, Radix astragali, Rhizoma atractylodis macrocephalae, Ramulus cinnamomi and Rhizoma zingiberis were used to supplement the Vital Energy, promote Yang, invigorate the Spleen, eliminate Wetness-Evil and stop diarrhea; Semen cuscutae, Fructus psoraleae and Fructus schisandrae to warm the Yang and invigorate the Kidney; Radix paeoniae alba was added to nourish the Liver and regulate the Spleen energy; Radix ledelouriellae to promote Spleen Yang; Pericarpium citri reticulatae to invigorate the Spleen and regulate the Vital Energy; and Concha margaritifera usta to soothe the Spleen and calm the Mind. This prescription has the properties of invigorating both the Spleen and Kidney, nourishing the Liver and regulating the Spleen. Its effect was evident in this case after administration of six doses. The patient had bowel movement with formed stool one to two times a day. Cornu cervi, Poria and Semen coicis were also used to invigorate the Spleen and Kidney and eliminate Wetness-Evil. After one year of treatment, his bowel movement became normal and the symptom of intolerance to cold was relieved.

In the prescription, we do not use Radix aconiti praeparatae and Cortex cinnamomi to promote Yang because the Xiao Ke disease is essentially due to the weakness of the Kidney. If they were administered, Radix aconiti praeparatae and Cortex cinnamomi are strong enough to damage the Yin body fluid. Should Radix aconiti praeparatae and Cortex cinnamomi be used in the prescription, prepared Rhizoma rehmanniae might be used to prevent their side effects. However, prepared Rhizoma rehmanniae could damage the Spleen-Yang. To avoid such side effects, we choose to use Semen cuscutae, which not only invigorates the Kidney and promotes the Yang but also strengthens Spleen-Yang and stops diarrhea.

As shown by studies on asthenia-syndrome, patients with Spleen deficiency and Kidney Yang have autonomic nervous system dysfunction, decreased function of the sympathetic nervous system and excess function of the parasympathetic nervous system. Such inequilibrium was manifested as poor appetite, increasing bowel movement and diarrhea. The patients had low concentration of DBH and cAMP/cGMP ratio and their body temperature regulation was also impaired. Patients with Kidney deficiency have a lower concentration of trace elements, especially Zn, Fe, Mn, etc. The Qi-supplementing and Yang-invigorating herbs had the effect of promoting the function of the sympathetic adrenal medulla and pituitary-cortico-adrenal system and of increasing the intracellular concentration of cAMP, thus elevating the cAMP/c-GMP ratio. In addition, these herbs are rich in essential trace elements, including zinc, iron and magnesium. In this particular case, the patient had diabetic gastrointestinal neuropathy and dysfunction of the autonomic nervous system manifested as deficiency of both Spleen- and Kidney-Yang. The therapy employing the principles to supplement the Vital Energy and invigorate the Yang was obviously appropriate in this case as evidenced by alleviation of the symptoms. Among the herbs administered, Radix astragali seu hedysari, Rhizoma atractylodis macrocephalae, Fructus psoraleae and Fructus schisandrae are rich in zinc and magnesium, while Semen cuscutae and Fructus schisandrae are rich in iron. Measures to enrich the essential trace elements may have played a therapeutic role in this case.

5.6 HEMATOCHYLURIA
(STRANGURIA)

Chen Kezhong and Zhang Jidong
Shandong Medical University Hospital, Jinan

Yin Shaotian, 30, male, Han nationality, married, shop assistant. Medical record number: 133924. Date of first consultation: August 17, 1976.

CHIEF COMPLAINT: Difficulty in passing urine; milky, white urine of one month duration.

HISTORY OF PRESENT ILLNESS: During the month prior to admission, the patient experienced milky urine with blood clots of various sizes, difficulty in urination and sometimes retention of urine. He had been treated for pyelonephritis in a local hospital and was given antibiotics and hemostatics and other medications but without much effect. Soon after, he was referred to our clinic for further treatment.

PAST HISTORY: History of filariasis in 1954 treated by hetrazan.

PERTINENT PHYSICAL EXAMINATION & LABORATORY FINDINGS: Dull complexion, percussion pain in the kidney area. Routine urinalysis: protein, (+++); RBC, (+++); chyluria, positive.

INSPECTION OF TONGUE: Red, thick and tender tongue with thin yellowish fur.

PULSE CONDITION: Deep and taut.

MODERN MEDICINE DIAGNOSIS: Hematochyluria.

TRADITIONAL CHINESE MEDICINE DIAGNOSIS: Stranguria.

THERAPEUTIC PRINCIPLES: Clear away Evil Heat and remove the stranguria; strengthen the Spleen and expel the Dampness.

PRESCRIPTION: Shiwei San and Bixiefenqingyin Jiajian (Modified Pyrrosia Leaf Powder and Yam Decoction for Clearing Turbid Urine). Rhizoma dioscoreae hypoglauae, 12 gm; Herba polygoni avicularis, 12 gm; Folium pyrrosiae, 12 gm; Spora lygodii, 12 gm; Rhizoma typhonii, 30 gm; Herba lysimachiae, 30 gm; Rhizoma atractylodis macrocephalae, 15 gm; Herba ecliptae, 15 gm; Polyporus umbellatus, 12 gm; and Liuyisang, 15 gm. To be decocted in water for oral ingestion. One dose per day. During the course of treatment, low-protein, low-fat diet was ordered so as to decrease the production of chyle.

FOLLOW-UP/COURSE OF TREATMENT:

Second consultation on August 21, 1976: After administration of four doses of the prescription, dysuria was partially relieved, but hematuria remained the same. In accordance with the principle of promoting Blood circulation to remove Blood stasis, Semen persicae, 9 gm, and Flos carthami, 9 gm, were added to the above prescription. Ten doses.

Third consultation on September 1, 1976: The patient's general condition was good. Hematuria had diminished gradually. Tongue was red with thin yellowish fur and pulse deep and wiry. Routine urinalysis: protein, (+++); RBC, (+); WBC, (+). Chyluria positive. In addition to the prescription, Sanqifen (Radix Notoginseng Powder), 3 gm, was taken at the same time. Ten doses.

Fourth consultation on September 11, 1976: The urine was transparent and routine urinalysis normal. Chyluria slightly positive. Tongue was pink with thin, yellowish fur and pulse deep and wiry. Discontinued Sanqifen. The same prescription was taken for another 30 days.

Fifth consultation on October 11, 1976: Urine was clear and routine urinalysis normal. Chyluria negative. The patient was discharged from hospital after being treated for more than 50 days. Ten-year follow-up has revealed no relapse of the symptoms.

DISCUSSION: The main cause of stranguria is accumulation of Dampness and Heat in the Lower Burner, resulting in obstruction of the flow of the Vital Energy, failure to distinguish the useful from the waste materials and failure to absorb the useful and excrete the waste materials. This condition gives rise to turbid urine and the urine can become thick as fat and creamy. In the early stage, the disease was characterized by presence of Dampness and Heat with burning pain in the urethra. *Danxi's Therapies* states that "though stranguria is of the Five Winds, they all belong to the syndrome of Heat." This indicates that the onset of stranguria results chiefly from retention of Heat and Dampness in the urinary bladder. And with the passing of time, the excess turns into deficiency. To treat the fundamental aspect of the disease, the therapeutic principle is to remove Heat and eliminate Dampness with febrifugal and diuretic herbs. In case of coexistence of deficiency and excess, both symptoms and cause can be treated at the same time by applying the principles of reinforcing the Spleen function and tonifying the Kidney.

Having been given hemostatics for treatment in a local hospital, the patient's condition failed to respond; this indicates that treatment by means of arresting the bleeding alone is not enough. Inspired by the TCM teaching that "long-time illnesses lead to pronounced Blood stasis" and "if Blood stasis is not removed, fresh blood will not be generated," Semen persicae, Flos carthami and Sanqifen (Radix Notoginseng Powder) were added to the prescription to effect the removal of the symptom of dysuria. From the point of view of modern medicine, the concept of Blood stasis relates not only to microcirculatory disturbance but also to metabolic disturbance as well as hyperplasia and atrophy of certain body tissues. For example, prolonged infliction by parasites, i.e., adult filariae in the lymphatic vessels of the human body, may result in hyperblastosis and cause obstruction of lymphatic vessels. The prescription of herbs for invigorating Blood circulation and eliminating Blood stasis can markedly decrease the degree of tissue edema and general anasarca during the inflammatory process, improve the permeability of capillaries, strengthen the phagocytic function of phagocytes and promote the digestion and absorption of hyperplastic tissues. During the period from 1965 to 1980, we treated 486 cases of stranguria, and excellent therapeutic effects were obtained in 178 cases. These successful cases were treated under the principles of clearing away Heat, eliminating Dampness and activating the Blood circulation to eliminate Blood stasis. Recent cure rate has reached 80.3%.

6. BLOOD DISEASES

6.1 IDIOPATHIC THROMBOCYTOPENIC PURPURA (ITP) (HEMORRHAGES IN SKIN AND MUCOUS MEMBRANES)

Zhou Zhongying
Nanjing College of Traditional Chinese Medicine, Nanjing

Chen Xilong, 42, male, Han nationality, married, worker. Medical record number: 819375. Date of first consultation: February 11, 1981.

CHIEF COMPLAINT: Subcutaneous bleeding for 75 days.

HISTORY OF PRESENT ILLNESS: Two and a half months prior to consultation, without apparent reason, the patient noticed that there were bleeding spots on his skin. He was then hospitalized in Nanjing and was diagnosed as having ITP. After being treated with corticosteroids for nearly 50 days, his condition improved and he was subsequently discharged. The patient was asked to continue taking the prednisone tablets, 10 mg, three times a day for two weeks, yet bleeding spots scattered on the skin of his extremities were still present. They were often caused by stroking or squeezing the skin. Accompanying symptoms experienced were lassitude, upper abdominal distention and sore sensation in the waist and knee joints.

PAST HISTORY: Measles complicated by pneumonia in childhood. Hospitalized for typhoid fever at age 20. Negative history of exposure to poisonous or chemical substances.

PERTINENT PHYSICAL EXAMINATION & LABORATORY FINDINGS: Examination of the heart and lungs negative. Petechiae observed on the upper extremities, each measuring 0.5-1.0 cm in diameter, two on the right and one on the left; dull reddish, or yellowish-green in colour. Platelet count, 52,000/mm³; WBC, 4,500/mm³; RBC, 4.01M/mm³; hemoglobin, 12.5 gm%.

INSPECTION OF TONGUE: Tongue proper reddish with thin fur.

PULSE CONDITION: Thready and rapid.

MODERN MEDICINE DIAGNOSIS: Idiopathic Thrombocytopenic Purpura.

TRADITIONAL CHINESE MEDICINE DIAGNOSIS: Subcutaneous Bleeding (Jinu).

THERAPEUTIC PRINCIPLES: Promote the Qi, nourish the Blood, soothe the Liver and tonify the Kidney.

PRESCRIPTION: A compound prescription was used, which was derived from two original prescriptions, Zhuogui Wan and Dang Gui Bu Xue Tang. Radix astragali seu hedysari, 10 gm; Radix codonopsis pilosulae, 12 gm; Fructus lycii, 12 gm; Rhizoma

177

rehmanniae praeparatae, 12 gm; Cornus cervi, 10 gm; Colla corii asini (melt), 10 gm; Herba ecliptae, 10 gm; Herba epimedii, 10 gm; Radix angelicae sinensis, 10 gm; Sprouted millet (baked and stirred), 10 gm; Malt (baked and stirred), 10 gm; Fructus corni, 5 gm; Pericarpium citri reticulatae, 5 gm; and Fructus ziziphi jujube, 5 pieces. Ten doses. Continued administration of prednisone at the same dosage. The patient was asked to refrain from taking alcoholic beverages and eating fried food. He was encouraged to take food such as soft-shell turtle, tortoise, pig's liver, jujube, longan, raw or boiled peanuts, Chinese yam, black soybean, sesame and fruits. Regular examination of platelet level was also advised and the patient should report to the doctor whenever petechiae appeared.

FOLLOW-UP/COURSE OF TREATMENT:

Second consultation on February 25, 1982: Platelet count 100,000/mm³. No purplish areas were noted and the patient had no particular complaint. Pulse thready. Apparently, the prescription has been effective. Continued another 30 doses and discontinued prednisone.

Third consultation on April 8, 1982: The patient's condition had improved. No purplish areas seen on the skin. Repeated examinations of blood platelet count were all over 100,000/mm³, though on the last two occasions, the platelet count did not reach this level; today's count was 72,000/mm³. In addition, the patient felt tired, had poor appetite and loose stools. Tongue substance red with thin coating. Pulse thready.

It was as though this disease was caused mainly by weakness of the Spleen and Kidney, thus leading to deficiency of the source for transformation of Qi and Blood. In light of this mechanism and in addition to the principles in use, i.e., nourishing the Liver and Kidney and tonifying Qi and Blood, herbs effective in reinforcing Spleen functions were added. The ingredients of this prescription were Radix astragali seu hedysari (stir-baked with adjuvants), 15 gm; Radix codonopsis pilosulae, 12 gm; Fructus lycii, 12 gm; Rhizoma rehmanniae praeparatae, 12 gm; Sprouted millet (baked and stirred), 12 gm; Malt (baked and stirred), 12 gm; Radix angelicae sinensis, 10 gm; Cornu cervi, 10 gm; Colla corii asini, 10 gm; Rhizoma dioscoreae, 10 gm; Rhizoma atractylodis macrocephalae (stir-baked with adjuvants), 3 gm; Fructus amomi, 3 gm, Endothelium corneum gigeriae galli (stir-baked with adjuvants), 6 gm; and Herba ecliptae, 10 gm. Thirty doses.

Fourth consultation on May 13, 1982: The latest platelet counts were all near the level of 100,000/mm³, and the patient did not complain of any discomfort. Tongue proper was normal and tongue fur seemed normal too. Pulse thready. Concerning the patient's present condition, the same principles of treatment could still be applied, thus 20 more doses were prescribed. In addition, in order to consolidate these effects, patent drugs such as Syrup for Nourishing Blood, 15 ml, b.i.d.; Shi Quan Da Bu Wan, 8 gm, b.i.d.; and Placenta Hominis Tablets, 4 tablets, b.i.d., were also prescribed along with the decoction.

Fifth consultation on June 7, 1982: Repeated platelet counts were all normal, between 110,000/mm³ and 150,000/mm³; 122,000/mm³ on the day of consultation. No purpuric spots were found. Tongue proper red and tongue fur thin. Pulse thready.

Discontinued the decoction but continued the patent drugs.

Sixth consultation on December 10, 1982: Last platelet count was 112,000/mm³. The patient had fully recovered. He was asked to continue the administration of patent medications to consolidate the therapeutic effects. During the next six months of follow-up, platelet counts were all over 100,000/mm³.

DISCUSSION: The main symptom of idiopathic thrombocytopenic purpura is hemorrhages in the skin and mucous membranes. This disease, belonging to the category of Blood syndrome, is called Jinu (Subcutaneous Bleeding) in traditional Chinese medicine. According to TCM theories, it is caused by perversion of Qi and flaring up of Fire, thus losing the control of Blood flow leading to its extravasation. Symptom-complex differentiation of traditional Chinese medicine classifies the disease into two categories, Shi (hyperactivity) and Xu (deficiency) syndromes. As to the deficiency syndrome, it is often caused by Qi weakness, lost control of Blood flow and flaring up of Fire leading to its extravasation. The patient in our case has had the disease for a long period of time, with accompanying symptoms of fatigue, lumbar soreness and upper abdomen distention, and his hemorrhagic spots in the skin were dull reddish or pinkish in colour. Tongue proper was reddish and the pulse felt thready. As such, these symptoms and signs were related to deficiency of Qi and Blood, especially the Vital Essence. In order to nourish Qi and essence and to tonify the Liver and Kidney in this case, a compound prescription derived from two prescriptions, Zhuogui Bolus and Modified Radix angelicae sinensis Decoction for Enriching Blood, was used. It is known that there exists an interdependence between Vital Energy (Yang) and Vital Essence (Yin) concerning the functions of transformation and promotion. In order to enrich the Essence and Blood, the Kidney is warmed first to flourish the Qi leading to the generation of a rich reservoir of Blood. This principle of treatment is known as reinforcing Yang, which is essential to the generation and enrichment of Yin. According to basic TCM teachings, the function of the Kidney is to master the bone marrow; therefore, reinforcement of the Kidney will certainly lead to nourishment of Vital Essence and Blood. The function of the Spleen is to digest and transform food and nutrients; thus, promotion of the Spleen will augment the source of Qi and Blood. Accordingly in treating this kind of disease, it is advisable to lay the stress on promoting the Spleen and reinforcing the Kidney. This patient, on the third visit after taking a lot of tonics, showed other symptoms due to deficiency of the Spleen. Apparently, these tonics have certain unfavourable influences on the Spleen. It is essential at this stage to promote the Spleen, and in this way the source of Qi and Blood will be enriched enabling a smooth course of recovery. In treating a case of this nature, medicinal materials derived from animal or human tissues may be more significant than those from herbs, woods, minerals and so on. In our prescription, Cornus cervi, Colla cori asini and Placenta hominis are animal or human tissues which have shown significant therapeutic effects, suggesting that these tissues contain a variety of nutrients and hormones which, on a large scale, seem responsible for the favourable outcome of this case.

6.2 CHRONIC MYELOGENOUS LEUKEMIA (QI AND YIN DEFICIENCIES WITH VIRULENT HEAT-EVIL BLAZING)

Lu Shiteng and Hu Guixuan

Hunan Academy of Traditional Chinese Medicine and
Materia Medica, Changsha

The patient was a 50-year-old peasant woman, who came to the Second Xinning County People's Hospital on April 2, 1973, with the chief complaints of weakness and gradually increasing fatigue for about two years and a fist-sized mass on the left upper abdomen of five months duration. The mass appeared to be increasing in size. It caused no pain and was accompanied by a sense of postprandial epigastric fullness, reduction in food intake, weight loss, frequent sensation of cold and low-grade fever in the afternoons, night sweats and constipation. During the past 10 days, the patient had light cough with a scanty amount of mucoid phlegm. Her urination was normal. No hemorrhage occurred in the course of the illness except two episodes of epistaxis about a year ago.

The patient enjoyed good health until onset of the present illness. There was no history of alcohol intake or smoking. Negative history of exposure to radiation or toxic materials.

PERTINENT PHYSICAL EXAMINATION & LABORATORY FINDINGS: Temperature, 38.5°C; pulse rate, 100/min; respiratory rate, 24/min; blood pressure, 120/80 mmHg. Pale and undernourished. No icterus, no hemorrhagic spots and petechiae on the mucosa and skin. Bean-sized auxiliary and inguinal lymph nodes palpable bilaterally. The neck was supple, with no thyroid abnormality. Sternum set medially with light tenderness in its lower portion. Harsh breath sounds on both lungs with a few moist rales appreciated at the right lower field. Heart with normal sinus rhythm and no murmur. The abdomen flat, negative for shifting dullness. Upper border of the liver on the fifth intercostal space by percussion, lower border palpable two finger-breadths below the right costal margin, moderate in consistency, smooth. Spleen markedly enlarged, descending two finger-breadths below the umbilicus, hard and nontender. No deformity of the spinal column and extremities. Neuropsychiatric examinations negative. Routine urinalysis normal. Chest fluoroscopy indicated accentuated lung markings on both sides and an ill-defined shadow in the right lower lung field. Blood: hemoglobin, 5.4 gm%; RBC, 2M/mm^3; WBC, 43,600/mm^3; myeloblasts, 3%; promyelocytes, 7%; myelocytes, 30%; metamyelocytes, 21%. Bone marrow biopsy showed polar hyperplasia, in which the granulocyte series was characterized by prominent hyperplasia with obvious proliferation at various stages, particularly the myelocyte and metalyelocyte. The numbers of basophils increased significantly. Erythrocyte and platelet in distribution was not decreased.

INSPECTION OF TONGUE: Dry with yellow fur.

PULSE CONDITION: Feeble, large, smooth and rapid.

MODERN MEDICINE DIAGNOSIS: Chronic Myelogenous Leukemia (CML).

TRADITIONAL CHINESE MEDICINE DIAGNOSIS: Qi and Yin Deficiencies with Virulent Heat-Evil Blazing.

PRESCRIPTION: Radix codonopsis pilosulae, 9 gm; Radix astragali seu heydysari, 12 gm; Radix paeoniae alba, 9 gm; Radix scrophulariae, 12 gm; Radix rehmanniae, 9 gm; Radix glycyrrhizae, 3 gm; Radix et rhizoma rhei, 9 gm; Viola yedoensis Makino, 9 gm; Herba taraxaci, 15 gm; Rhizoma anemarrhenae, 9 gm; Endothelium corneum gigeriae galli, 6 gm; and Shen Qu, 9 gm.

COURSE OF TREATMENT

Date	Signs & Symptoms	Prescription	Peripheral Blood			
			HB	RBC	WBC	Platelet
02/04/73	Same as previous	First prescription, eight doses	5.4 gm%	2,000,000	436,000	530,000
				juvenile leucocytes 61%		
10/04/73	Appetite improved, cough and rales disappeared	First prescription, ten doses	5.6 gm%	2,000,000	28,300	480,000
20/04/73	Tongue with thin white fur, constipation relieved	First prescription with Radix et rhizoma rhei, Endothelium corneum gigeriae galli and Shen Qu replaced by Radix angelicae sinensis, 9 gm; Folium mori, 12 gm; and Pericarpium citri reticulatae, 6 gm. Eight doses	6 gm%	2,100,000	161,000	460,000
				juvenile leucocytes 23%		
29/04/73	Temp.38°C	As above, ten doses	7 gm%	2,600,000	82,000	220,000
10/05/73	Temp.37.8°C, night sweating stopped	As above, ten doses	7 gm%	2,800,000	46,000	200,000
				juvenile leucocytes 14%		
20/05/73	Temp.37.5°C, spleen size reduced to below left costal margin 5 cm (3FB)	Above prescription minus Folium mori, eight doses	7.6 gm%	3,000,000	23,000	180,000
30/05/73	Same as above	As above, eight doses	8 gm%	3,200,000	20,000	200,000
				metamyelocytes 6%		

DISCUSSION: Based on clinical features and blood and bone marrow pictures, the diagnosis of CML was well established, though there was no detection of the Philadelphia chromosomes. The rales in the right lower lung might have been the result of infection or leukemia cell infiltration. As the blast count approaches 100,000 per litre, pulmonary-vascular leukostasis can occur.

By TCM theories, the human body has a vital energy termed Qi which is the moving force behind the activities of various organs. Deficiency of Qi will result in pallor and inadequate energy of organs. In addition, traditional Chinese medicine believes in the coexistence of Yin and Yang in the human body. Yang represents activity, external parts, etc., and Yin represents inertia, internal organs, etc. When one is healthy, these two are kept in balance. When Yin is deficient, Fire will be produced. This Fire may come from either exogenous evils or internal deficiency of Yin, leading to signs of dry tongue with yellow fur. Yin deficiency and accumulation of Fire could drive out the body fluids, as manifested by night sweating. In this case, deficiency of Qi and Yin and presence of virulent Heat Evil were evidenced by feeble, large, smooth and rapid pulse. This condition was treated with the therapeutic principles of invigorating Qi, nourishing Yin and clearing away Heat and toxins. In the prescription, Radix codonopsis and Radix glycyrrhizae invigorate the Qi; Radix paeoniae alba, Radix rehmanniae and Scrophulariae nourish the Yin; and Herba taraxaci, Rhizoma anemarrhenae, Radix et rhizoma rhei and Viola yedoensis clear away the Fire and toxins.

Pharmacologically, the effect of Radix codonopsis is on the hematopoietic process; Radix rehmanniae and Radix glycyrrhizae act in a way similar to glucocorticoids; Radix et Rhizoma rhei is one of the agents that enhances body immune functions; and Viola yedoensis and Herba taraxaci play an antiviral role. Moreover, Rhei and Radix glycyrrhizae have been demonstrated to be effective against some malignant neoplasms. Radix glycyrrhizae can also ameliorate the leukemia status in mice.

Treating the case according to TCM theories, the outcome saw an increase in appetite, remission of fever, disappearance of night sweating, cough and rales in the right lower lung and reduction in the size of the spleen. For two months, the patient's blood picture showed tremendous improvement. Leucocyte and juvenile leucocyte counts were reduced from $436,000/mm^3$ to $20,000/mm^3$ and 61% to 6%, respectively. This case recovered progressively until remission was reached. This was evidenced clinically by a significant reduction of the patient's peripheral leucocyte count. The mechanisms of these herbs in treating this case of CML need to be investigated further. Thomas found that in patients with blast phase of CML, a remission rate of 15% could be achieved by bone marrow transplantation, the indices of observation being absence of Philadelphia chromosome and a disease-free survival period of five to nine years. Those cases which receive bone marrow transplant in the remission period have a much better cure rate (approximately 60%). It is reasonable to believe that the TCM method of treatment described above might be able to transform the disease from blast phase to remission so as to allow enough time to identify a suitable donor and to arrange for the subsequent bone marrow transplantation.

This patient was treated in the outpatient department of a hospital located in the countryside, where the authors were sent for "ideological remoulding" during the infamous "cultural revolution." A follow-up was not possible in this case because the patient lived far away from the hospital and because the authors were transferred back to the city.

6.3 REFRACTORY ANEMIA
(SHU LOU)

Xie Renfu
Department of Hematology, Sino-Japanese
Friendship Hospital, Beijing

Han Aifeng, 13, female, student. Date of first consultation: March 7, 1987.

CHIEF COMPLAINT: Dizziness and palpitation for four months and gum bleeding for two months.

HISTORY OF PRESENT ILLNESS: One year prior to consultation, the patient was noted to be pale, though she felt well. Gradually, she experienced dizziness, lassitude and palpitation. Symptoms were usually aggravated by physical exertion in recent four months. In addition, there was a hemorrhagic tendency, manifested as gum bleeding, epistaxis, skin petechiae and menorrhagia for two months. She was found to have anemia at a local district hospital, where her condition did not respond to the treatment.

At the time of consultation, the patient complained of dizziness, tinnitus, fatigue, palpitations which were aggravated by physical activities, sensation of heat in her palms and soles, gum bleeding and skin purpura. She had a good appetite, and there was no abnormality in urination or bowel movement.

PAST HISTORY: Non-contributory.

PERTINENT PHYSICAL EXAMINATION & LABORATORY FINDINGS: Pale with scattering skin petechiae/purpura, especially prominent on the lower extremities. No lymphadenopathies. Lungs clear. Heart rate 92/min with blowing systolic murmur appreciated at the apex. Liver and spleen not palpable. Blood: hemoglobin, 6.4 gm%; WBC, 2,500/m^3; neutrophils, 45%; lymphocytes, 55%; platelets, 15,000/m^3; reticulocytes, 1%. Routine urinalysis normal. Rou's test, Ham's test, heat hemolysis, sucrose hemolysis and Coomb's test all were negative. Liver function tests normal. Bone marrow smear showed hypercellularity, erythroid hyperplasia with megaloblastoid erythropoiesis. There were hypogranulation, vacuoles, or nude nuclei in some myeloid cells; two megakaryocytes in one smear; sideroblasts 98%; no ring sideroblast observed.

INSPECTION OF TONGUE: Pale with white, thin fur.

PULSE CONDITION: Deep and small.

MODERN MEDICINE DIAGNOSIS: Refractory Anemia.

TRADITIONAL CHINESE MEDICINE DIAGNOSIS: Shu Lou; General Debility of Both Qi Xue and Yin Yang.

THERAPEUTIC PRINCIPLES: Tonify the Kidney.

Symptom-complex differentiation: The patient was afflicted by insufficiency of Qi-Blood and Yin-Yang. The fundamental pathogenesis was Kidney deficiency.

PRESCRIPTION: Radix polygoni multiflori, 15 gm; Herba ecliptae, 15 gm; Fructus ligustri lucidi, 15 gm; Fructus mori, 15 gm; Fructus leonuri, 15 gm; Rhizoma polygonati, 30 gm; Radix astragali, 30 gm; Caulis spatholobi, 30 gm; and Herba selaginellae, 15 gm

FOLLOW-UP/COURSE OF TREATMENT:

April 13, 1987: After taking 14 doses of the prescription, the patient's symptoms were alleviated. Hemoglobin, 7.8 gm%; WBC, 4,200/m³; platelet, 15,000/m³; reticulocytes, 3.2% Continued the same prescription.

April 27, 1987: The patient's condition was markedly improved. The tongue became redder and pulse was sinking and taut. Hemoglobin, 9 gm%; WBC, 4,300/m³; platelet, 35,000/m³. Minor modification of the prescription. Radix astragali, Herba selaginellae and Caulis spatholobi were removed from the prescription, while Fructus psoraleae, 15 gm, Herba cistanchis, 30 gm, and Herba agrimoniae, 15 gm, were added.

May 23, 1987: The patient did not complain of any symptom except a few petechiae on the skin. Hemoglobin, 12 gm%; WBC, 5,600/m³ and platelet, 80,000/m³. Prescription: Radix polygonati multiflori, 15 gm; Rhizoma polygonati, 30 gm; Fructus mori, 15 gm; Herba ecliptae, 15 gm; Herba agrimoniae, 15 gm; Radix rubiae, 15 gm; Herba cistanchis, 30 gm; Fructus psoraleae, 15 gm; and Fructus ligustri lucidi, 15 gm.

June 5, 1987: Blood examination showed improvement. Hemoglobin, 14.4 gm%; WBC, 5,500/m³; platelet, 76,000/m³. Modification: Herba cynomorii, 15 gm, and Folium pyrrosiae, 15 gm, were added and Herba cistanchis and Radix rubiae removed from the last prescription.

June 25, 1987: The patient felt well with a thin, white tongue coating and deep, taut pulse. Blood examination showed hemoglobin, 13.4 gm%; WBC, 4,100/m³; platelet, 74,000/m³. Hypercellularity of bone marrow with megaloblastoid erythropoiesis, nine megakaryocytes seen in a marrow smear. Prescription: Fructus mori, 15 gm; Herba ecliptae, 15 gm; Herba cynomorii, 15 gm; Radix moringae, 15 gm; Fructus ligustri lucidi, 15 gm; Rhizoma polygonati, 30 gm; Herba selaginellae, 30 gm; and Herba agrimoniae, 15 gm.

June 30, 1987: The patient was discharged from hospital with home medication (the same prescription) for another three months. She came back for a follow-up examination on February 5, 1988. Blood picture showed hemoglobin, 13.8 gm%; WBC, 6,200/m³; platelet, 102,000/m³. There was a hyperplasia marrow with mild megaloblastoid features of the erythroid series.

DISCUSSION: This was a case of pancytopenia with anemia and hemorrhagic manifestations. All tests on hemolysis were negative. Bone marrow showed hypercellularity with megablastoid erythropoiesis and some morphological abnormalities of the myeloid cells. Paroxysmal nocturnal hemoglobinurea and aplastic anemia could be ruled out and the diagnosis of refractory anemia was established.

Refractory anemia is a subtype of myelodysplastic syndromes according to FAB classification (Bennett JM, et al., 1982. *Brit. J. Hemat.* 51:189) and is generally difficult to treat. Androgens may be helpful in some cases but need a rather long time, i.e., from three to six months, to show any responsiveness. For this patient, therapeutic effect was first observed after 40 days of treatment with progressive improvement and clinical remission obtained in three months. She remained well after 11 months. The effect of herbal medicine in treating this case is unquestionable.

According to TCM theories, dizziness, general weakness and palpitation are signs of concomitant deficiency of Qi and Blood. Sensation of heat in the palms and soles and deep and fine pulse are signs of Kidney deficiency or deficiency of Kidney Yang or vital force, resulting in inadequacy of Vital Energy and insufficiency of Kidney Yin and leading to an insufficient quantity of Blood. It is clear that the fundamental pathogenesis was deficiency of the Kidney. One of the basic functions of the Kidney is to control the bone and the bone marrow which is the exclusive site for hematopoiesis in normal adults as interpreted by modern medicine. To replenish the Kidney Yin and Yang is therefore the primary goal of treatment for patients suffering from anemia or cytopenia.

Based on the author's more than 30 years of clinical experience, this prescription was given with modifications as dictated by the progress of her condition. Radix polygoni multiflori replenished the Vital Essence, marrow and Blood, Li Shizhen, the famous herbal medicine practitioner, indicated the effectiveness of Radix polygoni multiflori to tonify the Kidney as more superior than that of Radix rehmanniae and Asparagus root. The combination of Fructus ligustri lucidi and Herba ecliptae is a well-known ancient prescription called Er-Zhi Wan, which is both useful and economical for strengthening the bones and tendose, tonifying the loins and legs and nourishing Liver and Kidney essence. Fructus mori tonifies the Liver and Kidney by nourishing their essence. Fructus leonusi is able to intensify the Vital Energy or Qi and restores the essence and marrow. A large amount of Radix astragali, which is powerful in invigorating the Vital Energy and in turn promoting hemopoiesis, was also used. Rhizoma polygonati strengthens the essence and marrow, nourishes the Heart and Lung and calms and regulates the viscerae. All these herbs act together to tonify the Kidney. Since the patient has been afflicted by multiple hemorrhage for a long time, and because according to TCM teaching "once the Blood comes out of the vessels or channels, it is followed soon by Blood stasis," herbs such as Herba selaginellae and Caulis spatholobi were added to invigorate the Blood circulation and to remove Blood stasis in order to enhance hematopoiesis. In the latter stages, other tonics for replenishing the Kidney and promoting circulation were added or replaced some of the herbs used previously. Herba cistanchis and Herba cynomorii, which are warm but not dru in nature, can reinforce Kidney function without doing any harm to the essence. As it is very important to regulate the balance between Kidney Yin and Kidney Yang when replenishing or tonifying the Kidney, Fructus psoraleae and Radix morindae, which are helpful in strengthening the vital force or Kidney-Yang, were also used in the prescription.

From our laboratory studies in recent years, it has been shown that many Kidney-replenishing tonics, e.g., Radix polygoni multiflori, Fructus mori, Herba cistanchis, Herba cynomorii, Radix morindae and Fructus ligustri lucidi, can promote hemopoiesis *in vivo* and *in vitro*. Radix astragali, a powerful herb effective in invigorating the Vital Energy, can stimulate multipotent hemopoietic stem cells and granulocyte macrophage progenitors in mice. Huo Xue Hua Yu (Circulation Promoting and Stasis Removing) herbs cannot stimulate hemopoiesis directly, but they can enhance hematopoiesis by improving the function of marrow stroma.

CONCLUSION: Based on TCM theories, this complex prescription, which focuses on tonifying the Kidney to regulate Kidney-Yin and Kidney-Yang as well as replenishing the essence and marrow, was given as treatment in this case of refractory anemia. This prescription was supplemented by a large dosage of Radix astragali to invigorate the Vital Energy together with herbs effective in promoting Blood circulation in order to remove Blood stasis. An excellent clinical outcome was obtained. It is the author's belief, from his vast clinical experience, that this is the general principle indicated in treating cases of refractory anemia, aplastic anemia and other types of cytopenia.

6.4 EVAN'S SYNDROME
(*XUE ZHANG* HEMORRHAGIC DISORDER)

Xie Renfu

Department of Hematology, Sino-Japanese
Friendship Hospital, Beijing

Ma Zhunan, 54, female, married, cadre. Medical record number: 271182. Date of first consultation: August 20, 1985.

CHIEF COMPLAINT: Intermittent epistaxis and/or skin petechiae for more than 10 years.

HISTORY OF PRESENT ILLNESS: In 1972, the patient first experienced epistaxis and, occasionally, some skin petechiae or purpura was noted. Thereafter it reoccurred several times a year. A diagnosis of idiopathic thrombocytopenia (ITP) was given in a local hospital. The platelet count varied between 20,000-30,000/m³. This bleeding tendency was ameliorated by medications, but the platelet count remained low. In the last two years, the hemorrhagic manifestations exacerbated.

In January 1985, the patient suddenly developed chill and fever and was told she had a viral infection. The fever subsided after several days, though she still experienced lassitude and weakness. Blood examination revealed pancytopenia with reticulocytosis. Bone marrow smear showed a hyperplastic anemia picture. Antinuclear antibody, anti-DNA antibody tests were both negative, and no lupus erythematosus cell (LE cell) was found.

At the time of consultation, the patient complained of dizziness, headache, irritability and insomnia, poor appetite, dry stool and occasional epistaxis.

PAST HISTORY: Amenorrheic for four years.

PERTINENT PHYSICAL EXAMINATION & LABORATORY FINDINGS: Scattered skin petechiae and purpuric lesions. No superficial adenomegaly, nor icterus. Lungs clear. Heart rate 98/min. Liver and spleen not palpable. No edema detected. Blood picture: hemoglobin, 10.8gm%; WBC, 6,600/m³; neutrophils, 66%; lymphocytes, 34%; platelets, 17,000/m³; reticulocyte, 4.2%. Liver function tests and routine urinalysis normal. Serum bilirubin, 1.2 mg/dl; Rou's test, Ham's heat hemolysis and sucrose hemolysis test were all negative. Direct Coomb's test was positive. Auto-antibody test normal; normal range of IgG, IgA, IgM. Bone marrow examination showed hypercellyuarity with a M:E ratio of 1.38, hyperplasia of erythroid series, mainly polychromatic and normochromatic normoblasts.

INSPECTION OF TONGUE: Tongue substance red with a thin, white coat.

PULSE CONDITION: Taut and thread-like.

MODERN MEDICINE DIAGNOSIS: Evan's Syndrome (Auto-immune Hemolytic Anemia Complicated with Thrombocytopenia).

TRADITIONAL CHINESE MEDICINE DIAGNOSIS: *Xue Zheng* (Hemorrhagic Disorder) Secondary to Yin Deficiency.

THERAPEUTIC PRINCIPLES: Replenish the Essence to remove the Evil Heat and relax the irritation.

PRESCRIPTION: Modified Er-Zhi Wan and Can Mai Da Zao Tang. Fructus ligustri lucidi, 15 gm; Herba ecliptae, 15 gm; Fructus tritici levis, 30 gm; Radix astragali, 30 gm; Caulis spatholobi, 30 gm; Rhizoma smilacis glabrae, 30 gm; Folium pyrrosiae, 15 gm; Radix glycyrrhizae, 10 gm; and Fructus ziziphi jujubae, 15 gm. Decoct as one dose, q. i. d., and Wuji Baifeng Wan, a patent herbal pill, 10 gm, twice a day.

FOLLOW-UP/COURSE OF TREATMENT:

September 17, 1985: The patient took the herbal prescription and patent pills as advised. No epistaxis occurred, but she still complained of irritability, insomnia and lassitude. There was a small furuncle at the right side of the nose. Blood examination: hemoglobin, 13.5 gm%; WBC, 4,900/m³; platelets, 53,000/m³; reticulocyte, 1.6%. She was advised to keep on taking the last prescription with 15 gm of Semen coicis added. Pills of Flori Trollii were given for the furuncle.

The patient went to her hometown after this visit and was not able to return to the hospital until July 29, 1986.

July 29, 1986: She had taken the prescription of September 17, 1985, for 40 days and felt much better. The thrombocyte count varied between 39,000-49,000/m³. Then the prescription was discontinued. After a short period of time, she experienced vertigo and was admitted to a local hospital. Blood examination: hemoglobin, 78 gm%; WBC, 5,200/m³; platelets, 36,000/m³; reticulocyte, 8.6%. The vertigo was cured by medical treatment in a month. But dizziness, epistaxis and purpura remained in spite of active treatment with various medications.

At the time of consultation at our clinic, she complained of dizziness, lassitude, insomnia and irritation. She had bowel movement once every other day, tongue with red tip and white, thin fur; a sinking, weak and taut pulse.

PERTINENT PHYSICAL EXAMINATION & LABORATORY FINDINGS: Slightly jaundiced sclera, blowing systolic murmur at apex of heart, lungs clear, no hepatosplenomegaly, several petechiae or purpura scattered at lower extremities. Hemoglobin, 8.2 gm%; platelets, 41,000/m³; reticulocyte, 6.4%. Bone marrow smear showed a hyperplastic anemia picture. Coomb's test positive.

FOLLOW-UP/COURSE OF TREATMENT: According to TCM theories, she was diagnosed as having insufficiency of Vital Essence resulting in flaring up of Evil Heat. Modified Er-Zhi Wan was used to replenish the Vital Essence of the Liver and Kidney, to remove the Evil Heat and to serve as a sedative. Fructus mori, 15 gm; Fructus ligustri lucidi, 15 gm; Herba ecliptae, 15 gm; Radix polygoni multiflori, 15 gm; Herba cistanchis, 15 gm; Radix astragali, 30 gm; Herba selaginellae, 30 gm; Fructus tritici levis, 30 gm; Semen biotae, 15 gm; Semen nelumbinis, 15 gm. Decoct as one dose, q.i.d.

August 16, 1986: After two weeks, the patient felt better and could sleep for about four to five hours. There was no obvious change in the condition of the tongue and pulse. Hemoglobin, 9.4 gm%; platelet, 91,000/m^3; reticulocyte, 5.2%.

August 26, 1986: The sensation of ill-being was much ameliorated. The patient complained of dry throat. Thin fur over the tongue, pulse taut and slippery. Neither petechiae nor jaundice were noted. Prescription: Fructus mori, 15 gm; Fructus ligustri lucidi, 15 gm; Herba ecliptae, 15 gm; Semen nelumbinis, 15 gm; Rhizoma polygonati, 30 gm; Radix adenophorae strictae, 15 gm; Folium pyrrosiae, 15 gm; Radix ophiopognois, 15 gm, Radix scrophulariae, 15 gm. Wuji Baifeng Wan was also prescribed, one pill, twice a day.

September 16, 1986: The patient complained of bitterness in the mouth, dry throat, mild pain at both costal margins and some purpura in the skin. Hemoglobin, 10.9 gm%; platelet, 51,000/m^3; reticulocyte, 3.2%. Modified Yi Guan Jian was prescribed. Radix ophiopogonis, 15 gm; Radix adenophorae strictae, 15 gm; Fructus lycii, 15 gm; Fructus meliae toosendan, 10 gm; Rhizoma rehmanniae, 15 gm; Herba dendrobii, 10 gm; Fructus mori, 15 gm: Semen coicis, 30 gm; and Semen nelumbinis, 10 gm.

September 30, 1986: The patient's condition was better, tongue with fur and pulse taut. Hemoglobin, 10 gm%; platelet, 80,000/m^3; reticulocytes, 2%. Added Fructus ligustri lucidi, 15 gm, and Herba ecliptae, 15 gm, to the prescription.

October 21, 1986: General condition had been fine but in the last few days the patient suffered from common cold with headache, cough with scanty amount of sputum and sore throat. Tongue with white, thin fur. Pulse floating and taut. A prescription of Xin Su Yin was given to dispel pathogenic factors from exterior of the body. Folium perillae, 10 gm; Semen armeniacae amarum, 10 gm; Radix peucedani, 10 gm; Radix platycodi, 10 gm; Radix angelicae dahuriae, 10 gm; Radix ledebouriellae, 10 gm; Flos lonicerae, 30 gm; Pericarpium trichosanthis, 15 gm; Radix glycyrrhizae, 6 gm; and Radix tinosporae, 15 gm. Decocted and taken q.i.d.

November 5, 1986: The patient was well except for a little dizziness and occasional insomnia. Tongue with thin coat and pulse taut. No apparent abnormalities found in physical examination. Blood picture much improved: hemoglobin, 10.4 gm%; WBC, 8,500/m^3 with normal differentiation; platelets, 78×10^4/l; reticulocytes, 1.5%. The principle of treatment at this stage was to continue nourishing the Vital Essence of the Liver and Kidney. Prescription: Rhizoma polygonati, 20 gm; Herba ecliptae, 60 gm; Fructus ligustri lucidi, 60 gm; Fructus leonuri, 60 gm; Semen coicis, 60 gm; Herba cistanchis, 12 gm; Herba selaginellae, 60 gm; Folium pyrrosiae, 60 gm, and Radix astragali, 12 gm. Ground all ingredients into fine powders, made into pills by mixing with honey. Dosage at 10 gm, twice a day.

The patient went home in mid-December, 1986. We were informed later that she kept on taking the pills and felt much better. There had been no bleeding, hemoglobin, 10 gm% and platelet count in the range of 70,000-90,000/m^3. The pills were discontinued after a month.

DISCUSSION: This is a case of thrombocytopenia with bleeding tendency for more than 10 years. Later on in the course of the disease, there appeared anemia, reticulocytosis, mild jaundice of the sclera, elevated serum bilirubin and hypercellular bone marrow, in particular the erythroid hyperplasia with a majority of polychromatic and normochromatic normoblasts. There was no paroxysmal nocturnal hemoglobinuria as evidenced by negative Ham's test, nor collagen disease such as systemic lupus erythematosus as shown by negative anti-nuclear antibody tests. Based on positive Coomb's test and thrombocytopenia, the diagnosis of auto-immune hemolytic anemia complicated with thrombocytopenia, or Evan's syndrome, was established. There is no specific therapy for this disease entity except symptomatic relief. Cortico-adrenal steroids could be of benefit in some cases but usually need to be taken for a long time and complicate the situation with many severe side effects. For this patient, only traditional Chinese medications in the forms of decoctions and patent pills were given, and a satisfactory response was achieved.

Based on TCM theories, multiple hemorrhagic episodes, dry stool, red tongue and fine, taut pulse belong to the symptom-complex of insufficiency of the Vital Essence. The viscerae cannot be nourished properly and the Five Emotional Heats become exacerbated, resulting in irritability and insomnia. Er-Zhi Wan, composed of Fructus ligustri lucidi and Herba ecliptae, is economical and effective in replenishing the Vital Essence. Gan Mai Da Zao Tang is an ancient recipe recorded in *Jin Kui Yao Lue* for treating hysteria. Although there were no typical signs of hysteria, the symptoms of ill-being, irritability and restlessness had been constantly bothering the patient. Chen Xiuyuan once said that "the nature of viscerae is Yin, the viscerae will become dry or malnourished due to Evil Heat from deficiency of the Vital Essence, Gan Mai Da Zao Tang can replenish the Heart and Spleen and other viscerae as well." Gan Mai Da Zao Tang was therefore indicated for this patient. In addition, Radix astragali and Caulis spatholobi tonify the Vital Energy and Blood; Rhizoma smilacis glabrae and Folium pyrrosiae, which are effective in clearing away Heat and Dampness, are beneficial in elevating the thrombocyte level and enhancing the immune function. A satisfactory clinical outcome was obtained by administration of this prescription.

Vertigo is a disorder due to flaring up of excessive Heat secondary to deficiency of Liver and Kidney Essence. When the patient was seen in July 1986, the symptom of vertigo was still not present. Complaints of dizziness, restlessness, irritability combined with the conditions of tongue and pulse were all evidence of the symptom-complex of deficiency of Liver and Kidney Yin. Radix polygoni multiflori, Fructus mori and Herba cistanchis were added to Er-Zhi Wan to strengthen the effect of nourishing the Vital Essence; Fructus tritici levis, Semen nelumbinis and Semen biotae were added to clear away the Evil Heat and tranquilize the mental agitation; Herba ecliptae and Selaginellae were used to dispel noxious Heat from the Blood to promote hemostasis. With the administration of these herbs, the patient's symptoms were markedly relieved. There was also significant improvement of hematological findings.

In Septmeber 1986, other symptoms appeared, including bitterness in mouth, dry throat and subcostal region pain. These indicated hindrance of Vital Energy secondary to Liver and Kidney Essence deficiency. The prescription, Modified Yi Guan Jian, was given to relieve stagnation and replenish the essence. Radix ophiopogonis, Herba dendrobii, Fructus mori together with Er-Zhi Wan were applied to enhance this effect. The patient responded well to the treatment. Finally, ingredients from the prescription were made into pills in order to facilitate her recuperation.

Wuji Baifeng Wan, a patent herbal pill, was also prescribed. This is a prescription modified from Bai Feng Dan recorded in *Shou Shi Bao Yuan* which aids in replenishing the essence, nourishing the Blood and tonifying the Vital Energy. It has been reported that Wuji Baifeng Wan is also effective in treating leukopenic cases.

The author's experience shows that most of the hemopoietic disorders respond favourably to herbal medicines which emphasize tonifying the Kidney and regulating the Yin and Yang. In experimental studies, many Kidney-tonifying herbs are able to promote hemopoiesis and enhance immune functions, both *in vivo* and *in vitro*. These clinical and experimental findings once again illustrate the TCM theory that the Kidney controls the functions of the bone marrow.

7. NEUROLOGIC DISEASES

7.1 NEURASTHENIA
(INCOORDINATION BETWEEN THE HEART AND KIDNEY)

Xie Zhufan

Department of Traditional Chinese Medicine, Beijing Medical University
Teaching Hospital, Beijing

Xiao, 41, male, publishing house editor.
CHIEF COMPLAINT: Insomnia.

HISTORY OF PRESENT ILLNESS: Three months prior to consultation, the patient was assigned an urgent job that kept him working round the clock for one whole week. As a result of this intense mental and physical strain, he began to suffer from insomnia. There was marked difficulty in falling asleep which was usually preceded by three or four hours of tossing about in bed. The sleep was disturbed by dreams and frequent awakening. On the worse nights, he could only sleep for two or three hours. In the daytime, he felt dizzy and tired with particular weakness in the loins and knees. There were frequent night sweatings and his sexual activity was disturbed by premature ejaculation. He tried to take some tranquilizers and sedatives which in their usual dosages did not work while in double dosage made him drowsy in the daytime. He also rearranged his working schedule into a more relaxed one, but insomnia persisted.

PAST HISTORY: Non-contributory.

PERTINENT PHYSICAL EXAMINATION & LABORATORY FINDINGS: Essentially normal.

INSPECTION OF TONGUE: Red tip of tongue with thin coating.

PULSE CONDITION: Thready.

MODERN MEDICINE DIAGNOSIS: Neurasthenia.

TRADITIONAL CHINESE MEDICINE DIAGNOSIS: Incoordination between the Heart and Kidney.

THERAPEUTIC PRINCIPLES: Restore normal coordination between the Heart and Kidney.

PRESCRIPTION: Dihuang Wan (Rehmanniae Pills) and Jiaotai Wan (Pills for Restoring the Normal Coordination). Dihuang Wan is composed of Radix rehmanniae praeparatae, Poria, Chinese yam, Fructus schisandrae and Wolfberry bark which are ground into fine powder and mixed with honey and made into pills, 9 gm each, twice a day. Jiaotai Wan is an ancient prescription composed of two ingredients, Radix coptidis and Cinnamom bark. No patent preparation of this recipe is available at present. For the patient's convenience, the two ingredients were ground into powder and put into capsules to be taken at the dosage of 0.75 gm and 0.5 gm, respectively, once daily.

FOLLOW-UP/COURSE OF TREATMENT: After one week's administration of these herbal medications, the patient came back to the clinic with marked improvement. He could sleep for five hours or more each night and fell asleep easily in half an hour. After two weeks' administration, he slept normally for more than seven hours each night, the tongue was normal and other symptoms were also markedly improved.

DISCUSSION: According to TCM theory, sleep is controlled by the Heart where mental activities take place. If the Mind does not calm down after going to bed, usually due to disturbance in the Heart, insomnia ensues.

In most cases, the disturbance is caused by emotional factors, nervous strains, consumption of Yin, Blood or Qi by a chronic disease or loss of blood. Besides the Heart, other Zang Fu Organs, particularly the Liver, Spleen and Kidney, may be involved in the pathogenesis of insomnia.

In this case, overstrain was apparently the cause. The patient suffered both from dysfunction of the Heart as manifested by insomnia with dream-disturbed and wakeful sleep, and from Kidney symptoms, such as weakness in the loins and knees and sexual dysfunction. Further analysis showed that the imbalance was characterized by deficiency of Yin accompanied by excess of Heart-Fire evidenced by symptoms of night sweating, red tongue tip and thready pulse. However, as far as the Kidney was concerned, there was deficiency of both Yin and Yang as manifested by premature ejaculation. Since both the Heart and Kidney were involved in this case, the diagnosis pointed to incoordination between the Heart and Kidney.

Among the medications prescribed for this patient, Dihuang Wan was used for nourishing the Kidney-Yin and cinnamom bark contained in Jiaotai Wan for tonifying the Kidney-Yang. Cinnamom bark when used in combination with coptis root is said to have the effect of transmuting Fire from the Heart down to the Kidney. Coptis root is the most important ingredient used in this case. Although it is often used to remove toxic or Damp-Heat, as in the treatment of the inflammatory process due to infections and bacillary dysentery, it is also used for its action in reducing Fire of the Heart. Modern research studies have shown that coptis root enhances the inhibitory process of cerebral cortex while possessing an adrenolytic effect as well. This case serves as a good illustration of the teaching "to reduce the Fire of the Heart."

7.2 NEUROSIS
(DEPRESSION SYNDROME)

Qi Liyi

Guang'anmen Hospital, China Academy of Traditional Chinese Medicine,
Beijing

Zhang, 22, male, single, student. Medical record number: 163441. First consultation on January 12, 1988.

CHIEF COMPLAINT: Insomnia for five months and low spirits for one month.

HISTORY OF PRESENT ILLNESS: The patient started to have restless, dream-disturbed sleep and could only sleep for three to four hours every night after suffering from heavy mental upset in August of 1987. During the daytime, he experienced headache and sensation of head distention. In school, he was unable to concentrate and reacted slowly. His memory failed so sharply that he could not even understand and memorize simple things. His mood was depressed and his eyes dull. He took sedatives such as Valium and Oryzanol, but they did not afford any relief. In December 1987, the condition worsened and he could only sleep for one to two hours every night after unsuccessful attempts to do so for two to three nights successively. As a result, he became extremely giddy and felt frightened. He completely failed to concentrate in his classes. He lost confidence in himself to the extent that he was reluctant to do anything and became alienated from other people. He was skeptical about everything and almost lost his memory completely. He would soon forget what happened a few moments before. He felt dazed and unimaginative about everything around him. Speech was noted to be slow and incoherent at this point and he could not express himself well as there was only blankness in his mind. At night, when he heard a sound he would feel frightened and trembled and sweated all over. Auditory acuity declined and he could not distinguish sounds. The headache was so severe that he felt as if the head was splitting up. He was so nervous that he almost lost his mind. Sometimes he thought he would rather die. Earlier this year, he was suspended from the university because of inability to continue his studies. At the time of consultation, the patient was in a state of severe depression.

PAST HISTORY: Non-contributory.

PERTINENT PHYSICAL EXAMINATION & LABORATORY FINDINGS: The patient was depressed and low in spirits with dull eyes which winked very little. He was inactive, silent with pale face, low voice and slow reactions. He ate very little, but both urination and bowel movement were normal. Blood pressure, 110/80 mmHg. Examinations of the thyroid, heart, lungs, liver, spleen and nervous system were all normal. EEG findings were also within the normal range.

INSPECTION OF TONGUE: Pale tongue proper with red tip and thin, white coating.

PULSE CONDITION: Wiry, thready and slightly rapid.

MODERN MEDICINE DIAGNOSIS: Neurotic Depression.

TRADITIONAL CHINESE MEDICINE DIAGNOSIS: Depression Syndrome.

THERAPEUTIC PRINCIPLES: Disperse the stagnant Liver Qi and relieve depression, nourish the Heart, invigorate the Spleen and calm the Mind.

ACUPUNCTURE POINTS: Baihui (Du 20), Neiguan (P 6), Shenmen (H 7), Qimen (Liv 14), Taichong (Liv 3), Tanzhong (Ren 17), Fengchi (G 20), Sanyinjiao (Sp 6) and Upper Yintang (Ex).

FOLLOW-UP/COURSE OF TREATMENT:

Third consultation: After undergoing two courses of treatment, the patient could sleep for three to four hours every night. Sensation of fear had also disappeared. The headache with distending sensation still remained; he could not read more than an hour, and his memory was still poor. The patient appeared pale.

Fifth consultation: The patient started to smile and talk spontaneously. Headache was alleviated markedly and he could study for one to two hours every day. His sleep was disturbed for several days by the news of his grandfather's sickness but soon returned to normal.

Tenth consultation: The patient could sleep for six hours every night. He behaved and talked like normal people do. He talked more now and added more information to his medical history. Symptoms such as headache, irritation and restlessness had all disappeared.

Fifteenth consultation: His sleep had returned to normal. He was even able to nap for an hour at noon. All symptoms were gone completely. Apart from studying English at home, he was able to take two courses in the university, and he regained his memory.

Treatment was discontinued at this point in view of his complete recovery.

DISCUSSION: This is a case where the disease was caused by circumstantial and psychological factors. The patient was depressed, forgetful with slow reactions, taciturn, dull and low in spirits. Accompanying symptoms were severe insomnia, hidrosis and unrest. Although the patient thought he would rather die than seek treatment, he could still control himself and was willing to cooperate in the treatment. According to psychiatry classification, this was a case of neurotic depression.

In traditional Chinese medicine, this disease belongs to depression syndrome, which is different from depression spectrum disease. The former is caused by depression of mood and stagnation of Qi, while the latter is due to mental disorder in which the patient shows alternately Three-Yin symptoms, such as incoherent speech, catatonic-like behaviour and dull spirits, and Three-Yang symptoms, such as garrulous speech, restlessness, uncontrolled temperament and tantrums. In this case, the patient had stagnation of Liver Qi due to mental upset. The Liver Wood overwhelmed the Spleen Earth and caused deficiency of the Spleen which impaired the transformation and digestion of nutrition essence. Poor transformation and digestion of nutrients resulted in deficiency of the Blood which was unable to control the Heart and to house the Mind. Acupuncture applied to points of Neiguan, Shenmen and Baihui tranquilized the Heart and calmed the Mind; Fengchi point activated sense organs and improved both listening ability and vision. As a result of application of these measures, symptoms such as insomnia, forgetfulness and dull spirits were relieved. As stagnant Qi transforms into Fire which injures body fluids and causes formation of Phlegm and since both Fire and Phlegm disturb the Heart and Mind, the patient felt irritated, anxious and uneasy. Acupuncture applied to Qihai, Tanzhong and Qimen points restored the normal flow of Liver Qi; Sanyinjiao and Taichong points smoothed the circulation of Qi and Blood and pacified the Liver and alleviated the depression.

Upper Yintang point, 1 cm above Yintang, is good for insomnia. When needling this point, certain sensations must be obtained and the needles should be retained for 20 minutes. Acupuncture of this point is done once every other day. Treatment of neurotic depression by acupuncture is more effective than drugs. Acupuncture is believed to be able to regulate neurotransmitters and their moderators, but its actual mechanisms are still under study.

7.3 NEURASTHENIA
(DEFICIENCY OF THE LUNG AND KIDNEY, BREAKDOWN OF NORMAL PHYSIOLOGICAL COORDINATION BETWEEN THE HEART AND KIDNEY)

Yu Changzheng

Shandong Institute of Traditional Chinese Medicine and
Materia Medica, Jinan

Ji, 44, female, Han nationality, married, office worker. Medical record number: 52157. Date of first consultation: June 27, 1964.

CHIEF COMPLAINT: Severe insomnia, headache and giddiness.

HISTORY OF PRESENT ILLNESS: The patient frequently experienced symptoms of insomnia, frightful dreams, headache, giddiness, palpitation, restlessness and tinnitus. Severity of the symptoms was not stable and no obvious sedative or hypnotic effects were achieved by modern medications, and because of side effects these drugs had to be withdrawn. She had also taken several dozen doses of Chinese herbal decoctions but without any marked effect either. Recently, the symptoms became worse, and at times she was not able to get any sleep the whole night. However, her appetite was normal; urine and stool were also normal as well as her menstrual cycles.

PAST HISTORY: Non-contributory.

PERTINENT PHYSICAL EXAMINATION & LABORATORY FINDINGS: Medium development and nourishment. Yellow and sallow complexion. Heart and lungs normal. Liver and spleen not palpable. Chemical examinations unremarkable.

INSPECTION OF TONGUE: Tongue substance pinkish with white, thin fur.

PULSE CONDITION: Deep and fine, mildly taut and rapid.

MODERN MEDICINE DIAGNOSIS: Neurasthenia.

TRADITIONAL CHINESE MEDICINE DIAGNOSIS: Deficiency of the Lung and Kidney; Breakdown of Normal Physiological Coordination Between the Heart and Kidney.

THERAPEUTIC PRINCIPLES: Nourish Liver and Kidney Yin, restore physiological equilibrium between the Heart and Kidney.

PRESCRIPTION: Semen ziziphi spinosae, 45 gm; Radix glycyrrhizae, 3 gm; Rhizoma dioscoreae, 18 gm; Rhizoma atractylodis macrocephalae, 12 gm; Radix angelicae, 12 gm; Rhizoma cyperi, 12 gm; Radix polygala, 9 gm; Ramulus uncariae cum uncis, 6 gm; Periostracum cicadae, 9 gm; Concha haliotidis, 24 gm; Rhizoma acori graminei, 12 gm; Caulis polygoni multiflori, 12 gm; Flos chrysanthemi, 12 gm; Semen cuscutae, 30 gm; Fructus gardeniae, 9 gm; and Radix angelicae dahuricae, 9 gm. Mix the ingredients in adequate amount of water and boil for two periods of time. Remove the dregs from the liquid (about 250 ml). To be taken orally, 125 ml, b.i.d. Otherwise use Succinum, 3 gm, and Cinnabar, 0.9 gm, ground into fine powder; divide into two equal portions and take after mixing with water, three doses.

FOLLOW-UP/COURSE OF TREATMENT:

Second consultation on August 31, 1964: The patient had taken three doses of the prescription and could sleep better. She could sleep for about four hours each night. Headache and palpitation were also relieved. Tongue and pulse manifestations remained the same.

Prescription: The same as the last one except the dosage of Semen ziziphi was increased to 54 gm; also added Radix paeoniae alba, 15 gm, and Semen sojae praeparatae, 9 gm. Three doses.

Third consultation: The patient's sleep continued to improve. She could now sleep five hours or so every night and occurrence of dreams had decreased. Symptoms of palpitation, headache and restlessness were minimal, but the patient complained of weakness. Tongue fur white and thin. Pulse deep and fine, slightly taut; Chi Mai (Cubit) was weak. Modified the previous prescription by replacing Dandouchi with Radix codonopsis, 9 gm. This prescription replenished the Vital Energy in order to consolidate the patient's constitution. The dosage of Succinum was decreased to 1.5 gm. Nine doses.

Follow-up on November 12, 1964: The patient had taken fifteen doses of the prescription since her last consultation. Sleep essentially normal at this point. Headache, giddiness and tinnitus had all subsided and palpitation and restlessness been relieved. The patient was unable to sleep when she was exhausted both mentally and physically and at these times also suffered mild palpitation and restlessness. These symptoms were relieved significantly when a modified compound of Suanzaoren decoction was administered at a dosage of q.i.d. or q.o.d.

DISCUSSION: Over the years, the author has treated 209 cases of neurasthenia which had as their chief symptoms insomnia and restlessness. They were treated with Chinese medicinal herbs — Suanzaoren and compound Suanzaoren decoction. Among these cases, 129 were treated by decoction of compound Suanzaoren and a dose of Semen ziziphi, 15-60 gm; 60 were treated by Semen ziziphi (half stir-fried and half raw in 20 cases) and Radix glycyrrhizae praeparatae mixture. The dose of Semen ziziphi was 45 gm, single dose. Most of them did not show any untoward reactions, except in isolated cases where mild side effects were noted (one case showed drowsiness in the daytime and three others headache). These preliminary data indicate that Semen ziziphi possesses a short-term therapeutic effect on insomnia. In 20 cases, 20 gm of stir-fried Suanzaoren powder was administered h.s., which showed a tranquilizing effect.

Preliminary data gathered from the author's experimental studies on the pharmacological properties of aqueous extracts of Semen ziziphi have shown it to have both sedative and tranquilizing effects on the central nervous system. The aqueous extract contains mainly flavonoids, indicating that this ingredient is the principal agent for the sedative and tranquilizing effects. Results of these pharmacological experiments can be summarized as follows:

1) The active and passive movements of mice whose stomachs had been perfused with the aqueous extract of Semen ziziphi were decreased significantly;

2) Sleeping time of a group given Semen ziziphi extracts with sodium pentobarbital was significantly longer than the group given only sodium pentobarbital;

3) When given in small doses, the aqueous extract of Semen ziziphi was effective against convulsion induced by cardiazol and can eliminate the excitatory effect caused by caffeine;

4) The hypnotic effect of the aqueous Semen ziziphi extract was not significant by photoelectric method;

5) The toxigenicity of the aqueous Semen ziziphi extract was very low. This extract has been perfused into the stomachs of mice (1:2 solution, one gram of crude drug, 1 cc/20 gm weight) and there were no deaths among them; and

6) The crude and stir-fried Semen ziziphi also has sedative and hypnotic effects.

7.4 TRIGEMINAL NEURALGIA
(FACIAL PAIN)

Qi Liyi

Guang'anmen Hospital, China Academy of Traditional Chinese Medicine, Beijing

Cheng, 50, female, Han nationality, senior engineer. Medical record number: 191991. Date of first consultation: January 22, 1988.

CHIEF COMPLAINT: Right side facial pain of nine years duration, exacerbated in the last four months.

HISTORY OF PRESENT ILLNESS: The patient experienced sudden onset of pain on the right side of her face about nine years ago (at age 41) and thought its occurrence was due to overworking. The pain was located in the maxillary and mandibular regions, radiating from the zygomatic arch to the corner of the mouth, teeth and tongue. She described the pain as piercing, cutting and intense, occurring in bursts and lasting only for a few seconds. She related that the pain sensation was triggered by speaking, chewing, tongue movement and brushing of teeth. In the early stage, the pain occurred only two or three times a year, each time lasting about half a month until she took herbal medications (Calculus bovis bolus to clear away Fire from Brain and Radix gentianae Tablets to purge Liver Fire), 8 tablets each, twice a day. The pain was noted to disappear during summer and alleviated by sweating; it recurred when she got angry or ate ginger, dates or fried food.

Since 1985, the frequency of attacks had increased progressively, becoming intolerable four months ago. The frequency was about 20 to 30 times per day, each time lasting for from several seconds to one or two minutes. The interval between attacks was getting shorter as well. Because of the pain's severity, the patient could not open her mouth and could only take small amounts of semi-solid food. She also reported difficulty in falling asleep. When having difficulty falling asleep, she took diazepam (Valium), 10 ml, and three other analgesics which were able to help her sleep for only three to four hours. She was treated initially with Dilantin and carbamazepine (Tegretol) tablet at 200 mg daily, which was increased gradually to 800 mg each day. Relief was not very significant and side effects started to appear (weakness, lethargy and vertigo). A doctor suggested surgical treatment but the patient wanted to try acupuncture first.

PAST HISTORY: Hepatitis in 1981. Constipation since age 16, alleviated by taking cathartics (bowel movement once a week).

PERTINENT PHYSICAL EXAMINATION & LABORATORY FINDINGS: Painful expression, depression, difficulty in speaking; the patient pressed the area around the zygomatic arch with fingers to alleviate pain. Pain was noted to spread from the ears to the mouth with trigger point located in the medial region of the nasolabial groove. Facial and masseter muscular power not impaired and symmetrical. Superficial pain sensation more pronounced on the right side. Cornea reflex normal. Blood pressure, 130/90 mmHg. Neck supple, no cervical lymphadenopathy. According to VAS score by subjective assessment, based on the five parameters of pain intensity, frequency, analgesic, sleep disturbance and limitation, the patient had a score of 19 out of a maximum of 20. Her condition could be classified in the category of severe pain. Examination of the heart and lungs negative. Liver and spleen negative.

INSPECTION OF TONGUE: Red tongue proper with yellow, sticky coating.

PULSE CONDITION: Deep and thready.

MODERN MEDICINE DIAGNOSIS: Primary Trigeminal Neuralgia (Second and Third Branch Involvement).

TRADITIONAL CHINESE MEDICINE DIAGNOSIS: Facial Pain due to Invasion of Wind-Cold Combined with Heat in the Stomach and Large Intestine.

THERAPEUTIC PRINCIPLES: Select the local points in combination with distal points indicated for facial pain in the affected meridians to expel Wind and Cold and promote circulation of both Qi and Blood; eliminate Heat by purgation.

PRESCRIPTION: Xiaguan (St 7) and Taiyang (Ex 1) towards Jiache (St 6), Sibai (St 2), Ermen (SJ 21) and Jiacheng Jiang (Ex 5), towards Chengjiang (Ren 24) and Hegu (LI 4), using 100 Hz electric needle to combine Taiyang (Ex 1) and Chengjiang (Ren 24).

FOLLOW-UP/COURSE OF TREATMENT:
Second consultation: According to VAS assessment, the intensity of pain decreased

20% after acupuncture. Carbamazepine dosage lowered from four tablets to one daily at night. Amount of food taken increased (only liquid or semi-solid food).

Fifth consultation: VAS assessment score decreased 50%. The patient could take soft solid food (one steamed bun). She experienced enhanced ability to speak but not for too long.

Sixth consultation: The patient reported that pain and constipation had occurred for one week after eating fish. So Tianshu (St 25) point was added (Front Mu point of Large Intestine, used to regulate the Stomach and Intestines). Also in application were Shuidao (St 28) to disperse the Qi of Sanjian (LI 3) and Zhigou (SJ 6) and Zhaohai (K 6) to clear away the Heat and relieve constipation secondary to body fluid deficiency.

Ninth consultation: After three courses of treatment using these points, bowel movement was normal. Facial pain intensity decreased by 70%. Speech, food intake and face hyperesthesia improved but chewing or talking for long period of time could still induce pain. Carbamazepine discontinued.

Eleventh consultation: Carbamazepine had been discontinued for three days and pain decreased by 80%. The patient arrived at the clinic with a smiling face. Only the right pre-auricular area was still a little tender on pressure.

Sixteenth consultation: The pain had been alleviated completely. The patient did not experience pain while eating, drinking or talking. She complained only of a heavy sensation on the base of the nose. VAS score had decreased by more than 15. Reduction of such a scale indicates an excellent therapeutic effect.

DISCUSSION: According to the pain characteristics and evolution of this case, primary trigeminal neuralgia was diagnosed, though the etiology remains undetermined. Modern medicine postulates that the cause could be viral, hereditary, local ischemia, central nervous system defect, allergy or mechanical pressure on the trigeminal nerve.

Traditional Chinese medicine believes that facial pain is due to invasion of pathogenic Wind-Cold or Heat attacking the Three Yang Meridians of the face, especially the Yangming Meridian. Invasion by Wind-Cold or Wind-Heat leads to contraction of the meridians and collaterals, thus retarding the flow of Qi and Blood. Pain occurs when there is obstruction and is relieved when Qi and Blood can pass through. Other possible causes of facial pain are emotion, excess Heat in the Stomach and Liver, overwhelming Yang due to deficiency of Yin and flaring up of Fire.

This case of trigeminal neuralgia was accompanied by constipation of more than 30 years duration which suggests accumulation of Fire in the Stomach and Intestines. The Fire could damage the body fluid, and constipation resulted from deficiency of Yin-body fluid. This is an illustration of a combination of endogenous and exogenous evils.

High-frequency electrical stimulation was delivered through local acupuncture points of the pertinent meridian on the face to regulate the flow of Qi and Blood together with distal point stimulation in the same external and internal meridians. Excellent therapeutic effects were achieved through application of the principles of eliminating Evil Heat and nourishing Yin by purgation.

7.5 VERTEBROBASILAR ISCHEMIA (DIZZINESS)

Zhao Lunnai, Chen Ren and Wei Beihai
Beijing Traditional Chinese Medicine Hospital, Beijing

Xia Yanfan, 49, female, married, worker. Medical record number: 24399. Date of admission: July 4, 1985.

CHIEF COMPLAINT: Recurrent episodes of vertigo of more than 10 years duration.

HISTORY OF PRESENT ILLNESS: The patient had suffered from recurrent episodes of vertigo for more than 10 years. Lately, condition had worsened with increased frequency of attack. Accompanying symptoms were scotodinia, rotatory in character, loss of consciousness, numbness of upper extremities, convulsion, restlessness, feverish sensation in the palms and soles exacerbated in the afternoon or at night, epigastric fullness and pain with belching, nausea and vomiting, greasy taste in the mouth, thirst and preference for cold drinks and loss of appetite. The patient was high-strung and irritated. Sleep was disturbed by dreams, and she was also noted to be paranoid. Palpitation and shortness of breath were also experienced which were aggravated by physical exertion. She got tired easily. Colour of urine was yellow to clear; thick vaginal discharges also noted.

PAST HISTORY: She had a massive bleeding due to protracted labour 10 years ago.

PERTINENT PHYSICAL EXAMINATION & LABORATORY FINDINGS: Blood pressure, 100/70 mmHg; hemoglobin, 10.5 gm%; RBC, $3M/mm^3$; WBC, $5,500/mm^3$. Heart, lung, liver and spleen findings negative. Cervical vertebrae X-ray: proliferation of cervical joints, bony spur on vertebrae, lordotic cervical vertebrae and the possibility of ear as origin of vertigo was excluded. X-ray showed ischemia particularly evident in the area supplied by vertebrobasilar arteries.

INSPECTION OF TONGUE: Red tongue with yellow, greasy fur.

PULSE CONDITION: Taut and slippery.

MODERN MEDICINE DIAGNOSIS: Vertebrobasilar Ischemia.

TRADITIONAL CHINESE MEDICINE DIAGNOSIS: Dizziness (Yin Deficiency; Heat Stagnation with Phlegm).

THERAPEUTIC PRINCIPLES: Nourish the Essence, dispel pathogenic Heat and Phlegm.

Symptom-complex differentiation: Before admission, the patient was diagnosed as having vertebrobasilar ischemia. Various medications were given without obvious effects, so the patient turned to herbal medicine. According to traditional Chinese medicine symptom-complex differentiation, this case was classified as deficiency of Liver-Kidney Essence and hyperactivity of Fire. Treatment used initially was to soothe the Liver, stop the Wind and calm the Yang. Aside from a reduction in the frequency of attack, no other significant improvement of the condition was effected.

Canon of Internal Medicine states that "endogenous Wind marked by vertigo, spasm and convulsion is a pathological change related to the Liver" and "endogenous Dampness marked by water retention and edema is a pathological change related to the Spleen." Liver stores the Blood and is Yin by substance and Yang by function. Women are closely related to the physiological function of the Liver and Blood. In this case, the patient had deficiency of the Blood with functional disturbance of the Liver, manifested by irritability and flaring up of Liver Fire secondary to depression of Liver Qi resulting in impairment of Liver Essence. As such, the Yin failed to keep the Yang well and the endogenous Wind of the deficiency type stirred up as manifested by vertigo, convulsion and poor nourishment of tendons and muscles due to deficiency of the Blood leading to numbness of the extremities. Both the Liver and the Kidney are located in the lower part of the body cavity and have a common source. Essences of the Liver and Kidney reinforce each other, thus deficiency of one will lead to deficiency of the other. Deficiency of Kidney Yin leads to lassitude in the loins and knees as well as a sensation of heat in palms and soles. Deficiency of Five Organs Essence leads to depression and irritability. Deficiency of Heart Blood induces palpitation and shortness of breath. Hyperfunction of the Liver may affect the normal function of the Spleen. Dysfunction of the Spleen leads to failure of transportation and transformation resulting in accumulation of Phlegm-Dampness which further impairs the Spleen. Epigastric fullness, nausea and vomiting, poor appetite, greasy taste in the mouth and excessive vaginal discharge are all due to stagnation of Dampness. Stirring up of the Wind-Phlegm induces dizziness.

PRESCRIPTION: Modified Wendan Tang. Poria, 6 gm; Rhizoma pirellae, 6 gm; Exocarpium citri grandis, 6 gm; Rhizoma aurantii, 4.5 gm; Rhizoma acori graminei, 6 gm; Caulis bambusae in taeniam, 6 gm; Rhizoma cyperi, 3 gm; Concha margaritifera, 12 gm; Radix glycyrrhizae, 1.5 gm; Spica prunellae, 9 gm; Radix paeoniae alba, 6 gm; and Rhizoma gastrodiae, 9 gm. Three decoctions.

Rhizoma pirellae is used for its expectorant properties, while Exocarpium citri and Rhizoma aurantii are used as carminatives to dispel Phlegm; Poria strengthens the Spleen and removes Dampness; Caulis bambusae in taenian resolves Heat Phlegm. Rhizoma acori graminei, an aromatic stimulant, removes Wind-Phlegm. Radix paeoniae alba and Concha margaritifera calm the Liver and suppress the excessive Yang; Radix paeoniae alba nourishes Blood and Essence; Spica prunellae removes Heat from the Liver, while Rhizoma cyperi soothes the Liver and regulates the circulation of Qi. Rhizoma gastrodiae calms the Liver and suppresses the Wind; Radix glycyrrhizae coordinates the actions of various ingredients in this prescription. *Treatise on the Spleen and Stomach* states that "Rhizoma pirellae should be used to stop headache caused by Phlegm in the Spleen Channel of the Foot, and Rhizoma gastrodiae to treat dizziness and blurred vision induced by stirring up of endogenous Wind of the deficiency type."

FOLLOW-UP/COURSE OF TREATMENT:

Second consultation on July 7, 1985: After three doses, symptoms of greasy taste in the mouth, epigastric discomfort, nausea and vomiting had disappeared. Appetite had improved and the patient felt good and was in high spirits.

Third consultation on July 11, 1985: After taking another three doses, numbness and convulsion had disappeared, and sensation of heat in the palms and vertigo lessened significantly. Amount of vaginal discharge obviously reduced. Slightly red tongue proper with thin and greasy fur.

Fourth consultation: After another six doses, the symptom of vertigo was alleviated significantly. There was no more vaginal discharge, only mild heat sensation was felt in the palms. The patient was vigorous with good appetite and had normal urine excretion. Tongue manifestation was the same as before. Pulse taut and fine. Zhibai Dihuang Wan, 2 pills daily, was prescribed to nourish Liver-Kidney essence.

Fifth consultation on July 28, 1985: After a total of 23 doses, the patient was fully recovered and was discharged symptom-free. Her tongue and pulse conditions were normal. Ingredients of 20 prescriptions were mixed and ground into fine powder and divided into 20 gm packs. Prepared by boiling in water. There was no relapse after one year's follow-up.

DISCUSSION: This patient suffered from Liver-Kidney disease with secondary involvement of the Spleen. To dispel Phlegm-Dampness was the main therapeutic approach because of the close relationship between Liver and Spleen pathologies. "To treat Liver disease, emphasis should be put on treating Spleen pathology first." (*Canon of Internal Medicine*) The rationale is that the Spleen provides the material basis of the acquired constitution. The Spleen's function is to transport nutrients and Water-Dampness and to serve as the source of growth and development. When the Spleen function is normal, food is well digested, nutrients well absorbed and Qi and Blood generated abundantly to support and nourish all the viscerae, thus Phlegm-Dampness will not accumulate inside the body. This is the reason why Li Gao put so much stress on strengthening the Spleen and Stomach in treating various diseases.

Though the cause of this disease was deficiency of Essence and stagnation of Heat-Phlegm, the patient was treated mainly with herbs whose properties are those of dispelling Heat and Phlegm because herbs which nourish the Vital Essence are usually full of glutinous juice. This intrinsic herbal property can impair the function of the Spleen and Stomach and induce accumulation of Dampness and Phlegm, thus the principle applied to recover the Spleen function was instead that of dispelling Heat and Phlegm. Once the Spleen functions of transporting and transforming were robust, the consequent normal generation and circulation of Qi and Blood contributed to production of Liver-Kidney essence.

7.6 TIAS
(BLOOD STASIS SYMPTOM-COMPLEX)

Jean Yu and Chen Keji
Santa Barbara College of Oriental Medicine, California, U.S.A.
Xiyuan Hospital, China Academy of Traditional Chinese Medicine, Beijing

Anderson, 64, female, white, married, retired book-keeper. Medical record number: 3. Date of first consultation: March 12, 1986.

CHIEF COMPLAINT: Sudden paresthesias of the left arm with temporary partial loss of vision for four months.

HISTORY OF PRESENT ILLNESS: The patient suffered suddenly from weakness and numbness of the left arm with temporary loss of vision in both eyes (tunnel vision) since December 1985. The episodes usually lasted only a few minutes, two to three times a week. Occasionally intermittent difficulty in speech occurred simultaneously without any neurological residue, and consciousness remained intact throughout the episodes.

The patient's energy level was moderate to low. She complained of flatulence, incomplete, loose or soft stool and frequency of night urine (every two hours).

PAST HISTORY: Healthy retired woman. Hysterectomy in 1967. Positive history of osteoporosis.

PERTINENT PHYSICAL EXAMINATION & LABORATORY FINDINGS: On December 24, 1985, Doppler ultrasound examination showed that the patient's left carotid system had no significant narrowing, but there was a moderate amount of atheromatous plaques in the right carotid system. The narrowing was estimated to be in the range of 30-50%. On August 5, 1986, second Doppler ultrasound study was compared with that from December 1985. The impression was that the narrowing in the region of the right carotid bifurcation was in the range of 50-60%.

INSPECTION OF TONGUE: Slightly dark tongue proper with puffy edges and tooth marks and thin, white fur.

PULSE CONDITION: Deep wiry and slow (56-60/min).

MODERN MEDICINE DIAGNOSIS: Transient Ischemic Attacks and Atheromatous Disease.

TRADITIONAL CHINESE MEDICINE DIAGNOSIS: Qi Deficiency of the Spleen and Kidney and Blood Stasis.

THERAPEUTIC PRINCIPLES: Tonify the Spleen and Kidney Qi and move the Blood to relieve stagnation.

PRESCRIPTION: Yi Kun San, Dan Shen Yin and modified Sang Piao Xiao San. Radix codonopsis pilosulae, 9 gm; Poria, 9 gm; Rhizoma atractylodis macrocephalae, 9 gm; Ootheca mantidis, 9 gm; Fructus rubi, 9 gm; Cortex eucommiae, 15 gm; Morus alba, 15 gm; Radix salviae miltiorrhizae, 9 gm; Pericarpium citri reticulatae, 6 gm; Radix glycyrrhizae, 6 gm; and Fructus aurantii, 6 gm.

FOLLOW-UP/COURSE OF TREATMENT:

Twenty-third consultation on August 13, 1986: The patient took the herbs in three to four doses a week regularly, yet on August 5, Doppler ultrasound study showed no improvement, although her digestive function had much improved with completely formed stool. At this stage, it was apparent that the Spleen Qi needed to be strengthened in order to move the stasis. Blood-activating herbs were used predominantly. Radix codonopsis pilosulae, 9 gm, Radix salviae miltiorrhizae, 9 gm; Radix paeoniae rubra, 9 gm; Radix polygoni multiflori, 12 gm; Caulis spatholobi, 15 gm; Semen casiae, 12 gm; Radix curcumae, 9 gm; Radix paeoniae alba, 9 gm; Ramulus loranthi, 12 gm; Cortex eucommiae, 15 gm; and Radix glycyrrhizae, 6 gm.

Fiftieth consultation: Paresthesias of the left arm diminished to once in five to six weeks and night urine was less (one to two times per night). Digestion was better.

Because of a stressful situation, the patient had anxiety attack and palpitation daily.

Treatment principle: Move the Blood and benefit the Yin in order to pacify the Shen (spirit).

Prescription: Radix salviae miltiorrhizae, 12 gm; Caulis spatholobi, 9 gm; Radix paeoniae alba, 12 gm; Semen ziziphi spinosae, 12 gm; Fructus schisandrae, 12 gm; Radix glycyrrhizae, 10 gm; and fried honey, 6 gm.

Seventy-fifth consultation on November 12, 1987: The numbness and vision problem had disappeared for six months. Night urine frequency improved evidently (one to two times). The patient had good digestion, but still had anger palpitation attack from stressful relationship. November 11, 1987, radiology consultation reported that the Doppler ultrasound test showed no evidence of flow-restrictive disease involving the carotid arteries. Because of disparity of the results on the examination relative to suspicion of a 50-60% narrowing of the right internal carotid artery in the previous report, the study was repeated including a vasoscan arterial wave form analysis.

DISCUSSION: According to TCM theories, the patient had Spleen and Kidney Qi deficiency and Blood stasis symptoms (bad digestion, frequent night urination, numbness and weakness of the arm) with the corresponding tongue and pulse manifestations. Traditional sayings summarize the Qi and Blood relationship as "Qi is the commander of Blood" and "circulating Qi promotes the circulating Blood." Therefore, applying Qi tonic herbs will improve the symptoms and signs related to Blood stasis especially in combination with ABC (Activating Blood Circulation) herbs.

Recently, scientific research has proven that the Qi tonic herbs such as Radix astragali and Radix codonopsis pilosulae have definite effects on strengthening cardiac functions. Blood-activating herbs such as Radix salviae miltiorrhizae, Caulis spatholobi and Radix paeoniae rubra used in this case have the effect of decreasing atherosclerotic lesion and improving hemoreologic changes. So the therapeutic result in this case was reliable and convincing.

7.7 CHRONIC SUBDURAL HEMATOMA (HEADACHE DUE TO BLOOD STASIS)

Liu Yuzhao

Shandong Institute of Traditional Chinese Medicine and
Materia Medica, Jinan

Lin Jinhe, 42, male, Han nationality, married, cadre. Date of first consultation: March 14, 1988.
CHIEF COMPLAINT: Headache, nausea and blurred vision for one month.
HISTORY OF PRESENT ILLNESS: Three months prior to consultation, the patient fell off a motorcycle, hitting the right side of his head and suffering a temporary disturbance of consciousness. Two months later, he experienced severe headache, nausea, vomiting and blurred vision after catching a cold accompanied by

chills and fever. After treatment, the chills and fever were gone but recurrent headache, vomiting and blurred vision remained. The symptoms became worse when he had a cold with occasional occurrence of dyslalia, palpitation and hypomnesis.

PAST HISTORY: Positive history of arrhythmia.

PERTINENT PHYSICAL EXAMINATION & LABORATORY FINDINGS: Conscious, medium development and well-nourished. No phyma on the skull. EENT examination negative. Pupillary reflex normal and isocoric. Neck was supple. Heart and lung findings normal except for occurrence of premature beat (9-10/min). Liver and spleen not palpable. Neurological examination showed no abnormalities. Undistinguished optic papillary borders on funduscopic examination. Bleeding time, 2 min; clotting time, 3 min; platelet count, 100,000/mm^3. ECG showed ventricular premature contraction. CT scans of the brain and head: At 4-9 cm level, a dark crescent between the skull and the frontal, temporal lobes. CT value 59 Hm, 13 x 3 cm. The left lateral ventricle was obliterated with significant distortion of falx cerebri to the right.

INSPECTION OF TONGUE: Tongue substance dark red with yellowish, thick fur.

PULSE CONDITION: Slow pulse, irregular and rough.

MODERN MEDICINE DIAGNOSIS: Chronic Subdural Hematoma (CSH), Right Frontal and Temporal Lobes; Ventricular Extrasystole.

TRADITIONAL CHINESE MEDICINE DIAGNOSIS: Headache due to Blood Stasis; Palpitation.

THERAPEUTIC PRINCIPLES: Activate Blood circulation, eliminate stasis and promote the Collaterals for analgesia.

PRESCRIPTION: Radix salviae miltiorrhizae, 18 gm; Radix paeoniae rubra, 12 gm; Radix angelicae sinensis, 12 gm; Radix angelicae dahuricae, 9 gm; Semen persicae, 9 gm; Fried hirudo, 6 gm; Tabanus bivittatus, 6 gm; Fried Radix et rhizoma rhei with wine, 3 gm; Squama manitis, 9 gm; Radix glycyrrhizae, 6 gm; Bulbus allii fistulosi, 15 gm; and Rice wine, 25 gm. Method of preparation: mix the ingredients in an adequate amount of water and boil for two periods of time. Remove the dregs from the liquid (about 250 ml). Taken orally 125 ml b.i.d. Ten doses.

FOLLOW-UP/COURSE OF TREATMENT:

Second consultation on March 24, 1988: The patient had taken 10 doses of the decoction, but his headache had exacerbated and was accompanied by dizziness and blurred vision. His appetite had declined and stool was loose. Tongue and pulse manifestations essentially identical to last consultation.

Prescription: The same as the last one except that Radix et rhizoma rhei was decreased to 1 gm and Rhei, 0.05 gm, was added (taken after mixing with decoction), twelve doses.

Third consultation on April 7, 1988: Since the first consultation, the headache had been getting worse. Because the headache was too severe to bear, the patient went to visit a neurologist at a hospital. The diagnosis was the same, and he was advised to have craniotomy. Afraid of the operation, he preferred to take herbal medicine. During this month, his headache had shown signs of alleviation, and the occurrence was intermittent. He had a feeling of distention in the head while moving. Nausea and palpitation had disappeared and vision become clear and speech fluent. Examination of tongue essentially identical to the first consultation. Pulse was thin and rough.

Prescription: Added Platycodi, 9 gm, to the last prescription and increased the dosage of Radix glycyrrhizae to 9 gm. Twenty doses.

Fourth consultation on April 28, 1988: Symptoms had almost disappeared completely since last consultation. The patient caught common cold once but without any headache. He still complained of a feeling of distention in his head and fatigue. Tongue fur whitish, pulse small and weak. Bleeding time 1 minute and clotting time 3 minutes.

Prescription: Added Radix codonopsis pilosulae, 15 gm, and Radix astragali seu hedysari, 9 gm, to the last prescription. Twelve doses.

Fifth consultation on May 12, 1988: Fatigue and other symptoms had disappeared. The patient's appetite was good but his stool still loose, once a day. Tongue fur whitish, pulse small and wiry. Funduscopic examination showed clear-cut optic papilla borders and no pailloedema. CT scans of the brain and head normal.

Prescription: The same as the second one except increased the dosage of Danshen to 30 gm, removed Radix angelicae and Bulbus allii fistulosi and added Rhizoma ligustici Chuanxiong, 6 gm, and Radix platycodi, 9 gm. Twelve doses.

Follow-up on June 20, 1988: The patient had taken more than 60 doses of the decoction. Symptoms had disappeared for more than one and a half months. CT scans showed that the CSH had been absorbed completely.

DISCUSSION: CSH is due to hemorrhage in the drainage vein adjacent to the sagittal sinus after head injury resulting in capsule formation which adheres to dura mater firmly. Normally, drainage by craniotomy is the treatment of choice.

The disease is understood in traditional Chinese medicine as headache due to Blood stasis. *Errors of Medical Works* (Wang Qingren, 1839) of the Qing Dynasty states that "headache which lasts a long time is located at a definite place and is accompanied by dim and fawn tongue substance and rough pulse is the result of involvement of collaterals due to protracted pain. Treatment should deal with the Blood stasis." In our case, the Decoction for Promoting Blood Circulation, which removes the Blood stasis of the head and upper body was used. Since this case had a relatively long history, it was classified as obstinate Blood stasis, therefore Hirudo tabanus bivittatus, Rhei and Squama manitis were added to reinforce the effect of removing Blood stasis. It is notable that before the third consultation, the headache was severe which was a normal reaction and the prescription did not need to be modified.

Experimentally, Radix salviae has proven effective in improving the brain's microcirculation, increasing collateral circulation and repairing injured brain tissue. Rhizoma ligustici improves the brain's microcirculation and relieves cerebral edema significantly. Radix paeoniae rubra, Radix salviae and Radix angelicae have an anticoagulant effect and also reinforce fibrinolysis. Shuizhi enhances absorption of hematoma and reduces the inflammatory reaction of peripheral brain tissue, relieves cerebral edema and intracranial pressure, improves local circulation and therefore the nervous function and protects the brain tissue from ischemic and necrotic changes.

It has been reported that the therapeutic principles of promoting Blood circulation and removing Blood stasis are effective in treating cerebrovascular disease and acute brain impairment. This case used Radix salviae and Radix paeoniae rubra to nourish the Blood, and Hirudo, Tabanus, Taoren, Awuama manitis and others to remove Blood stasis. All of these herbs make up a compound which has a powerful action in removing Blood stasis and improving Blood circulation. Thus, with these herbs, the CSH was cured thoroughly within two months and without any side effects.

7.8 EPILEPSY
(OBSTRUCTION OF THE HEART CHANNEL BY PHLEGM AND ENDOGENOUS WIND STIRRING IN THE LIVER)

Yu Changzheng

Shandong Institute of Traditional Chinese Medicine and Materia Medica, Jinan

Chen Xinming, 26, male, Han nationality, married. Date of first consultation: May 8, 1987.

CHIEF COMPLAINT: Intermittent and paroxysmal convulsion and loss of consciousness for one year.

HISTORY OF PRESENT ILLNESS: On May 6 of last year, the patient experienced his first convulsive attack. He screamed suddenly, fell down on the ground and had a seizure. The fit stopped after five minutes, and the patient was noted to be in lethargy. One hour later, he was completely lucid and could not recall the incident. Since then, the seizure has happened once every two weeks or one month. In addition, he seemed to have disturbance of mental function which went without convulsion but lasted for only one to two minutes and occurred every day or every other day. EEG showed 3 Hz spikes. Cranial CT scan findings were negative. Taking Dilantin 0.1 gm t.i.d. and Diazepam 2.5 gm t.i.d. since June of the same year; frequency of grand mal was decreased to about once a month but condition of petit mal remained the same. In the last four months, after taking Tegretol, 0.2 gm t.i.d. and withdrawal of Diazepam, the petit mal was relieved significantly and frequency reduced to about once a week.

PAST AND FAMILY HISTORY: Non-contributory.

PERTINENT PHYSICAL EXAMINATION & LABORATORY FINDINGS: General condition good and body temperature normal. Heart and lungs findings negative. Liver and spleen not palpable. No abnormalities seen on neurological examination. Results of EEC done on the day of first consultation supported the clinical diagnosis.

INSPECTION OF TONGUE: Tongue substance pinkish in colour with white tongue fur.

PULSE CONDITION: Stringy and slippery.

MODERN MEDICINE DIAGNOSIS: Essential Epilepsy (Grand Mal and Petit Mal)

TRADITIONAL CHINESE MEDICINE DIAGNOSIS: Obstruction of the Heart

Channel by Phlegm and Endogenous Wind in the Liver.

THERAPEUTIC PRINCIPLES: Tonify the Kidney and subdue the Liver hyperactivity, subdue endogenous Wind and control the Yang exuberance, remove the Phlegm to effect resuscitation, nourish the Heart and soothe the nerves.

PRESCRIPTION: Ding Jian Pills. Stir-fried Semen ziziphi spinosae, 15 gm; Radix polygalae, Arisaema praeparatae, Lignum dalbergiae odoriferae, White fructus pipers, Bombyx batryticatus and Periostracum cicadae, 9 gm each; Scolopendra, 3 pieces; Rhizoma acori graminei, 30 gm; Lignum aquilariae resinatum, 6 gm; medicated leaven and Rhizoma dioscoreae, 12 gm each; Concha margaritifera usta, 30 gm; Succinum, 3 gm; and Cinnabaris, 1 gm. Place 10 doses of this prescription in water, mix and make into small pills; 6 gm, b.i.d.

FOLLOW-UP/COURSE OF TREATMENT:

Second consultation on July 24, 1987: The patient had taken the above pills for two months. Grand mal only occurred once 10 days ago and frequency of petit mal had decreased to once every two weeks. Tongue condition same as last visit. Pulse string-like and mild, slippery. Continued Ding Jian Pills.

Follow-up on May 27, 1988: After continuous administration of the pills, grand mal had subsided since last October and petit mal stopped since early November and had not recurred since then. Dosage of Tegretol had changed to 0.2 gm q.i.d. and Diazepam been withdrawn since January of this year.

Both grand mal and petit mal conditions of this case had been successfully controlled by administration of Ding Jian Pills. At present, Tegretol is given at a maintenance dosage of 0.2 gm, q.i.d., while the patient continues to take Ding Jian Pills. Both these medications should be discontinued if there is no recurrence of the seizures for two years.

DISCUSSION: The therapeutic strategy of this case was mapped out based on the author's many years of clinical experience as well as those working with the late Dr. Liu Huimin, a famous herbal medicine practitioner. References to works by other scholars were also taken into account and the most important therapeutic principles in this case were those of tonifying the Kidney and subduing the Liver hyperactivity, subduing the endogenous Wind and controlling the Yang exuberance. Also applied in this case were the principles of removing Phlegm to effect resuscitation, nourishing the Heart and soothing the nerves. The patent medication Ding Jian Pills (Pills for Curing Epilepsy) were prepared in our hospital. During the past 10 years, the author treated 60 cases of grand mal with these pills and achieved excellent clinical results. All cases were followed up for one year after taking the pills. In this series, nine cases (15%) were essentially cured (from frequent attacks to remission), 36 cases (60%) showed marked reduction in the frequency of epileptic seizures, 15 cases (25%) were not responsive. These 60 cases had been treated by Dilantin initially with no or little response. Ding Jian Pills are usually administered at a dosage of 6 gm, b.i.d., in adults and with appropriate reduction in children. They should be withdrawn gradually one year after commencement of administration as the symptoms progress towards remission.

7.9 MYASTHENIA GRAVIS
(SPLEEN-KIDNEY YANG DEFICIENCY)

Yu Changzheng

Shandong Institute of Traditional Chinese Medicine and
Materia Medica, Jinan

Gao Baoqin, 18, female, Han nationality, single. Medical record number: H41726.
Date of first consultation: February 15, 1978.

CHIEF COMPLAINT: Weakness of the extremities and alternate ptosis of both eyelids for five months; difficulty in swallowing for two weeks.

HISTORY OF PRESENT ILLNESS: Five months prior to consultation, the patient experienced weakness in all extremities, and she was unable to sustain or repeat muscular contractions. Soon afterwards, alternate ptosis of the eyelids occurred with obvious narrowing of palpebral fissues. These symptoms were less evident in the morning or after rest but aggravated at night or when tired. The patient reported occasional diplopia and cold sensation of the extremities. Neostigmine Methosulfate Test positive. No enlarged shadow of the mediastinum revealed on chest X-ray. After taking Neostigmine bromide, 15 mg, t.i.d., the symptoms decreased temporarily for about four hours initially, but the relief period was shortened gradually to about two hours. For the last two weeks the patient could only swallow slowly. Pridostigmine was added, 60 mg, t.i.d., AC.

PAST HISTORY: Non-contributory.

PERTINENT PHYSICAL EXAMINATION & LABORATORY FINDINGS: Palpebral fissure: right, 0.7 cm; left, 0.5 cm. Eyeballs half fixed. Muscle Strength Testing on the extremities are graded as approximately three and more than four distally. Determination of cellular and humoral immune factors showed generalized decreased levels. EMG showed neuromuscular fatigue, decremental responses to repetitive nerve stimulation.

INSPECTION OF TONGUE: Tongue substance pinkish in colour with fur.

PULSE CONDITION: Deep and small.

MODERN MEDICINE DIAGNOSIS: General Myasthenia Gravis.

TRADITIONAL CHINESE MEDICINE DIAGNOSIS: Spleen-Kidney Yang deficiency.

THERAPEUTIC PRINCIPLES: Strengthen the Spleen and reinforce the Qi, replenish the Kidney and strengthen the Yang.

PRESCRIPTION: Bu Zhong Yi Qi and Fu Zi Li Zhong Decoctions. Radix codonopsis, 30 gm; Radix astragali, 30 gm; Rhizoma cimicifugae, 9 gm; Rhizoma atractylodis macrocephalae, 12 gm; Radix bulpleuri, 9 gm; Radix aconiti praeparatae, 36 gm; Pericarpium citri reticulatae, 9 gm; Radix angelicae, 12 gm; Radix glycyrrhizae, 6 gm; Lumbricus, 9 gm; Herba ephedrae, 6 gm; and Radix puerariae, 30 gm. Place the ingredients in adequate amount of water, boil for two periods of time and remove the dregs from the liquid to obtain 250 ml of decoction. One hundred twenty-five ml orally, b.i.d.

FOLLOW-UP/COURSE OF TREATMENT:

Fourth consultation on March 15, 1978: The patient had taken 24 doses of the prescription since first consultation. Weakness of the extremities were significantly relieved. Degree of ptosis was lessened but still occurred alternately with occasional diplopia. Mild warm sensation was felt after taking the prescription. Neostigmine bromide was decreased by half a tablet, t.i.d. Occasional loss of appetite. Tongue and pulse condition remained the same.

Modified the original prescription by increasing the dosage of both Radix aconiti and Radix astragali to 60 gm and adding Charred triplet, 9 gm. Administration same as before.

Eighth consultation on August 5, 1978: The patient had taken the prescription successively for two months since the fourth visit. The dosage of administration was decreased to q.i.d. Because of significant alleviation of the symptoms, Neostigmine bromide was discontinued one month ago. Pridostigmine was decreased to one tablet q.i.d. or b.i.d. Swallowing seemed normal, though the extremities weakness and ptosis (right or left) still appeared when the patient was tired. No diplopia. Tongue and pulse condition remained the same. Palpebral fissure 1.0 cm on both sides. Eyeball movements normal. There was a mild weakness of the adductors on the right side and transient diplopia occurred which recovered spontaneously after a few minutes.

Modified the last prescription by decreasing the dosage of Radix aconiti to 36 gm and that of Radix astragali to 45 gm. Two doses per week.

Fifteenth consultation on July 5, 1982: The patient got married in January 1980 and gave birth to a healthy baby girl in April 1981. Mild degree of weakness of the extremities experienced when the patient was tired. Pridostigmine was decreased to one tablet p.r.n. Cellular and humoral immune factor levels were all normal. Tongue and pulse conditions same as before.

Prescription: Place 10 prescriptions together and mix with water, then make into small pills, 6 gm, t.i.d.

Follow-up in May 1987: The patient had taken two preparations of the pills. Condition had been in remission for more than three years. All medications were discontinued. However, the patient still takes one or two decoctions when she is under strain. She had been gaining weight in the past years. At present she weighs about 80 kg. She was diagnosed as having simple obesity. Chest X-ray performed six months ago showed evidence of thymoma. Thymusectomy was suggested but the patient refused surgical treatment because she had no symptoms of myasthenia gravis.

DISCUSSION: This author and his associates have reported on a series of 73 cases of myasthenia gravis treated by a combination of modern and traditional Chinese medicine. Results of studies done on Fuzi, both its clinical application and experimental studies, have also been reported. Since 1972, the chief ingredients of myasthenia gravis prescription, Radix aconiti and Radix astragali, have been used in large dosages in accordance with the principles of promoting the Spleen to restore its normal function, nourishing the Kidney and enhancing the Yang. Treating myasthenia gravis with a combination of traditional Chinese and modern medicine, the author has

achieved comparatively satisfying clinical results. Of the 6,
medications, 15 cases (22.39%) were cured, 27 cases (40.30%
20 cases (29.85%) improved, four cases (5.94%) unresponsive ar
due to the onset of another disease during the course of treatm
of cases cured and cases with significant improvement was 42 (62.0
suffering from bulbus type of myasthenia gravis, four cases were
cases improved significantly, nine cases improved, three cases were
one case died. Fifteen clinically cured cases were followed up for fro
nine months to four and a half years. Of these 15 cases, 14 cases rema
remission without any relapse, while one died from myasthenic crisis.

The chemical components of prepared Radix aconiti are appraised primarily by thin-layer chromatography which show absence of aconitine. Pharmacological research on boiled extracts of Radix aconiti indicates that it has an anti-curare effect in rabbits. Using load swimming test in mice, the results demonstrate the antifatigue properties of Radix aconiti. Radix aconiti is also effective in increasing the contraction of rectus abdominis muscles in toads and diaphragmatic muscles in rats. Other experimental observations are increased peristalsis of isolated mice's intestines and increased contractility of isolated toad's heart. If concentration of the extract is increased, it can cause inhibition because the dosage was so large that it produced no polarization at muscular endplates.

These experimental findings proved primarily that Radix aconiti enhances the function of both the voluntary and involuntary muscles. Clinically, there were no toxicity or side effects observed even when large doses were applied. It is probable that the effective element of this herb is not aconitine as generally believed previously but other low-toxicity elements. Occasional reports of allergic cases to Radix aconiti are basically due to individual differences. In our two groups of cases treated by medicinal herbs, both had lowered cellular and humoral immune factor levels before treatment. These chemical indices as well as clinical signs and symptoms all improved after treatment.

7.10 MYASTHENIA
(ASTHENIA OF BOTH THE SPLEEN AND KIDNEY)

Liu Shenqiu
Department of Traditional Chinese Medicine, Beijing Hospital, Beijing

Qin Zhenyin, 46, female, Han nationality, married, cadre. Medical record number: 60943. Date of admission: September 11, 1978.

CHIEF COMPLAINT: Difficulty in swallowing, chewing and dysarthria, aggravation of weakness of limbs for 15 days.

HISTORY OF PRESENT ILLNESS: The patient was admitted in June 1977 because of diplopia and ptosis. Myasthenia gravis was diagnosed. Pyridostigmine 240

...ly in divided doses was administered but did not afford significant relief of the ...ptoms. Difficulty in chewing and proximal limbs weakness in accentuation appeared later on. It caused some difficulty in daily activities. Azathioprine, 50 mg, thrice daily, was given for two months. After that, radiotherapy of thymus was done with a total dose of 4,500 rads in 33 days. These treatments did not achieve the expected effect. Pyridostigmine was increased to 360 mg/day and symptoms gradually improved. The patient was discharged in December of 1977. She was admitted to a TCM hospital from March to May, 1987 for treatment of myasthenia gravis, but the results were not satisfactory.

Fifteen days prior to admission, symptoms of difficulty in chewing, dysphagia, dysarthria and increasing weakness of the lower extremities developed gradually without a particular precipitating factor. Pyridostigmine was increased from 360 mg to 480 mg daily without significant effect. She was admitted to neurological department. Bowel movement two to three times daily with watery stool.

PAST HISTORY: History of tuberculous pleuritis.

MENSTRUAL HISTORY: Menstruation irregular since last year and usually lasted more than 10 days with a small amount of discharge. Patient in menstrnation now.

PERTINENT PHYSICAL EXAMINATION & LABORATORY FINDINGS: Physical examination essentially normal except bilateral ptosis. Peripheral blood count, routine examination of urine and stool were normal. ESR, 6 mm/hr; SGPT within normal range; TTT, 2 u; blood cholesterol, 225 mg%; blood potassium, 4.57 mg/L; sodium, 148 mg/L; chloride, 105 mg/L; A/GM = 4.05 gm/2.5 gm; IgA, 120 IU/ml; IgG, 1,000 IU/ml; IgM, 125 IU/ml; antinuclear antibodies fluorescent test negative. Thyroid absorption of I_{131} normal. Electromyography confirmed the diagnosis of myasthenia gravis; ECG, normal; chest X-ray and UGIS findings negative.

INSPECTION OF TONGUE: Tongue substance red with thin, white fur.

PULSE CONDITION: Fine pulse.

MODERN MEDICINE DIAGNOSIS: Myasthenia Gravis.

TRADITIONAL CHINESE MEDICINE DIAGNOSIS: Athenia of Spleen Qi.

THERAPEUTIC PRINCIPLES: Replenish Qi to invigorate the function of the Spleen.

PRESCRIPTION: Modified Shen Ling Bai Zhu San. Radix codonopsis pilosulae, 15 gm; Atractylodis macrocephalae, 15 gm; Semen dolichoris, 15 gm; Poria, 15 gm; Rhizoma dioscoreae, 15 gm; Semen nelumbinis, 10 gm; Fructus amomi, 3 gm; Radix platycodi, 5 gm; and Radix glycyrrhizae, 3 gm. Decoction; one dose daily.

Other management: Pyridostigmine, 60 mg, q.i.d.; Ambenoniun, 5 mg, q.i.d.; Atropine, 0.3 mg, q.i.d. (Original regimen which the patient had been taking for seven years).

FOLLOW-UP/COURSE OF TREATMENT:

Follow-up on September 21, 1987: The patient reported that she could speak better. Symptoms of weakness in chewing and dysphagia remained unchanged. She had soreness of the waist and weakness of the legs. Bowel movement was normal. Menstrual bleeding had stopped. Observations of tongue and pulse were the same as before.

Therapeutic principles were to warm the Kidney and activate the Spleen.

Prescription: Modified Er Xian Tang plus Si Jun Zi Tang. Rhizoma curculiginis, 10 gm; Herba epimedii, 10 gm; Radix angelicae, 10 gm; Radix rehmanniae, 10 gm; Radix rehmanniae praeparatae, 10 gm; Radix codonopsis pilosulae, 15 gm; Rhizoma atractylodis macrocephalae, 10 gm; Poria, 10 gm; Radix pipsaci, 10 gm; Fructus lycii, 10 gm; and Fructus psoraleae, 10 gm.

This prescription with minor modifications was used for about four months. Prednisone, 60 mg, q.i.d. was added beginning on November 8, 1987.

Dysphagia, difficulty in chewing, soreness of the waist, limb weakness and fatigue gradually improved though with frequent fluctuation. In addition, the patient complained of shortness of breath, palpitation, night sweating and insomnia frequently.

The patient was inspected on November 10. Corpulent tongue, red tongue tip with thin white fur. Pulse taut and fine. Therapeutic principles: reinforce the Qi of the Spleen, warm and nourish Yang and Yin of the Kidney.

Prescription: Modified Bu Zhong Yi Qi Tang; Er Xian Tang and Er Zhi Wan. Radix astragali, 30 gm; Radix codonopsis pilosulae, 25 gm; Rhizoma atractylodis macrocephalae, 10 gm; Rhizoma cimicifugae, 10 gm; Fructus ligustri lucidi, 10 gm; Herba ecliptae, 10 gm; Herba epimedii, 10 gm; Rhizoma curculiginis, 10 gm; Radix rehmanniae praeparatae, 15 gm; Semen cuscutae, 15 gm; Fructus psoraleae, 10 gm; Semen ziziphi spinosae, 15 gm; Fructus amomi, 3 gm; and Radix glycyrrhizae, 3 gm. Decoct for oral ingestion; one dose daily.

All other treatments remained unchanged. Symptoms had disappeared gradually or significantly reduced though with mild fluctuation occasionally. The patient was discharged on April 6, 1979, and rested at home.

Follow-up on April 28, 1979 in outpatient department: The patient's condition was fairly good. She reported a mild sensation of heaviness on the shoulders and slight ptosis. Occasionally she had palpitation and insomnia. She got excited easily. Bowel movement normal. No menstruation for six months. Reddened tip of the tongue with thin, white fur. Pulse fine and rapid. Therapeutic principles: reinforce Spleen Qi and nourish Kidney Yin.

Prescription: Modified Bu Zhong Yi Qi Tang plus Er Zhi Wan. Radix astragali, 45 gm; Radix codonopsis, 18 gm; Rhizoma atractylodis macrocephalae, 10 gm; Poria, 15 gm; Radix aucklandiae, 8 gm; Fructus amomi, 3 gm; Rhizoma rehmanniae, 30 gm; Rhizoma anemarrhenae, 15 gm; Fructus ligustri lucidi, 15 gm; Herba ecliptae, 15 gm; Semen cuscutae, 15 gm; Caulis polygoni multiflori, 30 gm; Concha margaritifera usta, 15 gm; and Radix glycyrrhizae, 3 gm. Decoct for oral ingestion; one dose daily initially. The dose was changed gradually to q.i.d. and once in three days later on. Huang Qi (Root of Mongolian Milkvetch), 30-50 gm, was given alternately with the prescription. During this period, the dose of prednisone was reduced gradually from 60 mg to 10 mg, q.i.d. She increased from part- to full-time work in April 1980. The patient's condition remained fairly good. On three occasions, attempts were made to discontinue the herbal medications, but each time symptoms aggravated within two weeks. Therefore, honey pills were made by using the last prescription to consolidate the therapeutic effect beginning in 1982; 9 gm pills, 2 pills, twice daily. The patient worked abroad beginning in the autumn of 1983 in fairly good condition by using the above management.

DISCUSSION: Myasthenia gravis, a disease of unknown origin due to humoral antibodies to acetylcholine receptor, is considered as neuromuscular function disorder and auto-immune disease. It is characterized by general weakness with particular predilection for the ocular and other cranial muscles, a tendency to fluctuate in severity, no signs of neural lesion and amelioration of weakness by cholinergic drugs.

Myasthenia gravis is similar to flaccidity-syndrome or paralysis due to apoplexy in the teachings of traditional Chinese medicine. It may seem similar to flaccidity or paralysis, but actually it is not. Therefore it shouldn't be treated as such. By symptom-complex differentiation, the patient usually has ptosis, diplopia and fatigue in the early stage of the disease. In traditional Chinese medicine, eyelids belong to the Spleen, and the eyes the orifice to the Liver. The majority of patients with myasthenia gravis at this stage are treated as asthenia of Spleen Qi or deficiency of Liver Yin. As the disease progresses, patients have soreness of the waist, weakness of the extremities or heaviness of the neck. Deficiency of Spleen and Kidney Yang, deficiency of Qi and Spleen and Kidney Yin should be thus recognized. They may be further complicated with Phlegm or Blood stasis leading to asthenia-syndrome accompanied by sthenia-syndrome. All these signs and symptoms of various stages of the illness should be differentiated carefully during treatment.

Our case was of the ocular muscles type initially which soon progressed to weakness of the extremities and difficulty in chewing. Previously, the patient had received pyridostigmine in combination with azathioprine and radiotherapy. She had also received a period of Chinese herbal treatment. Condition of the patient deteriorated later on; oropharyngeal symptoms such as dysphagia, dysarthria and difficulty in chewing developed. The patient was admitted at this stage.

TCM treatment was given in combination with pyridostigmine, ambenonium chloridum and prednisone. The patient had weakness, fatigue, symptoms of muscular disorder, mild diarrhea and menstruation disturbance. Asthenia of Spleen Qi and the failure of the Spleen in keeping Blood circulating within the vessels were diagnosed and treated. Diarrhea ceased and menstrual bleeding stopped. At this juncture, the principle of replenishing Yang of the Spleen and Kidney was applied for about four months but with minimal improvement of the symptoms. In February 1979, the patient had night sweating, insomnia, reddened tongue tip and other symptoms and signs of Yin deficiency. Impairment of Yang would impede generation of Yin caused by prolonged disease. Er Zhi Wan was added to replenish Yin. The dosage of Mongolian Milkvetch Root was increased to strengthen the Qi. The patient was discharged from hospital.

About 20 days after discharge, the patient's condition was noted to be good, but deficiency of Yin was still evident. Based on the last prescription, the herbs for warming the Kidney Yang were withdrawn and the dosage of Radix rehmanniae and Radix astragali increased. Henceforth, the dose of prednisone was reduced successfully without fluctuation of symptoms. Finally, pills made from the previous prescription stabilized and consolidated the therapeutic effect successfully.

In recent years, the author has treated 10 cases of myasthenia gravis. The therapeutic effect of replenishing Qi and Yin of the Spleen and Kidney was used in combination with cholinergic drugs in all cases with satisfactory results (with minor modification in different patients). Among these cases, traditional Chinese medications could be used alone without cholinergic drugs to treat simple ocular muscle type myasthenia gravis. E.C. Zhao summed up the reports of the treatment of nearly 300 cases of myasthenia gravis with Chinese herbal medications; 83.5% of these were treated by replenishing both the Kidney and Spleen. The total effective rate was 92% (*J. of Zhejiang Traditional Chinese Medicine*, 1986, [2]: 92-93). These results agree with those of the author.

Pharmacological and clinical investigations have shown that the herbs used to treat this case, such as Radix astragali, have extensive influence on the immune system; Radix codonopsis pilosulae, Rhizoma atractylodis, Rhizoma rehmanniae, Fructus ligustri lucidi and Herba ecliptae regulate the immune function; and some of the other herbs have diphasic actions in regulating the immune function.

In addition, Rhizoma curculiginis, Herba epimedii, Semen cuscutae and Fructus lycii regulate the functions of the pituitary-gonadal axis. They helped to control concurrent menopausal syndrome symptoms in this case.

8. SKIN DISEASES AND CONNECTIVE TISSUE DISEASES

8.1 URTICARIA
(PEILEI)

Zhang Zhili
Beijing Traditional Chinese Medicine Hospital, Beijing

Gu, 40, female, Hui nationality, married, technician. Medical record number: 834263. Date of first consultation: July 10, 1986.

CHIEF COMPLAINT: Rubella all over body for 14 years, aggravated recently.

HISTORY OF PRESENT ILLNESS: Fourteen years prior to consultation, the patient felt itchiness all over the body with appearance of large red areas on the skin, some of them elevated. These episodes occurred on and off during the past years and became more frequent during spring and autumn, especially on cloudy or rainy days. Ten days ago, the patient experienced the same condition and the itchiness aggravated with lesions spreading all over the body. This condition was accompanied by abdominal pain and dry stool.

PAST HISTORY: Denied having parasitic and allergic diseases.

PERTINENT PHYSICAL EXAMINATION & LABORATORY FINDINGS: Red or elevated skin lesions all over the extremities and trunk. Of various sizes, from as small as the finger tip to as large as a coin, irregular in shape. In some locations, the lesions were in fusion and occupied a large area. Skin scratch test positive; leukocyte count 7,200/mm³. Stool examination for parasite ovum negative.

INSPECTION OF TONGUE: Slightly red tongue with white fur.

PULSE CONDITION: Deep, thready and fast pulse.

MODERN MEDICINE DIAGNOSIS: Acute Attack of Chronic Urticaria.

TRADITIONAL CHINESE MEDICINE DIAGNOSIS: Peilei.

Symptom-complex differentiation: Internal Heat caused by deficiency of the Blood, vulnerability of tendon-muscle attacked by pathogenic Wind factor.

THERAPEUTIC PRINCIPLES: Refresh the Blood, dispel the Wind and eliminate the Heat.

PRESCRIPTION: Modified Xia Xue Xiao Feng Powder. Radix angelicae sinensis, 10 gm; Radix rehmanniae, 30 gm; Herba schizonepetae, 10 gm; Radix ledebouriellae, 10 gm; Radix sophorae flavescentis, 15 gm; Fructus tribuli, 15 gm; Cortex dictamni radicis, 15 gm; Cortex mori radicis, 15 gm; Periostracum, 5 gm; Cicadae, 10 gm; Herba spirodelae,

10 gm; Cortex moutan radicis, 10 gm; and Rhizoma anemarrhenae, 10 gm. Seven doses.

FOLLOW-UP/COURSE OF TREATMENT:

Second consultation on July 17, 1986: The patient reported that the itch had been alleviated, rubella lesions got smaller and she could sleep well at night. She complained of feeble and heavy limbs. Tongue proper light red with white fur. Pulse string-like and slippery. Continued to treat using the principle of refreshing the Blood, dispelling the Wind and eliminating the Dampness. The prescription was composed of Radix angelicae sinensis, 10 gm; Caulis polygoni multiflori, 15 gm; Radix paeoniae alba, 10 gm; Radix rehmanniae, 15 gm; Cortex moutan radicis, 10 gm; Fructus tribulli, 15 gm; Radix ledebouriellae, 10 gm; Cortex mori radicis, 10 gm; Herba spirodelae, 10 gm; Semen coicis, 15 gm; Semen plantaginis, 15 gm; and Cortex benincasae, 15 gm. Seven doses.

Third consultation on July 24, 1986: The rubella had disappeared and no new lesions appeared since. The patient felt well and was given five doses of the same prescription to regulate the symptom-complex. She wrote to the clinic in May of 1987 to express her gratitude for a speedy recovery using only 20 doses to cure a protracted disease of 14-year duration. There has not been relapse.

DISCUSSION: Urticaria, known as Peilei or Feng Chen Yan in traditional Chinese medicine, is an allergic skin disease which often occurs because it is difficult to find the allergen. Traditional Chinese medicine regards it to be caused by unstable emotions or unusual diet which results in imbalance between the Yin and Yang, dysfunction of the Qi, vulnerability of the Qi and tendon-muscles attacked by pathogenic Wind. The disease can be divided into following types: Wind-Heat, Wind-Cold, Heat and deficiency of Blood and attack by Wind pathogenic factor. Accordingly, the patient was given Radix angelicae sinensis, Radix rehmanniae and Fructus tribulli to refresh the Blood; Cortex mori radicis, Cortex moutan radicis and Rhizoma anemarrhenae to eliminate the Heat in the Blood; Cortex dictamni radicis and Radix sophorae flavescentis to eliminate the Heat and Dampness; Radix ledebouriellae, Herba schizonepitae, Periostracum, Cicadae and Herba spirodalae to dispel the Wind and eliminate the Heat. All these herbs are capable of dispelling the Wind and eliminating the Heat from the Blood. At the second consultation, Heat symptoms had been alleviated, but the patient showed symptoms due to the presence of pathogenic Dampness, i.e., heavy limbs, so Cortex benincasae, Semen plantaginis and Semen coicis were added to the prescription. Seven more decoctions were administered to make the rubella disappear. The patient took a total of 19 decoctions and was cured. There was no relapse in the following six months.

8.2 ZOSTER
(CHAN YAO HUO DAN, FIRE AROUND THE WAIST)

Zhang Zhili

Beijing Traditional Chinese Medicine Hospital, Beijing

Chang, 30, female, Han nationality, married, worker. Medical record number:

875098. Date of first consultation: October 14, 1987.

CHIEF COMPLAINT: Water blister on the left chest and back with severe pain for five days.

HISTORY OF PRESENT ILLNESS: Five days prior to consultation, the patient felt prickly pain on the left back but paid no attention to it. Later, small water blisters appeared on the site of the pain and gradually diffused to the front of the chest with severe pain that affected her sleep. She also felt thirsty and craved for water. The condition was accompanied by constipation of several days duration and yellow-reddish urine.

PAST HISTORY: Non-contributory.

PERTINENT PHYSICAL EXAMINATION & LABORATORY FINDINGS: The pain was along the course of the seventh and eighth ribs on the left chest and back. Skin appeared light red in colour with piles of blisters of different sizes (some as small as a grain of rice, others the size of beans). The blisters were arranged in a strip configuration, with no fusion nor rupture. Most of the blisters were filled with clear and light material, some with blood. Leukocyte count 8,700/mm^3 (neutrophil, 72%, lymphocytes, 27% and eosinophil, 1%); routine urinalysis normal; and hepatic functions normal.

INSPECTION OF TONGUE: Red tongue substance with dense, slippery and yellow fur.

PULSE CONDITION: String-like and slippery.

MODERN MEDICINE DIAGNOSIS: Zoster.

TRADITIONAL CHINESE MEDICINE DIAGNOSIS: Chan Yao Huo Dan.

Symptom-complex differentiation: Stagnation of Dampness and Heat, attack by toxic pathogenic factor.

THERAPEUTIC PRINCIPLES: Eliminate Heat and detoxicate, discharge Dampness.

PRESCRIPTION: Modified Long Nan Xie Gan Tang. Radix gentianae, 10 gm; Radix scutellariae, 10 gm; Fructus gardeniae, 10 gm; Gallis akebiae, 10 gm; Radix rehmanniae, 30 gm; Folium isatidis, 80 gm; Radix arnebiae seu lithospermi, 15 gm; Semen plantaginis, 15 gm; Semen coicis, 30 gm; Rhizoma corydalis, 10 gm; Radix paeoniae rubra, 15 gm; and Radix et rhizoma rhei, 6 gm. Five doses, once daily.

External application using Xiong Huang Jie Du Powder (made up of Realgar, 30 gm; Calcite, 30 gm; Alumen, 20 gm; and 100 ml of Radix stemonae Wine prepared by using 60 gm of Radix stemonae in 120 ml of 75% alcohol).

FOLLOW-UP/COURSE OF TREATMENT:

Second consultation on October 19, 1987: The patient reported alleviation of much of the pain. Part of the blisters had become dry and formed a scab. She still complained of thirst, yellowish discolouration of urine, red tongue substance with slippery fur and string-like, slippery pulse. The bowel movement was normal. Continued to take another five doses of the same prescription, replacing Radix et rhizoma rhei with Rhizoma coptidis, 10 gm.

Third consultation on October 24, 1987: Scab formation on most of the blisters and part of them healed. The patient felt no pain and was not thirsty, though still had light red tongue substance and thin, white fur and deep and tardy pulse. Continued to treat following the principles of reinforcing the Spleen and eliminating Dampness, activating Blood and detoxicating and eliminating Heat. Prescription: Rhizoma atractylodis macrocephalae, 10 gm; Poria, 10 gm; Semen coicis, 10 gm; Semen plantaginis, 10 gm; Rhizoma alismatis, 30 gm; Fructus trichosanthis, 15 gm; Radix angelicae sinensis, 10 gm; Radix paeoniae rubra, 15 gm; Radix salviae miltiorrhizae, 10 gm; Radix isatidis, 15 gm; Herba portulacae, 15 gm; and Cortex moutan radicis, 15 gm. Following seven doses of this prescription, the patient recovered fully.

DISCUSSION: Zoster, referred in traditional Chinese medicine as Chan Yao Huo Dan (Fire Around the Waist) and Sha Dan, is an acute skin disease with blisters caused by zoster virus infection. It often appears on the chest and waist, extremities and face, and shows a strip-like configuration along the course of a nerve. Traditional Chinese medicine regards the cause of the disease as unstable emotions resulting in stagnation of Damp-Heat in the Spleen coupled with attack by toxic pathogenic factors. The pathogenesis of zoster is made up of Liver Fire and toxic pathogenic factor, accumulation of Damp-Heat leading to stagnation of Qi and Blood and blockade of Channels. Subsequently, the patient experiences fever and pain. Accumulation of Dampness toxin leads to blister formation. To tackle the cause of the disease, traditional Chinese medicine employs the therapeutic principle of eliminating Dampness and Heat while applying the principles of Blood activation, stasis dissolution and Qi invigoration to treat the symptoms. By following these therapeutic principles, good results were obtained.

For external application, it was important to detoxicate and eliminate the Heat. Xiong Huang Jie Du Powder in Radix Stemonae Wine was applied to the lesion area for this purpose. In this prescription, Realgar and Radix stemonae were used to effect detoxication, Calcite to eliminate Heat and Alumen to eliminate Dampness and to dry the blisters.

8.3 ACUTE ECZEMA
(FENG SHI YANG, WIND-DAMP INJURY)

Zhang Zhili
Beijing Traditional Chinese Medicine Hospital, Beijing

Li, 28, male, Han nationality, married, administration officer. Medical record number: 367034. Date of first consultation: September 2, 1985.
CHIEF COMPLAINT: Papules and water blisters all over body for 10 days.
HISTORY OF PRESENT ILLNESS: Red papules with severe itching and pain on the extremities were first noted 10 days prior to consultation. Upon scratching, the papules ruptured with watery secretions. Lately, the papules had become generalized. The patient felt thirsty and craved for water. Stool was dry and urine yellowish-red in colour.

PAST HISTORY: There were similar papules on the left leg several years previously and rupture of the papules led to exudations and erosions.

PERTINENT PHYSICAL EXAMINATION & LABORATORY FINDINGS: Needletip-like or ricegrain-like red papules or water blister covering the face, neck, extremities and trunk. Some of the papules were in fusion and formed erosive areas with exudation in surface. Body temperature 37.7°C; leukocyte count 9,700/mm^3.

INSPECTION OF TONGUE: Red tongue tip with white fur.

PULSE CONDITION: String-like and slippery.

MODERN MEDICINE DIAGNOSIS: Acute Eczema.

TRADITIONAL CHINESE MEDICINE DIAGNOSIS: Feng Shi Yang; Stagnation of Dampness and Damp-Heat.

THERAPEUTIC PRINCIPLES: Eliminate Heat and Dampness.

PRESCRIPTION: Modified Long Dan Xie Gan Tang. Radix gentianae, 10 gm; Radix scutellariae, 10 gm; Cortex phellodendri, 10 gm; Fructus gardeniae, 10 gm; Herba artemisiae scopariae, 15 gm; Rhizoma alismatis, 10 gm; Semen plantaginis, 15 gm; Radix rehmanniae, 15 gm; Herba lophatheri, 10 gm; Folium isatidis, 30 gm; Liu Yi Powder (consisting of Talcum and Radix glycyrrhizae) 30 gm; and Cortex benincasae, 15 gm. Five doses, once daily.

FOLLOW-UP/COURSE OF TREATMENT:

Second consultation on September 7, 1985: The skin was drier and not as red, fewer blisters as well. The patient still complained of thirst and itchiness. Continued to take the prescription with addition of 30 gm each of Herba portulacae and Cortex dictamni radicis. Five decoctions.

Third consultation on September 12, 1985: Desquamation of most lesions, no exudation. No complaint from the patient except slight itchiness. Continued administration of the same prescription. After a total of 20 dosages, the patient recovered completely.

For external treatment, applied Extract of Herba Portulacae (boiled in water) on areas with erosions, and Coptis Root Ointment on the dry areas.

DISCUSSION: Acute eczema, as diagnosed by modern medicine, often shows symptoms and signs such as hyperemic skin, blisters with exudations, dry stool, short stream of reddish, discoloured urine, thirst and craving for water. According to these manifestations, the condition was one that suffers from accumulation of Damp-Heat which turns into Fire. Its manifestation was Heat (Fire), while the root was Dampness. Therefore, the main therapeutic approach was to eliminate the Heat and Dampness by administering medicinal herbs with appropriate properties.

In this case, a satisfactory outcome was obtained. In the prescription, Radix gentianae was used to eliminate Liver Fire; Radix scutellariae to eliminate Fire of the Lower Burner and Kidney; Fructus gardeniae to eliminate Heat of the Three Burners and Heart; Radix rehmanniae to eliminate Heat and refresh Blood; Herba lophatheri to facilitate Fructus gardeniae and Radix gentianae in eliminating Fire from the Liver and Heart; Herba artemisiae scopariae, Rhizoma alismatis, Semen plantaginis and Liu Yi Powder to eliminate Heat and dispel Water to keep the Dampness out; and Folium isatidis to eliminate Heat and detoxicate to prevent secondary infection. All these herbs can eliminate Heat (Fire) from the Three Burners and at the same time dispel Dampness and effect the disappearance of the blisters. The function of this prescription is analogous to taking the coal out of the stove.

In addition, external application of Extract of Herba Portulacae (60 gm boiled with 3,000 ml of water, filter before use) on the lesion site eliminated Fire, relieved itching and improved growth of skin. This extract is even more effective in treating acute exudative eczema.

8.4 TRICHOMATOSIS
(SHEDDING OF HAIR)

Hu Longcai
Department of Traditional Chinese Medicine, First Affiliated
Hospital of the Suzhou Medical College, Suzhou

Liu, male, Han nationality, married, accountant. Medical record number: 21876. Date of first consultation: May 7, 1976.

CHIEF COMPLAINT: Gradual shedding of hair, aggravated in the past month.

HISTORY OF PRESENT ILLNESS: The patient's hair began to shed after Spring Festival, 1976. In recent months, he suffered from intolerable itching of the scalp. Upon scratching, much scurf was noted. The hair on the vertex and occiput shed en masse and did not regenerate. He received treatment in the Dermatology Department of Xunyi County People's Hospital and was given cystine orally and some medical solutions for external application. But condition remained the same. He took some Radix Polygoni Multiflori Longevity Bolus but to no avail either.

PAST HISTORY: Non-contributory.

PERTINENT PHYSICAL EXAMINATION & LABORATORY FINDINGS: Temperature, 37°C; pulse, 72/min; and blood pressure, 110/70 mmHg. Conscious, in fairly good spirits. Non-icteric sclera; pupils round and regular. Hair dry and lustreless. Scratching or combing caused the hair to shed easily in large amounts. Heart and lungs negative. Abdomen soft. No hepatomegaly nor splenomegaly. Neurological examination negative.

INSPECTION OF TONGUE: Slightly purplish with thin fur.

PULSE CONDITION: Fine and taut.

MODERN MEDICINE DIAGNOSIS: Trichomatosis.

TRADITIONAL CHINESE MEDICINE DIAGNOSIS: Shedding of Hair.

THERAPEUTIC PRINCIPLES: Activate Blood Circulation and eliminate Blood stasis to facilitate hair growth.

PRESCRIPTION: Tongqiao Huoxue Tang.

FOLLOW-UP/COURSE OF TREATMENT:

First consultation on May 7, 1976: The patient enjoyed good health in the past but his hair started to shed in the past four months. As stated by Wang Qingren

(1768-1831), "Shedding of hair without illness is caused by Blood stasis." Tongqiao Huoxue Tang was adopted in this light. Radix paeoniae rubra, 6 gm; Rhizoma ligustici Chuanxiong, 6 gm; Semen persicae, 9 gm; Flos carthami, 3 gm; Fructus ziziphi jujubae, 7 gm; Allium fistulosum, 3 gm; Rhizoma zingiberis recens, 3 gm; and Moschus, 0.15 gm. Three doses. Method of preparation: place the first seven herbs in 250 ml of wine and boil down to 50 ml. Filter and add Musk. Boil twice. Take the decoction before bedtime, once a day for three days.

Second consultation on May 10, 1976: No significant response was observed after the first dose. After administration of the second dose, the patient felt warmth on the scalp and shedding of hair reduced. After the third dose, shedding of hair stopped and fine hair began to grow. Since the prescription was effective, the patient requested another five doses.

After taking eight more doses, loss of hair stopped and new hair began to grow. Half a year later his hair was as black and lustrous as it used to be.

DISCUSSION: Hair is nourished by Blood, hence the saying: "Hair is the sign of the Blood's condition." This case was caused by Blood deficiency due to Blood stasis and the hindered generation of new Blood. Hair without nourishment will fall out. Among the herbs used in this prescription, Radix paeoniae rubra, Rhizoma ligustici Chuanxiong, Semen persicae and Flos cathami eliminate Blood stasis and promote Blood circulation, while Fructus ziziphi jujubae and Rhizoma zingiberis recens regulate Ying and Wei. Allium fistulosum activates Yang, and the wine helps to activate Blood circulation. Moschus also facilitates the elimination of Blood stasis. Since the prescription is the medication of choice for this disease, the therapeutic effect was therefore evident and immediate.

8.5 RHEUMATIC RASH
(CHRONIC, PROTRACTED RASH SECONDARY TO BLOOD-WIND)

Chen Keji
Xiyuan Hospital, China Academy of Traditional Chinese Medicine, Beijing

Lu Jin, 29, female, Han nationality, married, cadre. Admitted on November 2, 1962. Medical record number: 161861.

CHIEF COMPLAINT: Recurrent rashes on all extremities for the past eight years, and low-grade fever for the past two years.

HISTORY OF PRESENT ILLNESS: For the past eight years, the patient noticed recurrent appearances of rashes on the lateral aspects of her extremities. The rash was described as reddish in colour, irregular in size and circular or irregular in shape. The rash tended to increase gradually in size after its appearance with accentuation of colour in the centre that faded at the borders; borders were elevated, and the rash was accompanied by a mild degree of itchiness. No marks or just a slight discolouration of the skin remained after the rash subsided, and occasionally scaling was observed. The rash appeared at irregular intervals ranging from a minimum of three to five days to as many as 30 days or more. The interval between appearances was from a few days at the shortest to 13 days at the longest. The tissue biopsy of the wheals showed only "hyperemic changes." For the past two years, the patient also noted that she had a low-grade fever (temperature between 37-37.8°C). Condition could be controlled effectively with Salpital retention enema or taking steroids. Nevertheless, symptoms recurred after cessation of these treatments. Other accompanying signs and symptoms were palpitation, shortness of breath, body numbness, hand tremor, epistaxis and occasional pinpoint epidermal bleedings.

PAST HISTORY AND FAMILY HISTORY: History of malaria and pain of the knee joints; frequent throat pain and susceptibility to influenza attacks. In 1950, the patient's job subjected her to exposure to Trichloroethylene and acetone. In 1956, due to "fever and heart murmur" the patient was diagnosed in one of the hospitals in Nanjing as having "rheumatic fever" and "endomyocarditis." The patient's assignment in 1959 exposed her to Stibium (Sb), Cesium (Cs) and Tin (Sn). She was noted to have hepatomegaly after delivery of her child, but hepatic function tests then were found to be within normal limits. SGPT level recorded in February of 1961 was 150 units and 215 units in March of 1962. Normal menstrual cycle. Her husband was diagnosed as having "hepatitis" in 1961. Family history non-contributory.

PERTINENT PHYSICAL EXAMINATION & LABORATORY FINDINGS: On admission, temperature (axillary) was 37.3°C; pulse rate 82/min; blood pressure 124/80 mmHg; of average build and health status. Hypertrophy of posterior laryngeal wall lymphatic tissues and tonsils. Normal cardiac borders; apical grade II blowing systolic murmur with occasional third heart sound. Accentuation of the pulmonary aortic cusp second sound. Cardiac rhythm normal. Lungs negative. Abdomen soft; liver palpable one centimetre below the right costal margin, soft and non-tender. Spleen likewise palpable about one centimetre below the left costal margin. Medial aspects of both thighs had several round or semilunar-shape wheals. No deformity nor evidence of edema of the joints; no skin nodules; no epidermal bleeding. No enlargement of superficial nodes. CBC normal. Hepatic function test (SGPT, TTT, TFT) normal (on five occasions); anti-'O' test negative (twice). Bleeding time, 1'30"; Howell's prothrombin time, 3'30"; platelet count normal. Sedimentation rate, 11mm/2hrs (November 5, 1962) and 2 mm/2hrs (March 5, 1963). ECG normal. Scratch test positive. Liver ultrasonogram showed dense microformation (November 9, 1962) and scattered wave (January 14, 1963). Chest X-ray did not reveal any abnormal findings on the shape and size of the cardiac shadow. Barium esophagogram did not show any significant depression or deviation; both lungs clear; UGIS normal.

INSPECTION OF TONGUE: Tongue fur clear.

PULSE CONDITION: Soft and weak.

MODERN MEDICINE DIAGNOSIS: 1) Rheumatic Disease; Chronic Rheumatic Fever; Rheumatic Heart Disease; Bicuspid Valve Failure; Rheumatic Rash; 2) Chronic Active Hepatitis (?); Hepatitis Secondary to Chemical Intoxication (?); 3) Chronic Tonsillitis; Chronic Laryngopharyngitis.

TRADITIONAL CHINESE MEDICINE DIAGNOSIS: General Debility and Deficiency of Body Functions; Chronic Protracted Rash Secondary to Blood-Wind.

FOLLOW-UP/COURSE OF TREATMENT:

First stage of treatment: During her five-month confinement to the hospital, the same rash recurred several times. Temperature was recorded to be 37.5°C on seven occasions and on more than five occasions the temperature was over 37.5°C. Based on signs on admission, such as palpitation, shortness of breath, low-grade fever, rash, soft and weak pulse and clear tongue fur, the patient was considered to be suffering from symptom-complex of general debilitation and deficiency, Qi-Deficiency, Blood Stasis and Rash Secondary to Blood-Wind. Therapeutic strategy was to follow the principle of "relieving fever by administering sweet and warming-up herbs" by giving the patient a prescription similar to that of Danggui Jianzhong Decoction. She was also given herbal preparations to revitalize the Blood. After taking 18 decoctions of this prescription, the patient did not experience significant alleviation of the symptoms. Taking into consideration other signs, such as diarrhea, soft and weak pulse, yellowish tongue fur with dark tongue substance, the prescription was changed to Buzhong Yiqi Decoction with additional herbs of Radix paeoniae alba, Danpi and Sanzhi Fructus gardeniae. After another 18 doses of this prescription, there was an apparent drop of temperature, but the rash stayed on. Thereafter, "Qi-replenishing and Blood-revitalizing" herbs, such as Radix codonopsis pilosulae, Rhizoma atractylodis macrocephalae, Radix angelicae sinensis, Radix salviae miltiorrhizae, Herba lycopi, Radix paeoniae alba, Fructus lycii, Radix cynanchi atrati, Cortex dictamni radicis and Cortex albiziae, were used in order to treat the disease by replenishing the Qi and Blood simultaneously. This new prescription was administered for 17 doses; there was no new rash noted, but the old one persisted. Two treatment courses of penicillin and streptomycin were undertaken in addition to the existing herbal medicines but to no avail. One week later, the rash recurred with its distribution similar to the previous occasion. The patient displayed recurrent fever and palpitation easily induced by minimal physical activities. Examination of her pulse showed it to be weak and rapid, tongue substance was purplish with very thin, almost absent tongue fur. Further analysis of the case concluded that the illness was quite deep-seated and such a chronic disease called for a milder and more prudent approach. Thus, Yuepi Decoction and Danggui Buxue Tang (Blood-Tonifying Decoction with Chinese Angelicae) together with the additional herbs Flos lonicerae, Radix rehmanniae, Fructus forsythiae and Radix isatidis were given accordingly. Temperature was lowered and the rash subsided slightly after one week of administration of this regimen. Dexamethasone was given at this juncture, and all the rashes disappeared six days later, but the low-grade fever still remained (37.2-37.5°C). Temperature finally subsided with administration of Salpital retention enema. After one therapeutic course, dexamethasone was replaced with prednisone, which was administered for 48 days. Three days after cessation of prednisone administration, the ring-shape rash recurred, distributed on medial aspects of the thighs, the poplitial fossas and axillas. The wheals were of different sizes, circular in shape and red in colour with elevated borders. Steroid therapy no longer could contain the symptoms.

Second stage of treatment: To further enforce the approach of "replenishing the

Qi, revitalizing the Blood and dispelling the pathogenic Wind," two prescriptions, Fangji Dihuang Decoction from the *Jin Kui Yao Lue (Synopsis of Prescriptions of the Golden Chamber)* and Hongnanhua Jiu were administered. The prescription, made up of Raw Radix astragali, 15 gm; Radix ledebouriellae, 10 gm; Radix stephaniae tetrandrae, 10 gm; Ramulus cinnamomi, 10 gm; Radix glycyrrhizae, 6 gm; Radix puerariae, 12 gm; raw Radix rehmanniae, 30 gm; Flos carthami, 12 gm; and Huang Jiu (yellow rice wine), 60 ml, was taken one dose per day.

No new rash appeared after administration of the new prescription and the old rash subsided gradually with total remission achieved on April 30. Condition remained unchanged for the next two months. Sedimentation rate reading on May 28 was mm/2hrs, and findings of liver functions, CBC and routine urinalysis were all within normal limits. At the beginning of June, the patient had a few days of low-grade fever which was due to common cold and stomatitis, but there was no recurrence of the rash. Condition was generally stable. At the beginning of July, the patient had common cold again with fever, cough, throat pain; the rash reappeared but only to a mild degree. She was consequently given a prescription, the main characteristic of which was intended to "dispel pathogenic factors from the exterior of the body with herbs pungent in flavour and warm in property." After administering several doses, other "Heat-ventilating" herbs, such as Radix platycodi, Periostracum cicadae and Herba schizone-petae, were added to the original prescription. Treatment reverted to the original prescription after fever had subsided and throat pain disappeared. Penicillin and tetracycline were also added to more effectively control the infections. The common cold and its complications brought about reappearance of rashes but severity and duration of the rash proved to be much milder than that of the previous ones. Recent therapeutic regimen also proved to be more effective than all the other medications used to control the rash, both traditional and modern.

DISCUSSION: Fangji Dihuang Decoction has its provenance in *Jin Kui: Concise Synopsis of Pathological Pulses and Symptom-Complexes of Apoplexy*. The prescription relies heavily on the "Blood-nurturing and cooling" effects of Radix rehmanniae as well as the "Wind and Dampness dispelling" effects of Radix ledebouriellae and Radix steogabuae and the "Blood-invigorating and Resistance-strengthening" effects of Gly-cyrrhizae and Ramulus cinnamoni. This prescription is indicated in cases where the illness manifests signs of "Wind and Dampness in the Jin and Pulse" and also those with "Blood Deficiency." Hongnanhua Jiu was first seen in *Jin Kui: General Diseases of Women*. It utilizes Flos carthamia to generate Blood and induce its regeneration. It is decocted in wine to further enhance its pharmacological properties and to remove all the obstructions so that the flow of Qi and Blood can move without hindrance in the body. It is particularly effective in treating women's diseases caused by "pathogenic Wind." This thrappeutic regimen, which is composed of Fangji Dihuang Decoction, Hongnanhua Jiu, the "Qi-replenishing and exterior-consolidating" effects of Huangqi and the febrifugal and detoxicating effects of Gegneg, exerts its force not only in correcting Qi-Blood Deficiencies of the patient but also in dispelling the evils and pathogens from the body. It follows closely the principle of "in order to remove pathogenic Wind, one must straighten out the Blood first; once the Blood moves smoothly and without hindrance, the pathogenic Wind will be gone by itself." There was no precedent recording ring-shaped rashes in traditional medicine literature, but in view of the fact that this case responded favourably to the therapeutic regimen, it comes close to what the *Jin Kui: Concise Synopsis of Pathological Pulses and Symptom-Complexes of Apoplexy* describes as "pathogenic Wind encroaches on the Jin resulting in itchiness of the body and manifesting with menacing patches." After one year of follow-up, the patient's condition was shown to be stable and the effect of the prescription consistent.

8.6 SKIN RASH, HYPOCHONDRIAC PAIN (DAMP-HEAT AND BLOOD STASIS)

Jean Yu

Santa Barbara College of Oriental Medicine, California, U.S.A.

Kinnebrew, 63, female, white, single, real estate broker. Medical record number: 898. Date of first consultation: October 19, 1987.

CHIEF COMPLAINT: Itchy rash on the face, hypochondriac and abdominal pain, diarrhea.

HISTORY OF PRESENT ILLNESS: The patient experienced an itchy rash on her face that she had not been able to clear up. She had blood tests done, and they indicated presence of yeast in the blood. The cells were elongated rather than round. She complained of chronic pain and soreness in the hypochondriac and intercostal regions. She had left-side pain especially when turning to the left. She reported soreness of the sternum and pain directly below the ribs. When moving, the pain traversed from below the navel upward and laterally. She also had diarrhea four times every morning which was loose to watery. She had distention in the abdomen and a slight amount of gas. She reported that she occasionally felt drained of energy with recurring bouts of tiredness. She did not report feelings of warm sensation in her body but preferred not to drink cold fluids. She reported a tendency of spontaneous sweating. She normally got up once a night to urinate. Urine colour was normally slightly yellow. Her sleep was often interrupted. She felt that her abdominal and hypochondriac pain was stress related.

PAST HISTORY: Positive history of skin irregularities and recently had two biopsies on her left forearm and below the outer canthus. The patient was prescribed tetracycline for her skin condition by a dermatologist but did not take the prescription.

INSPECTION OF TONGUE: Dark and puffy tongue body with no coating.

PULSE CONDITION: Deep, wiry, slightly slippery and slightly rapid (80/min).

MODERN MEDICINE DIAGNOSIS: Undifferentiated Dermatitis; Undifferentiated Abdominal Pain.

TRADITIONAL CHINESE MEDICINE DIAGNOSIS: Damp-Heat in the Surface; Stagnant Qi and Blood; Spleen Qi Deficiency.

THERAPEUTIC PRINCIPLES: Clear away Dampness and Heat, move the Blood and Qi, and tonify Qi.

PRESCRIPTION: Four doses, Rhizoma smilacis glabrae, 12 gm; Cortex dictamni radicis, 6 gm; Cortex moutan radicis, 6 gm; Cortex alismatis, 12 gm; Radix curcumae, 6 gm; Semen ziziphi spinosae, 9 gm; Radix codonopsis pilosulae, 9 gm; and Radix glycyrrhizae, 9 gm.

FOLLOW-UP/COURSE OF TREATMENT:

Second consultation on October 26, 1987: The patient reported that the rash had disappeared as well as the itchiness. She had no pain on her left side or hypochondriac areas. She reported that she had loose stools in the morning and sometimes immediately after eating. She reported her energy as being normal and did not experience tiredness. Abdominal distention and intestinal gas still present. Sleep was still interrupted with the patient waking up about twice each night, usually around 4 to 5 a.m. Her tongue was dark with tooth marks and had a thin yellow coat in the centre. Pulse weak and slippery. The prescription was modified to increase the Qi-tonifying and sedating herbs and to eliminate herbs that were specifically for the rash. Modification: Three doses. Radix codonopsis pilosulae, 9 gm; Poria cocos, 12 gm; Rhizoma atractylodis macrocephalae, 6 gm; Fried Semen coicis, 12 gm; Cortex alismatis, 12 gm; Radix salviae miltiorrhizae, 9 gm; Radix curcumae, 6 gm; Semen ziziphi spinosae, 9 gm; Caulis poligoni multiflori, 9 gm; Cortex alhizziae, 9 gm; and Radix glycyrrhizae, 6 gm.

Third consultation on November 2, 1987: The patient reported continued absence of rash and itching and continued absence of abdominal or hypochondriac pain. She was able to sleep soundly through the night. She continued to suffer from distention and intestinal gas and loose stools in the morning and after eating. The prescription was changed to work on Spleen Qi deficiency and chronic diarrhea. Prescription: Modified Shen Ling Bai Zhu San (Powder of Ginseng, Poria and White atractylodis). Four doses. Radix codonopsis pilosulae, 9 gm; Poria cocos, 12 gm; Rhizoma atractylodis macrostemae, 6 gm; Semen coicis, 12 gm; Rhizoma dioscoreae, 9 gm; Semen nelumbinis, 9 gm; Semen euryales, 9 gm; Massa fermentata medicinalis, 9 gm; and Radix glycyrrhizae, 6 gm.

Fourth consultation on November 9, 1987: The patient reported continued absence of rashes and hypochondriac pain. Sleep remained good. Appetite was good and she reported no abdominal distention with normal, well-formed stools. She still had some intestinal gas but without pain. She reported absence of spontaneous sweating.

DISCUSSION: This case displayed three disorders in the body, namely, stagnation, presence of pathogenic factors and deficiency. Despite the inner connections, the stagnation and pathogenic factors were concentrated at first. Rhizoma smilacis glabrae and Lortox dictamni radicis are two herbs that act on the skin by eliminating Dampness. Cortex moutan radicis moves the Blood and cools it. Radix curcumae is especially indicated for pains of the chest and abdomen. Once the less constitutional disorders were removed rather quickly, the intent became that of tonifying the Spleen Qi. Shen Ling Bai Zhu San is an excellent formula for replenishing the Qi and tonifying the Spleen and Stomach. This formula also dispels Dampness in the body resulting from Spleen Qi deficiency and is made stronger in this respect by the addition of Cortex alismatis which effectively removes Dampness but does not act on the Spleen.

(Collator: Brock Haines)

8.7 RHEUMATIC ARTHRITIS
(ARTHRALGIA SYNDROME)

Chen Kezhong and Zhang Jidong
Shandong Medical University Hospital, Jinan

Cheng Yuejie, 26, female, Han nationality, single, worker. Medical record number: 269533. Date of first consultation: June 7, 1982.
CHIEF COMPLAINT: Generalized joint pain.
HISTORY OF PRESENT ILLNESS: The patient stated that she developed a fever abruptly on May 5 of this year with body temperature reaching 37.6°C and joint pain all over the body, especially the knee joints. The onset was accompanied by sore throat, thirst and fatigue. Antibiotic was given in local hospital without satisfactory effect. She consulted our clinic and was subsequently admitted.
PAST HISTORY: Positive history of bronchitis.
PERTINENT PHYSICAL EXAMINATION & LABORATORY FINDINGS: Difficulty in flexion and extension in her joints; ESR, 100 mm/hr; ASO, 800 units.
INSPECTION OF TONGUE: Red tongue substance with yellow fur.
PULSE CONDITION: Wiry and rapid.
MODERN MEDICINE DIAGNOSIS: Rheumatic Arthritis (Active Stage).
TRADITIONAL CHINESE MEDICINE DIAGNOSIS: Arthralgia Syndrome.
THERAPEUTIC PRINCIPLES: Remove Heat and obstruction in the Channels, remove Wind and overcome Dampness.
PRESCRIPTION: Modified Guizhishaoyaozhimu Tang. Ramulus cinnamomi, 6 gm; Radix paeoniae alba and rubra, 12 gm each; Rhizoma anemarrhenae, 9 gm; Gypsum fibrosum, 30 gm; Poria, 24 gm; Herba ephedrae, 4.5 gm; Radix astragali, 15 gm; Pollen typhae, 20 gm; Caulis spatholobi, 20 gm; Rhizoma ligustici, 9 gm; Caulis sinomenii, 20 gm; Caulis piperis futokodaurae, 20 gm; and Radix clematis, 20 gm. To be taken in decoction form. Four doses, one dose per day.
FOLLOW-UP/COURSE OF TREATMENT:
Second consultation on June 11, 1982: Perspiration followed intake of the decoctions. Pain at the joints were relieved. The patient had a good appetite and could sleep well. The tongue was red with thin, yellowish fur and wiry and rapid pulse. Seven more doses of the same prescription were prescribed.
Third consultation on June 18, 1982: Slight pain in the right knee joint still troubled the patient. Tongue was pink with thin and white fur. Pulse was wiry and rapid. Modified the prescription by reducing the dosage of Gypsum fibrosum and Poria to 20 gm each and added Radix achyranthis bidentate, 20 gm. Five doses.
Fourth consultation: Joint pains alleviated markedly. General condition was good. Re-examination of ESR, 3 mm/hour; ASO normal. Continued administration of the

prescription. Rest and follow-up were suggested on her discharge from hospital so as to maintain the therapeutic effect.

DISCUSSION: The pathogenesis of arthralgia syndrome is retention of pathogens in the Channels and Collaterals and disturbance of the relationship between Vital Energy and Blood characterized by joint pains. Onset of the disease is sudden, with symptoms of fever, thirst, red tongue and rapid pulse, etc., as manifestations of the internal accumulation of Dampness and Heat. Modified decoction of cinnamon twig, peony and rhizoma of Wind-Wood combined with herbs effective in clearing away Evil Heat and Wind and in promoting diuresis were selected to remove both the exogenous and endogenous Dampness and Heat and to clear and activate the Channels and Collaterals. The degree of Dampness in this case was quite extensive and difficult to overcome. In our prescription, the medicinal herb Poria was used to reinforce the function of the Spleen to eliminate Dampness. With Heat removed and Dampness eliminated, we saw a favourable outcome.

8.8 ACUTE RHEUMATIC FEVER (ARTHRALGIA DUE TO HEAT)

Chen Wenbin and Zhang Taihuai

First Affiliated Hospital of the West China University of Medical Sciences, Chengdu

Li Changlin, 19, male, Han nationality, single, student. Medical record number: 161394. Date of first consultation: February 16, 1966.

CHIEF COMPLAINT: Fever with sore throat for 16 days.

HISTORY OF PRESENT ILLNESS: About 16 days prior to admission, the patient had a severe bout of common cold accompanied by chill, fever, sore throat, headache, perspiration and anorexia. A diagnosis of "acute tonsillitis" was given in the school clinic, and penicillin C was used for three days without effect. One week prior to admission, he began to experience severe pain in the lumbar area. Hip and knee joints did not swell or become red. Two days prior to admission, he experienced sudden palpitation and sharp precordial pain which appeared to be sporadic in nature. There was no history of skin lesions, weight loss, epistaxis, shortness of breath, ankle edema or hematuria.

PAST HISTORY: About three years prior to admission, the patient felt for the first time sore throat with fever, and since then the attacks occurred one to two times every year, each lasting for about a week.

PERTINENT PHYSICAL EXAMINATION & LABORATORY FINDINGS: Temperature, 38°C; pulse, 46/min; respiratory rate, 20/min; and blood pressure, 100/50 mmHg. The patient looked pale. A lymph node 1.5 × 1.0 cm in size palpated at the right submandibular region with tenderness. Pharynx was engorged and the tonsils enlarged covered by whitish secretion. Neck veins were markedly distended. On percussion, heart borders appeared to be normal. Heart rate was 46/min with irregular rhythm. First heart sound at the apex was weak and a third heart sound was heard. There was systolic soft blowing apical murmur radiating to the axilla; P2 › A2. Lungs clear. Liver palpable 1.5 cm below right costal margin with tenderness. There was no subcutaneous nodules or erythema marginatum present, nor was there any pain, swelling or tenderness present over the joints. WBC: 13,050/mm³; ESR: 3 mm/hr. Pharyngeal swab culture positive for Streptococcus viridans growth. Electrophoresis of serum protein showed albumin, 37.9%; α_1, 8.55%; α_2, 11.1%; ß, 12.3% and γ, 39.15%. Chest film was normal. ECG showed grade III A-V block.

INSPECTION OF TONGUE: Tongue substance appeared reddish with thick, white fur.

PULSE CONDITION: Moderate rate; sinking with irregularity.

MODERN MEDICINE DIAGNOSIS: Acute Rheumatic Fever; Rheumatic My-ocarditis and Arthritis.

TRADITIONAL CHINESE MEDICINE DIAGNOSIS: Arthralgia due to Heat.

THERAPEUTIC PRINCIPLES: Remove toxic Heat and dispel Dampness.

PRESCRIPTION:

1) Basic recipes for oral administration: Decoction of White Tiger plus Ramulus Cinnamomi. Gypsum, 60 mg; Rhizoma anemarrhenae, 15 gm; Ramulus cinnamomi, 9 gm; Cauli lonicerae, 30 gm; Fructus forsythiae, 15 gm; Radix scutellariae, 15 gm; Radix sophorae subprostrae, 15 gm; Fructus chaenomelis, 30 gm; Radix tetrandrae, 30 gm; Semen oryzae stative, 15 gm; and Radix glycyrrhizae, 9 gm. Two doses per day.

2) Recipes for external use:

(i) Bingpeng Powder.

(ii) Plum Flake, 0.3 gm; Realgar, 0.3 gm; and Borax 0.24 gm. Mixed and ground.

Applied on pharyngeal walls two to three times per day, (i) and (ii) alternately.

FOLLOW-UP/COURSE OF TREATMENT: Two days after treatment, sore throat and precordial chest pain subsided. Pulse rate went up to 60/min. Six days later, temperature was down to 36.5-37.5°C. Cardiac rhythm regular. ECG examination showed grade II and grade I A-V block. Tongue substance appeared to be whitish and covered with slimy and greasy fur. Pulse slow and moderate. These signs indicated that the Wetness-Evil were still overwhelming; 15 gm of Atractylodis rhizome were added to the basic prescription, two recipes per day. The patient was discharged after two months of treatment. At that time, pharyngitis had subsided and heart rate was 74/min with regular rhythm. WBC, ESR, serum mucous protein and electrophoresis of serum protein were all within normal limits. ECG examination, inspection of the tongue and pulse were also normal.

DISCUSSION: The etiological factors of Heat arthralgia in this case are three atmospheric influence, i.e., Wind, Cold, and Dampness invasion of the body. The pathological changes are results of Heat-transformation. Pathogenesis of this disease follows attack by exogenous pathogenic factors from exterior to interior and blocking the Channels of the body. As a result, Blood and Vital Energy transportation was disturbed. Consequently, pathogenic Dampness lingered in the secondary defensive system and caused deficiency of the vital function of the Heart. This was evidenced by the major clinical manifestations of this case, i.e., bradycardia and pulse weakness.

Rheumatic fever is an allergic disease. The patient had a history of hemolytic streptococcic infection followed by development of serious myocarditis. In management of this kind of case, it was important to reduce the allergic reaction. Accordingly, Decoction of White Tiger plus Ramulus Cinnamomi was selected to remove toxic Heat, dispel Dampness and remove the obstruction of the Channels. Using White Tiger Decoction as a base, we added Caulis lonicerae, Fructus forsythiae, Radix scutellariae and Radix sophorae subprostrae for management of specific symptoms. Simultaneously, herbs effective in dispelling Dampness and removing obstruction of the Channels, such as Fructus chaenomelis, Radix lonicerae and Atractylodis rhizoma, were employed to achieve a more comprehensive therapeutic approach.

In view of the seriousness of the patient's condition, a larger than usual dosage was used in this case, i.e., two doses instead of one per day. On the other hand, attention was also drawn to the management of pharyngitis by application of external medications. The required blood concentration of these herbs, therefore, could be maintained for a desired period of time, and the local foci as well as the general symptoms could be put under control in due time. Following the lowering of temperature, the pulse rate went up to normal range rapidly and ECG abnormalities were effectively corrected.

Twenty-two years of following up on this case have shown that the curative effects of traditional Chinese medicine are satisfactory. We would like to suggest here that the therapeutic methods employed in the management of this case not only could arrest the development of rheumatic fever but also could prevent damage to the heart valves.

8.9 PRIMARY CUTANEOUS AMYLOIDOSIS (BLOOD STASIS DUE TO WIND-COLD

Bian Tianyu

Dermatological Institute of Integrated Traditional Chinese
and Western Medicine, Tianjin Changzheng Hospital, Tianjin

Gao, 63, male, Han nationality, married, worker. Date of first consultation: July 7, 1977.

CHIEF COMPLAINT: Verrucous, itchy and lichenoid lesions on extensive areas of the extremities for three years.

HISTORY OF PRESENT ILLNESS: At the beginning, itchiness was experienced on an extensive surface of the lower extremities. Gradually, plain papules appeared on the affected skin followed by involvement of the upper extremities and trunk. These lesions fused to form large plagues, verrucous in appearance and intensively pruritic. This condition, especially pruritis, usually worsened in winter and in cold weather. Sleepless nights resulted from this intense pruritus.

PAST HISTORY: No history of specific contagious disease. No habits of smoking and alcoholic drinking.

PERTINENT PHYSICAL EXAMINATION & LABORATORY FINDINGS: Development and nutrition status good. Blood pressure, 120/80 mmHg. No GGE; heart and lungs normal; no enlargement of the liver and spleen. Motor activity normal. Except for skin of the head, face, palms and soles, crusted bloody papules with hyperpigmentation were noted over the body. Large plagues of verrucous hypertrophic lesions over an extensive surface of the extremities. Presence of numerous small grayish papules on the back and thorax. Histopathology: epiderma showed hyperkeratosis, acanthosis and hyperpigmentation of basal cells; dermal layer with papules dilated and infiltrated with pinkish and homogenous substances which in methyl-purple preparation revealed purple amyloid protein.

INSPECTION OF TONGUE: Purplish tongue proper.

PULSE CONDITION: Floating and slippery.

MODERN MEDICINE DIAGNOSIS: Primary Cutaneous Amyloidosis.

TRADITIONAL CHINESE MEDICINE DIAGNOSIS: Blood stasis due to Wind-Cold.

THERAPEUTIC PRINCIPLES: Relieve Blood stasis and eliminate Wind and Cold.

PRESCRIPTION: Herba ephedrae, 6 gm; Herba schijonepetae, 9 gm; Radix ledebourielae, 9 gm; Bombyx batryticatus, 6 gm; Rhizoma atractylodis, 9 gm; Herba menthae, 6 gm; Radix angelicae, 6 gm; Radix paeoniae rubra, 9 gm; Flos carthami, 9 gm; Rhizoma zedoriae, 9 gm; and Radix glycyrrhizae, 6 gm. Decoct and to be taken once daily.

FOLLOW-UP/COURSE OF TREATMENT: Beginning in August 1977, the patient took the medication once every one to three days and applied 0.05% terimesone cream locally for three months. A total of 40 doses of medicine were administered and the skin lesions disappeared completely. Pigmentation also diminished markedly. The disease was cured essentially except for some follicular, small black points on the back. Some itching still occurred at night.

DISCUSSION: Physical examination revealed sporadic areas of hyperpigmentation with verrucous papules. Tongue proper purplish in colour. These are all signs of Blood stasis. Presence of Wind-Cold was evidenced by the patient's sensation of cold and his pulse manifestations. The therapeutic prescription was prepared to overcome these pathologies, and a good result was obtained.

8.10 DERMATOMYOSITIS
(SPLEEN DEFICIENCY AND BLOOD STASIS)

Qin Wanzhan, Shan Yijun and Gu Wenzhen
Zhongshan Hospital, Shanghai Medical University, Shanghai

Chen Yingfang, 35, female, Han nationality, married, worker. Medical record number: 85-43120. Date of first consultation: May 28, 1986.

CHIEF COMPLAINT: Fever, muscle pain, skin lesions and arthralgia.

HISTORY OF PRESENT ILLNESS: For the past six months, erythema appeared on and off on the face and back of hands accompanied by irregular, often low-grade fever. Severe muscular pain and weakness and arthralgia developed frequently which involved proximal muscles of the extremities and resulted in difficulty in locomotion. Other signs and symptoms were dizziness, swelling of the face, anorexia, abdominal distention, insomnia, loss of body weight, spontaneous perspiration, menoschesis and light-coloured and copious amount of urine. Loose bowel movement always developed. She was diagnosed as a case of connective tissue disease. Symptoms improved after using indomethacin and tripterygil hypoglauci. Two weeks ago, muscular pain and weakness aggravated because of exposure to cold accompanied by fever and excessive fatigue. She consulted our clinic because her facial lesions had become worse, now involving the eyelids.

PAST HISTORY: General body weakness and gastric ulceration.

FAMILY HISTORY: Mother died from intestinal cancer; sister with positive history of rheumatoid arthritis.

PERTINENT PHYSICAL EXAMINATION & LABORATORY FINDINGS: Temperature, 37.5°C. Erythema and swelling with pinkish-violet and minute telangiectases on the face and upper eyelids were obvious. Poikiloderma-like hyperpigmentation and hypopigmentation spots spread on the thorax and back. Violet erythema-covered scales were seen symmetrically on the back of the finger joints. Gripping power of both hands was poor. Difficulty in raising the arms and standing up from squatting position. Lymph nodes swollen in cervical and axillary regions. Liver palpable 1 cm below the right costal margin and slightly tender. WBC, 10,200/mm^3; RBC, 2.5M/mm^3; ESR, 32 mm/hour. Routine urinalysis normal. SGOT, 72 u; SGPT, 48 u; LDH, 800 u and CPK, 50 u, and 24-hr urinary creatine, 720 mg. Electromyography suggested myogenic change. Electrocardiogram, chest X-ray and CT scan normal.

INSPECTION OF TONGUE: Light, white, slimy and greasy fur of the tongue; purplish tongue substance with tooth prints at its borders.

PULSE CONDITION: Fine and soft.

MODERN MEDICINE DIAGNOSIS: Dermatomyositis.

TRADITIONAL CHINESE MEDICINE DIAGNOSIS: Spleen Deficiency and Blood Stasis; Pain, Swelling and Stiffness of Muscles.

THERAPEUTIC PRINCIPLES: Invigorate Spleen functions, reinforce Vital Energy and activate Blood circulation to eliminate Blood stasis.

PRESCRIPTION: Ba Zhen Decoction (Decoction of Eight Precious Ingredients) and prescription for invigoration of blood circulation. Radix codonopsis pilosulae, 15 gm; Radix astragali, 15 gm; Rhizoma atractylodis, 9 gm; Radix rehmanniae, 15 gm; Caulis et radix sargentodixue, 15 gm; Caulis spatholobi, 15 gm; and Tripterygium wilfordii Hook F (TWHF), 25 gm. Boiled and taken orally twice a day. Triamcinolone acetic cream applied externally two times a day.

FOLLOW-UP/COURSE OF TREATMENT:

Second consultation: Fever, arthralgia and muscular pain took a favourable turn after two weeks of treatment, but fatigue remained. The coating and purplish discolouration of the tongue substance were still present. Pulse was soft and fine. Radix angelicae, 12 gm, was added and the dosage of Radix astragali increased to 30 gm in the prescription.

Third consultation: Facial erythema lightened, muscle pain and tenderness alleviated. Myasthenia lessened, WBC count declined to 8,000/mm^3 and ESR to 16 mm/hr, SGOT 40 u. Continued administration of the same prescription.

Fourth consultation: Muscle pain, tenderness and myasthenia had disappeared and pinkish-violet erythema of the eyelids gone down. Lymph nodes not palpable on the cervical and axillary regions. Pulse and tongue inspection, routine CBC and urinalysis were normal. ESR also normal. GOT, 40 u; LDH and CPK had declined to normal range. Urinary creatine had decreased to 100 mg. Discontinued the prescription. Instead, TWHF syrup in the dosage of 10 ml and Far-Reaching Tonic Pill, 9 gm, were taken orally, twice a day in order to consolidate the therapeutic effect.

Fifth consultation: Half a year later, her condition was stable. TWHF syrup was taken intermittently. She was engaged in normal work.

DISCUSSION: A definite diagnosis of dermatomyositis was established based on signs of fever, muscle pain and tenderness, myasthenia, pinkish-violet erythema and swelling of the face and eyelids. Other pertinent findings were flat-topped violaceous papules over the knuckles (Gottron's sign), increased WBC count, elevated serum level of GOT, GPT, LDH, CPK, elevated 24-hr urinary creatine and myogenic change in electromyogram. According to TCM diagnosis and symptom-complex differentiation, this case was one of debility, combining congenital defect with weakness in a chronic morbid state. On the other hand, signs of myosthenia, dizziness, fatigue, facial swelling, anorexia, abdominal distention, loose bowel, white, slimy fur of the tongue with tooth marks at its borders and fine and soft pulse were also evident. All of these suggested deficiency of the Spleen. Purple colour of the tongue substance, menoschesis, erythematous or pinkish-violet patches indicated Blood stasis.

Etiology and Pathogenesis: The etiology of dermatomyositis, an auto-immune disease, is unknown. It has been suggested that heredity, infection and allergy might be implicated as causative agents. In traditional Chinese medicine, the Spleen determines the muscles, the Lung determines the skin and the Kidney determines the bones. The cause of this disease is likely to be dysfunction of the Spleen, Lung and Kidney associated with Yin deficiency. The three pathogenic factors (Wind, Cold and Dampness) enter the body, accumulate in the muscles, Channels and Collaterals and joints, resulting in obstruction of the Channels with derangement of anabolic and defensive energy, disturbed circulation of the Vital Energy and Blood and muscle dysfunction, such as myoapathy, myalgia, amyosthenia as well as facial erythema. Spleen deficiency and Blood stasis resulting from a congenital defect combined with a prolonged course of illness undermined the Vital Energy and enabled the pathogenic factors to prevail.

Treatment: According to TCM symptom-complex differentiation, this was a typical case of Spleen deficiency and Blood stasis. The therapeutic principles of invigorating Blood circulation, reinforcing Spleen functions and replenishing the Vital Energy were used to regulate the flow of the Vital Energy and Blood, strengthen the patient's resistance, dispel invading pathogenic factors and invigorate the function of the Middle Burner. Decoction of Eight Precious Ingredients, capable of activating Blood circulation, was the basic vehicle to achieve these goals. To activate Blood circulation and eliminate Blood stasis, the herbs used were Radix salviae miltiorrhizae to nourish the Blood and stimulate the Channels; Radix angelicae to nourish the Blood and activate Blood circulation; Caulis spatholobi and Caulis et radix sargentodoxue to remove toxic Heat, promote normal flow of the Vital Energy and eliminate the nodule; and TWHF to remove toxic Heat, eliminate swelling, inhibit antigen-antibody reaction, enhance immune functions and effect anti-inflammation and analgesic functions similar to corticosteroids. Herbs for activating Blood circulation and eliminating stasis were combined with herbs for strengthening the patient's resistance, e.g., Radix codonopsis pilosulae to reinforce the Middle Burner and replenish the Vital Energy to invigorate the function of the Spleen, replenish the Vital Energy and body fluid; Radix astragali to replenish the Vital Energy to strengthen superficial resistance, enhance cellular immunity and rectify the immune disturbance; and Rhizoma atractylodis macrocephalae to invigorate functions of the Spleen and normalize Stomach functions.

Decoction is the main form of administration in treating patients suffering from the active stage of dermatomyositis, while pills and syrup are used as maintenance measures during recovery periods. Moreover, corticosteroids are applied externally on skin lesions. A satisfactory effect was achieved by this combined traditional Chinese and modern medicine approach to treatment.

8.11 DERMATOMYOSITIS
(WEI ZHENG)

Bian Tianyu and Yu Xichen

Dermatological Institute of Integrated Traditional Chinese
and Western Medicine, Tianjin Changzheng Hospital, Tianjin

Li, 16, female, Han nationality, student. Medical record number: 36961. Date of admission: February 8, 1964.

CHIEF COMPLAINT: Chills and fever, erythema and facial swelling, muscle pain and weakness of the extremities and difficulty in swallowing for more than 20 days.

HISTORY OF PRESENT ILLNESS: At the onset of the disease, the patient experienced chills and fever, erythema of the face, sore throat and weakness and pain of the muscles of the whole body. She was diagnosed as having "tonsillitis" and treated by APC, Penicillin, etc. A week later, erythematous lesions were evident over the upper eyelids accompanied by minimal pitting edema on the neck, shoulder and upper extremities. Pain and weakness of muscles generally became worse and she could not rise from the bed. When she attempted to swallow water or fluid, it flowed out through the nostrils. Constipation and malodorous breath were also noted. She was treated as a case of Fengshui Zheng with herbal medications such as Yue Pi Tang, Bai Hu Tang, Wu Ling San and Chi Xiao Dou Tang. No satisfactory effect was obtained.

PAST HISTORY: Positive history for sore throat and tonsillitis. No habits of smoking or alcohol ingestion. Cycles of menstruation 15/3-4/30 days. Amount of menstruation normal. No history of Raynaud's syndrome. No history of arthralgia.

PERTINENT PHYSICAL EXAMINATION & LABORATORY FINDINGS: Acute facies, bedridden, conscious and cooperative. Temperature, 38°C; pulse rate, 120/min. No GCE. Face puffy and erythematous in appearance. Slight pitting edema on palpebral fissures. Diffuse erythematous eruptions over the eyelids and around the nose. The demarcation of erythema was not clearly visible. Tenderness of muscles of the whole body exacerbated during movement of the extremities. Flexion and extension ability of the extremities lost. Gripping power of both hands very weak. Unable to raise her legs from supine position and unable to raise her hands and head. Liquid flowed out through the nostrils during swallowing. Voice with a distinct nasal twang. Light reflex of the eye normal. Congestion of mucosa on the throat with enlarged tonsils. Contracted, flowing murmur detected on the apex of the heart; regular cardiac rhythm. Lung findings negative. Liver and spleen not palpable. No pathological reflex elicited. Hemoglobin, 12 gm%; RBC, 3.6M/mm^3; WBC, 10,200/mm^3; polymorphs, 80%; and lymphocytes, 20%. Urinary creatinine, 100 mg/24hrs. ESR, 40 mm/hr; LE cell (-). Biopsy of epidermis: liquid degeneration of basal layer. Dermis: edematous superficial layer with focal infiltration of mononuclear cells and edematous degeneration of muscle fibres. Loss of transverse striation, infiltration of mononuclear cells between the muscular fibres.

INSPECTION OF TONGUE: Tongue proper red in colour with yellowish, rough coating.

PULSE CONDITION: Superficial and slippery.

MODERN MEDICINE DIAGNOSIS: Dermatomyositis.

TRADITIONAL CHINESE MEDICINE DIAGNOSIS: Wei Zheng (Gan Re Yin-xue Zheng).

THERAPEUTIC PRINCIPLES: Smooth the Liver, remove the pathogenic Heat, nurture the Yin and benefit the Qi (Shugan Qingre Yangyin Yiqi).

FOLLOW-UP/ COURSE OF TREATMENT: The patient was diagnosed initially as a case of "Wen Du Zheng' and treated with Qingre Jiedu (Heat Removing and Detoxicating) Composition plus Radix panacis quinquefolii, Zi Jin Dan, Cornu ante-lopis, Cornu Rhinoceri, etc., but no significant effect was obtained by this regimen.

On February 15, 1964, the patient's temperature was between 37°C and 38°C; she complained of nausea, easy fatigability, sore throat and bitter taste in the mouth. Tongue substance was red in colour with yellow, greasy coating. Gan Mai Chai Hu Tang was prescribed. Fructus tritici levis, 60 gm; Fructus ziziphi jujubae, in pieces; Radix glycyrrhizae, 6 gm; Radix bupleuri, 9 gm; Radix trichosanthis, 9 gm; Herba dendrobii, 9 gm; Radix rehmanniae, 15 gm; Radix astragali, 15 gm; and Rhizoma cimicifugae, 3 gm. Decocted and taken twice daily. On the third day of administration, temperature returned to normal and the patient's general condition improved. Symptoms of muscle pain and tenderness much relieved. Ten days after administration, the symptom of difficulty in swallowing disappeared. The patient could raise her head. She brightened up. Skin edema had disappeared, too. Tongue substance red with thin, yellow fur. The patient continued to take the prescription with additional tonifying herbs. Continued for about six months. She recovered completely from the illness and was discharged. On discharge, ESR was 20 mm/hr and urine creatinine level 3.1 mg/24 hr.

The patient was last seen in 1972; there had not been a relapse of the condition.

DISCUSSION: This case of dermatomyositis was treated initially with Qingre Jiedu Composition for about a week and there was no improvement. With administration of the Shugan Qingre Yangyin Yiqi prescription, favourable therapeutic results were obtained. Most of the symptoms and signs disappeared promptly. Later in the course of the treatment, tonifying herbs were added to the prescription and administered for a period of six months to consolidate the therapeutic effect. The patient recovered fully from the illness.

Since then, the authors have prescribed Ganmai Chaihu Tang for the early stage of dermatomyositis and tonifying herbs for the later stage of the disease. Of the 12 cases treated, nine recovered completely and the conditions of two improved.

8.12 SYSTEMIC LUPUS ERYTHEMATOSUS (QI-XUE LIANG FENG ZHENG)

Bian Tianyu and Ding Suxian
Dermatological Institute of Integrated Traditional Chinese and Western Medicine, Tianjin Changzheng Hospital, Tianjin

Ding, 17, female, Han nationality, single, student. Medical record number: 110. Date of first consultation: January 10, 1975.

CHIEF COMPLAINT: Fever, butterfly erythematous markings on the face and arthralgia for one month.

HISTORY OF PRESENT ILLNESS: One month prior to consultation, the patient suffered from fever almost every day, with body temperature varying between 38°C-39.8°C, which generally elevated in the afternoons. Butterfly erythematous markings appeared on the face and around the edges of the ears. These erythematous lesions were well outlined, painless and non-pruritic. Also present was migrating arthralgia of the extremities. There was no swelling or erythema of the joints. Accompanying symptoms were weakness, anorexia, thirst and constipation. Amenorrheic for 40 days. No treatment received.

PAST HISTORY: Positive history of chronic tonsillitis; no specific infectious disease and no history of connective disease in family. Menstruation 13/3-4/26-30.

PERTINENT PHYSICAL EXAMINATION & LABORATORY FINDINGS: Acute facies and pale. Nutritional status and development fair. Evident butterfly and edematous erythema on face. Purplish patches on fingers and roots of nails. No GGE. Tonsils enlarged, grade II, with no inflammation or pus point. Neck supple. Heart and lungs negative. Abdomen soft, liver and spleen not palpable. No malformation of extremities. Hemoglobin, 11 gm%; RBC, 4M/mm³; WBC, 3,900/mm³; polymorphs, 70%; lymphocytes, 30%. Urinalysis: protein, (++); WBC/RBC, 3-5/hpf. No cast. ESR,

33 mm/hr; LE cell, (-).

INSPECTION OF TONGUE: Purplish tongue proper with thin, yellowish coating.

PULSE CONDITION: Slippery, rapid and forced.

MODERN MEDICINE DIAGNOSIS: Systemic Lupus Erythematosus (SLE).

TRADITIONAL CHINESE MEDICINE DIAGNOSIS: Qi-Xue Liang Feng Zheng.

THERAPEUTIC PRINCIPLES: Cool the Blood and clear away the Heat, promote Blood circulation and remove stasis.

PRESCRIPTION: Qi-Xue Liang Feng Tang. Radix rehmanniae, 30 gm; Radix Scrophulariae, 9 gm; Radix paeoniae alba, 12 gm; Gypsum fibrosum, 30 gm; Flos lonicerae, 12 gm; Fructus arctii, 9 gm; Herba schizonepetae, 9 gm; Radix ledebouriellae, 9 gm; Rhizoma imperatae, 30 gm; Rhizoma anemarrhae, 3 gm; Radix glycyrrhizae, 6 gm; Radix angelicae, 9 gm; and Flos carthami, 9 gm. Decocted and taken once daily.

FOLLOW-UP/COURSE OF TREATMENT:

Second consultation on January 17, 1975: Fever subsided after taking six doses of this prescription. Erythema on the face became dark red in colour. Arthralgia relieved, though the patient still complained of general weakness. Pulse slippery and red colour on the sides of the tongue. Shugan Huoxue Tang was prescribed. Radix bupleuri, 9 gm; Herba menthae, 6 gm; Fructus gardeniae, 9 gm; Radix scutellariae, 9 gm; Radix angelicae, 9 gm; Flos carthami, 9 gm; Radix paeoniae, 9 gm; Rhizoma zedoariae, 9 gm; Pericarpium citri reticulatae, 9 gm; Radix glycyrrhizae, 6 gm; Flos lonicerae, 9 gm; and Fructus forsythiae, 9 gm. Decocted and taken once daily.

Third consultation on January 23, 1975: Eruptions on the face diminished markedly. Amenorrheic for two months. Pulse deep and small. Tongue pale in colour with minimal fur. Additional herbs for the prescription: Radix salviae, Rhizoma atractylodis macrocephalae and Poria.

Fourth consultation on March 1, 1975: Treatment continued. Menstruation reappeared in mid-February 1975. Eruptions on the face had disappeared completely. General condition was fair. Continued administration of the prescription. The patient was admitted to study in school.

Fifth consultation on June 1, 1975: Itchy erythema on the face appeared after exposure to sunlight. Low-grade fever (37.5°C-38°C) was noted and the patient complained of weakness. Urine protein (++). WBC: 2-3/hpf; ESR, 30 mm/hr. Pulse taut and tongue proper red with yellow coating. Shugan Huoxue Tang prescribed for 30 days and all symptoms disappeared. Routine urinalysis negative. ESR, 10 mm/hr.

The patient was followed-up by mail in February 1978. Her condition was well except that her menstruation cycle was delayed for one to two weeks.

DISCUSSION: SLE is a disease difficult to treat. We have reported 42 cases of subacute SLE treated by traditional Chinese medicine, 80% of which obtained favourable therapeutic outcomes. The usual prescription used is Modified Shugan Huoxue Tang. For this particular case, the patient was treated initially with Qi-Xue Liang Feng Tang, which was able to obtain a satisfactory result. Shugan Huoxue Tang was prescribed after the high fever subsided and was also able to obtain a satisfactory outcome.

Experimental studies on the effects of Shugan Huoxue Tang prescription on mice have been reported by the author. It has been shown that these herbs are effective in inhibiting testosterone and increasing the activity of stilbestrol. It is a well-known fact that SLE is a disease of the young female and that imbalance of hormonal levels could be one of the causes of SLE. Shugan Huoxue Tang prescription is effective in treating SLE probably through its action in regulating the balance and equilibrium of sexual hormones.

8.13 SYSTEMIC LUPUS ERYTHEMATOSUS (DEFICIENCY IN YIN OF THE KIDNEY)

Qin Wanzhan and Gu Wenzhen
Zhongshan Hospital, Shanghai Medical University, Shanghai

Zhang Xuezhen, 37, female, Han nationality, married, teacher. Medical record number: 87-5324. Date of first consultation: April 25, 1987.
CHIEF COMPLAINT: Fever, skin lesions and joint pain of three months duration.
HISTORY OF PRESENT ILLNESS: Erythema occurred on and off during the three-month period prior to consultation. Low-grade fever was a common accompanying sign. High-grade fever was rarely seen. General joint pain was serious, especially in the shoulders, knees, waist and back. Weakness, dizziness and tinnitus, flushed face, sensation of heat felt in the chest, palms and soles, thirst and preference for cold food, pain in the heels, insomnia, darkened urine colour, constipation, shortening of menstruation period and alopecia were often present. She was diagnosed as having connective tissue disease in a hospital and treated by both modern (e.g., antibiotics and indomethacine) and traditional Chinese medicine, but the treatments were not effective. Skin lesions of the face aggravated after exposure to sunlight two weeks ago. Joint pain became worse and swelling appeared on the eyelids and lower extremities, with dull pain felt on the hepatic region. The patient thus consulted our clinic.
PAST HISTORY: Episodes of fainting; positive history of PTB cured by Rimifon regimen.
FAMILY HISTORY: Mother suffered from Sjorgren's syndrome and sister from Raynaud's disease.
PERTINENT PHYSICAL EXAMINATION & LABORATORY FINDINGS: Oral temperature, 37.6°C; butterfly erythema marking evident on the face. Puffy swelling of the eyelids and edema of the lower extremities. Erythema multiforme on the back of her hands. Cervical lymph nodes enlarged and tender. Leukocyte count, 4,000/mm^3; RBC, 3M/mm^3. Routine urinalysis: urinary protein (++), WBC: 1-2/hpf; 24-hour urinary protein 2.35 gm. ESR, 35 mm/hr. Serum antinuclear antibody titer was positive and at dilution of ›1:1280. Anti-dsDNA, Sm and rheumatoid factor (RF) antibody tier and lupus erythematosus (LE) cells positive; Serum γ-globulin, 26.5 gm/dl; hemolytic complement, 3.55 u/ml; and IgG, 2,600 mg%. Circulating immune complex (CIC):

0.081. Hepatic function test: ZnT, 20 u. Electrocardiogram and chest X-ray findings essentially normal.

INSPECTION OF TONGUE: Red tongue edge and tip, fine cracks on the body.

PULSE CONDITION: Thready and rapid, and faint in the cubit place.

MODERN MEDICINE DIAGNOSIS: Systemic Lupus Erythematosus.

TRADITIONAL CHINESE MEDICINE DIAGNOSIS: Deficiency of Kidney Yin.

THERAPEUTIC PRINCIPLES: Tonify the Kidney and nourish Yin, remove toxic Heat.

PRESCRIPTION: Modified Luiwei-Dihuang Pill and Zhengyi Tang. Radix ophio-pogonis, 15 gm; Fructus ligustri lucidi, 15 gm; Cortex moutan radicis 12 gm; Rhizoma anemarrhenae, 9 gm; Fructus corni, 15 gm; Tripterygium wilfordii Hook, 20 gm; Caulis sargentodocuae, 20 gm; Rhizoma alismatis, 9 gm; and Radix glycyrrhizae, 3 gm. Decocted in water and taken twice a day. Cream triamcinole was used externally on the face and the handbacks, twice a day. Corticosteroid was not taken orally.

FOLLOW-UP/COURSE OF TREATMENT:

Second consultation: Fever and joint pain improved after two weeks of medication. Cervical lymph node sizes diminished. Skin lesions began to subside. Weakness still evident. Red tongue tip with white and thin fur, pulse soft and weak in the cubit place. The patient continued to take the prescription with the addition of Radix astragali.

Third consultation: Swelling on the eyelids and lower extremities had gone down after one month of treatment. Skin lesions subsided gradually, which can now be seen as areas of slight hyperpigmentation. Symptoms of weakness, dizziness, flushed face, tinnitus and sleeplessness were partially alleviated. Joint pain had disappeared. Urinary protein had decreased to (+) and WBC increased to 5,000/mm³. ESR, 16 mm/hr. No LE cells were found. Continued administration of the same prescription.

Fourth consultation: After eight weeks of medication, all symptoms had disappeared except for sensation of heat felt in the palms. Physical signs and results of laboratory findings had also improved. Lymph nodes were not palpable in cervical and axillary regions. Skin lesions had almost completely regressed except some areas of slight hyperpigmentation. Inspection of the tongue and pulse showed no abnormality. Routine urinalysis negative. RBC, 3M/mm³, ESR, 12 mm/hr; serum ANA titer had declined to 1:64; serum ds-DNA, Sm antibody and RF negative. No LE cells were found. γ-globulin, 21.2%; ZnT, 12 u; IgG, 1,600 mg%. Hemolytic complement 80 units/ml. Prescription was replaced by 6 gm of Pills of Six Drugs with Rehmanniae, twice a day.

Fifth consultation: The patient was followed-up six months later. Her condition was stable. Pills of Six Drugs with Rehmanniae and TWHF Syrup were taken intermittently. She was engaged in full-time work.

DISCUSSION: This was a case of a middle-aged woman, sensitive to sunlight with joint pain, butterfly erythema and enlarged lymph nodes. Hepatic and renal functions were impaired and RBC and WBC counts had decreased. ESR was noted to have increased while CIC and IgG, ANA, ds-DNA and Sm antibody titers had elevated and C3 decreased. She was tested positive for LE cells and RF. A diagnosis of systemic lupus erythematosus was thus established.

Symptom-complex differentiation: There is a positive family history of connective tissue disease; the patient's mother suffers from Sjorgren's syndrome and her sister from Raynaud's disease. The patient herself has a positive history of pulmonary tuberculosis. This is due to a congenital defect. When first seen, the patient was weak due to a protracted course of the disease, with accompanying signs and symptoms such as menstrual disturbance, alopecia, tinnitus, pain in heels and faint pulse in the cubit place. These all indicated deficiency of the Kidney. Additional findings, such as flushed face, sensation of heat felt in the chest, palms and soles, thirst and preference for cold food, darkened urine colour with increased frequency and decreased amount, constipation, red skin lesions, reddened tongue edge and tip with fine cracks and thready and rapid pulse, further indicated the presence of Kidney Yin deficiency.

Pathogenesis and Etiology: SLE is a representative entity of auto-immune diseases. It manifests many immune abnormalities. Presence of auto-antibodies, such as LE cells, RF, ds-DNA, Sm, ANA, CIC, etc., indicates that SLE is a disease of immune disturbance, though its definitive etiology is still unknown. Genetic and endocrinological elements have been considered contributing factors. Taking into consideration the theories of traditional Chinese medicine, we believe it to be basically a disturbance of the Kidney as evidenced by the waxing and waning of Kidney Yin and Yang during the course of the disease. The main clinical manifestation of this case is exuberance of Yang due to deficiency of Yin. A vicious cycle is thus formed with Yang exuberance leading to Yin deficiency and Yin deficiency further causing the Yang exuberance. Fundamentally, deficiency of Yin is the trigger of this vicious cycle and exuberance of Yang its manifestation. Such a pathogenesis could be endocrine in nature. Disturbance of Kidney Yin was established based on symptom-complex differentiation as well as the patient's positive history of pulmonary tuberculosis and positive family history of connective tissue disease. The long course of the disease and positive family history point to the influence of congenital defects and could also be considered the pathogenesis of SLE. In TCM teaching, Kidney is the essence of life. When Kidney is consumed, Yin deficiency accompanied by flaring up of Evil-Fire leads to accumulation of internal Heat manifesting itself in a clinical pathology, such as SLE.

Treatment: As analyzed by symptom-complex differentiation, the patient presented typical symptoms of Kidney Yin deficiency. The main vehicle of treatment was Pills of Six Drugs with Rehmanniae plus other secretion-promoting decoctions which tonify the Kidney and nourish Yin. Large doses of Radix rehmanniae, Radix scrophulariae and Radix ophiopogonis were used to nourish the Yin and remove toxic Heat. Dogwood fruit, Rhizoma anemarrhenae, Unci ligustrum fruit, Cortex moutan and Rhizoma alismatis were used to tonify the Kidney, nourish the Yin and dispel pathogenic Heat from the Blood. In addition, one major clinical manifestation of SLE is vasculitis. Experimental and clinical studies have shown that the Chinese herb TWHF and Caulis sargentodoxue (CRS) have anti-inflammatory and immunity-enhancing properties. Accordingly, TWHF and CRS, which remove toxic Heat and eliminate inflammation and swelling, were also used in the treatment of this case. The decoction was administered orally as well as applied externally. Pronounced therapeutic effects were obtained by integrating traditional Chinese and modern medicine in treating systemically and externally both the symptoms and the cause of the disease.

8.14 SYSTEMIC SCLERODERMATOSIS (XUEYU ZHENG)

Bian Tianyu and Ding Suxian

Dermatological Institute of Integrated Traditional Chinese
and Western Medicine, Tianjin Changzheng Hospital, Tianjin

Chang, 39, male, Han nationality, married, cadre. Medical record number: 93141.
Date of admission: June 9, 1978.

CHIEF COMPLAINT: Coldness of hands and feet, hardness of skin of the face and extremities for 18 months.

HISTORY OF PRESENT ILLNESS: In the winter of 1976, the patient began to experience cold sensation of hands and feet. The skin of his hands was pale to purplish and painful when exposed to cold. Gradually, the skin of his face and hands became edematous and was noted to have hardened. Similar changes occurred in the forearms, neck and chest. Deep respiration was found to be difficult. The condition improved in summer. Swallowing, appetite and general condition were normal. He had taken about 20 doses of the traditional Chinese drug Huoxue Huayu. There was no evident improvement.

PAST HISTORY: Non-contributory.

PERSONAL HISTORY: The patient is a smoker and lives in Inner Mongolia, where the average air temperature is -10°C in winter.

PERTINENT PHYSICAL EXAMINATION & LABORATORY FINDINGS: Development and nutritional status normal; face swollen, shiny, indurated and expressionless. Nose appeared sharp and pinched. The lips were thin, with difficulty in opening the mouth. Diffused involvement of skin over the hands, feet, arms, forearms, legs and chest noted, more severe on the hands and forearms. No pitting edema. No tenderness. The mobility of the fingers was limited and unable to close the hand completely. Heart and lung findings negative. Abdomen soft, liver and spleen not palpable. Hemoglobin, 13 gm%; RBC, 5.2M/mm³; WBC, 8,000/mm³; neutrophils, 70%; lymphocytes, 30%. Routine urinalysis negative. ESR, 7 mm/hr. Chest X-ray, ECG and UGIS negative.

INSPECTION OF TONGUE: Corpulent with little coat.

PULSE CONDITION: Slippery.

MODERN MEDICINE DIAGNOSIS: Systemic Sclerodermatosis.

TRADITIONAL CHINESE MEDICINE DIAGNOSIS: Xueyu Zheng.

THERAPEUTIC PRINCIPLES: Tonify the Spleen and Kidney, activated Blood circulation.

PRESCRIPTION: Radix astragali, 30 gm; Cortex cinnamomi, 10 gm; Ramulus cinnamomi, 10 gm; Radix aconiti praeparatae, 9 gm; Radix polygoni multiflori, 10 gm;

Caulis spatholobi, 24 gm; Rhizoma corydalis, 12 gm; Resina boswelliae carterii, 6 gm; Resina commiphorae, 6 gm; Herba lycopi, 24 gm; Flos lonicerae, 24 gm; Radix salviae, 21 gm; Radix bupleuri, 15 gm; Radix scrophulariae, 21 gm; and Radix curcumae, 12 gm. Decocted and taken once daily. Maodong Qing (Root of Hairy Flower Actinidia) ampule, 2 ml, IM once a day.

FOLLOW-UP/COURSE OF TREATMENT: Two weeks after treatment, the patient could feel that the extremities were becoming warm. Raynaud's sign diminished and the hardened skin began to soften and sweat reappeared. The therapeutic regimen was continued for about six months. The patient was discharged from hospital after the skin pathology had completely disappeared. The prescription was made into prepared form (pills) and administered for another several months.

The patient was contacted two years later by mail. No recurrence of symptoms.

DISCUSSION: Patients with systemic sclerodermatosis often complain of coldness, Raynaud's sign and hardened skin of hands, feet and face. This prescription was effective in treating the disease. Of course, other cases may not follow a similar clinical course and physicians-in-charge should prescribe the medications in accordance with the symptom-complex differentiation.

8.15 MIXED CONNECTIVE TISSUE DISEASE (DEFICIENCY OF KIDNEY YANG AND BLOOD STASIS)

Qin Wanzhang and Gu Wenzhen
Zhongshan Hospital, Shanghai Medical University, Shanghai

Zhu Jinmei, 45, female, Han nationality, married, worker. Medical record number: 84-5657. Date of first consultation: July 30, 1984.

CHIEF COMPLAINT: Joint pain, acrocyanosis for one and a half years.

HISTORY OF PRESENT ILLNESS: Joint pain first appeared in 1983, especially in large joints. There had been no redness and swelling. The fingers became white and violet when exposed to cold water and the patient experienced sensation of numbness. Symptoms aggravated gradually and developed progressively. Later, the fingers were constantly a violet discolouration and seldom recovered normal colouring. Initially, the symptoms were prominent only in winter seasons and later even in summer. The extremities were painful, the back of the hands and fingers swollen. Last year, she felt tightness in her face and pain on proximal muscles of all extremities. Since the onset of the disease, she often had low-grade fever, fatigue and difficulty in swallowing as well as spontaneous perspiration. She could not tolerate cold. There was also dull pain on the hepatic region and intermittent appearance of red nodules and petechiae on the lower extremities. Urine was normal and bowel movement loose. Her hair fell out easily. She was diagnosed as having a collagen disease. The therapeutic effect of indomethacin, long-action aspirin and chloroquine was not satisfactory. Her condition worsened recently.

PAST HISTORY: Frequent bouts of pneumonia and chilblain in winter. Menstruation period usually delayed. She had been amenorrheic since she was ill.

FAMILY HISTORY: Positive history of rheumatoid arthritis (father).

PERTINENT PHYSICAL EXAMINATION & LABORATORY FINDINGS: Pale, swelling and induration of the face and hands with tapered, sausage-like fingers. Pain and tenderness prominent at proximal muscles of the extremities and gastrocnemius muscle. More than 10 red, marble-sized nodules scattered on the lower extremities. Raynaud's phenomenon was severe. Lymph nodules the size of broad beans were palpable and tender in the axillary and inguinal regions. Liver palpable 2 cm below the right costal margin. The hair was sparse. CBC and routine urinalysis examination were normal. ESR, 26 mm/hr. ANA titer was positive and a speckled staining pattern was seen with a dilution of ⟩ 1:1280. Anti-dsDNA and Sm antibody titer negative. RNP antibody titer elevated significantly. Presence of LE cells positive. Serum γ-globulin level 30.2 mg/dl; IGG, 3,500 mg; IgA & IgM normal. CIC, 0.082. Hepatic function test: ZnT, 26 u. 24-hour urine creatine, 380 mg. Urinary 17-hydroxylsteroid, 4.6 mg. Barium meal fluoroscopy of esophagus suggested slow peristalsis. The electrocardiogram and chest X-ray negative.

INSPECTION OF TONGUE: Plump, soft, light-coloured tongue with slight violet discolouration; tooth marks seen at its borders.

PULSE CONDITION: Deep and slow, and faint in the cubit place.

MODERN MEDICINE DIAGNOSIS: Mixed Connective Tissue Disease (MCTD).

TRADITIONAL CHINESE MEDICINE DIAGNOSIS: Deficiency of Kidney Yang and Blood stasis.

THERAPEUTIC PRINCIPLES: Tonify the Kidney and invigorate Yang, activate the Blood circulation to eliminate Blood stasis.

PRESCRIPTION: Modified Two Xian Decoction and Prescription. Herba leonuri, 30 gm; Ramulus cinnamomi, 9 gm; Rhizoma curenliginis, 9 gm; Herba epimedii, 9 gm; Fructus psoralea, 9 gm; Chuanxiong rhizome, 9 gm; Herba cistanches, 9 gm; Cortex phellodendri, 9 gm; Tripterygium wilfordii Hood F, 15 gm; Caulis spatholobi, 30 gm; and Radix glycyrrhizae, 6 gm. Oral decoction, twice a day. Corticosteroid discontinued.

FOLLOW-UP/COURSE OF TREATMENT:

Second consultation: Joints and muscular pain alleviated after two weeks of treatment. Fatigue took a turn for the better. Her spirits improved. Pain on the hepatic region disappeared. Tightness of the face and hands ameliorated. There was no complaint of spontaneous perspiration. Lymph node size diminished. Frequency of Raynaud's phenomenon decreased. White, thin fur of the tongue. The deep fine pulse remained, as well as the weak pulse in the cubit place. Continued administration of the prescription.

Third consultation: Joint pain and Raynaud's phenomenon disappeared. Symptoms improved significantly after two months of treatment. Muscular tenderness was minimal in the extremities. Induration and swelling of the face and hands lessened. The face looked flushed. No difficulty in swallowing. Lymph nodes not palpable and red nodules disappeared from the lower extremities. LE cells rheumatoid factor (RF) detection negative. ESR declined to 14 mm/hour; serum ANA titer was positive with speckled pattern in a dilution of 1:160; IgG, 2,600 mg%. γ-globulin, 20%; ZnT, 12 u. 24-hour urine creatine, 80 mg. Urine 17-hydroxylsteroid, 8 mg. Tongue remained red and pulse soft. Medication was changed to Three Lianas Syrup (TLS) which composed of TWHF, Caulis spatholobi and Caulis et radix saegentodoxue instead of the past prescription; 10 ml of TLS was taken three times a day.

Fourth consultation: Induration and swelling of the face and hands disappeared after four months of treatment. Raynaud's phenomenon greatly diminished except when the patient came in contact with cold water; then, the hands turned white and felt numb. There was no cyanosis. Her general condition was good. Serum anti-RNP antibody was slightly positive. Thin and white fur on the tongue with strong pulse. TLS was taken intermittently.

Fifth consultation: The patient was checked in May 1985. Joint pain seldom occurred. Her general condition was stable and well. She was engaged in normal work.

DISCUSSION:

Diagnosis and Symptom-complex differentiation: MCTD was first noticed in the 70's. It represents an overlap of collagen diseases. This entity is characterized by symptoms mimicking those of systemic lupus erythematosus (SLE), scleroderma and dermatomyositis or polymyositis, but none of them can be diagnosed independently as a single disease entity. Raynaud's phenomenon, arthralgia or arthritis, swelling of the hands and face and sausage-like fingers are distinctive symptoms. Renal involvement is rarely seen or only to a mild degree when present. Immune-serology revealed positive fluorescent ANA test with a speckled staining pattern. All MCTD patients have high titers of RNP while Sm antibody test remained negative. Diagnosis of MCTD was established in this particular case. Signs and symptoms in this case which indicate Deficiency of Kidney Yang were mid-section pain, alopecia, menstruation disturbance, faint pulse in the cubit place, plump, soft, light-coloured tongue, decreased 24-hour urine 17-hydroxylsteroid level, intolerance to cold, cold sensation on the extremities, spontaneous perspiration and loose bowel movement. Signs pertaining to Blood stasis were Raynaud's phenomenon, violet discolouration of the tongue, swelling and induration of the face and hands, enlarged lymph nodes and petechiae on the lower extremities, digital and hepatic region pain, and hepatomegaly. In the past 10 years, this clinic has seen 65 cases of MCTD manifesting signs and symptoms congruent with Deficiency of Kidney Yang and Blood stasis.

Treatment: Since MCTD patients are usually deficient in Yang and have Blood stasis, the therapeutic principles would naturally be to tonify the Kidney, invigorate Yang and activate the Blood circulation to eliminate Blood stasis. Two Xian Decoction, a product of our research prepared in our clinic which possesses properties to activate Blood circulation, was the main vehicle of treatment. Satisfactory therapeutic effects have been obtained based on TCM symptom-complex differentiation. Curculigo rhizome, Epidemdium, Herba cistanches and Psoralea fruit are used to tonify the Kidney and invigorate Yang; Motherwort, Chuanxiong rhizome, Red age root and Ramulus cinnamomi are used to nourish and activate the Blood to communicate with Yang; while Caulis spatholobi and Phellodendrom bark nourish the Blood to relieve symptoms of dryness.

MCTD is a typical representation of auto-immune diseases. Several positive antibody detection and immunological abnormalities were seen in this case. TLS, a compound prescription prepared by our clinic, controlled inflammation and regulated swelling. It is our belief that, in MCTD cases, prescriptions effective in activating Blood circulation and invigorating Yang can be used in place of corticosteroids as a mode of treatment. Satisfactory and long-lasting remission can be achieved this way.

8.16 ANKYLOSING SPONDYLITIS (STUBBORN ARTHRALGIA)

Zhao Runlai, Qi Yan and Wei Beihai
Beijing Traditional Chinese Medicine Hospital, Beijing

Yan, 35, male, married, cadre. Date of first consultation: April 19, 1986.

CHIEF COMPLAINT: Intermittent lumbosacral pain and stabbing pain in the neck associated with limited movement of the spine and extremities of 10 years duration.

HISTORY OF PRESENT ILLNESS: In winter of 1971, the patient's knee joints suddenly developed sharp pain. He was treated as a case of "acute rheumatic fever" in hospital. Treatment then afforded him relief from the symptoms. Two years later, he felt stiffness in the lumbosacral region, backache and limited spine movement. A diagnosis of "rheumatoid spondylitis" was given based on X-ray analysis of the lumbar and sacroiliac joints. The patient received treatment in the forms of antirheumatics, herbal medicine, acupuncture and massage, but no satisfactory result was achieved. In July of 1985, the condition worsened with severe neck pain and limitation of spine movement. Temporary relief was obtained when he was given dexamethasone. The dosage needed to continue to afford relief had to be steadily increased, and side effects started to appear.

At the time of present consultation, the patient complained of persistent stabbing pain in his spine and limited movement, more marked in the cervical and lumbar sections. General fatigue, sweating and morning stiffness were pronounced. His face and back were fat and hirsute. Condition usually exacerbated during nighttime and cold weather. The daily requirement of dexamethasone now was 0.75 mg x 6 together with nine tablets of tripterygium hypoglaucum. His right ankle was swollen. The condition had progressed to such an extent that the pain was too severe to bear and he was unable to care for himself.

PERTINENT PHYSICAL EXAMINATION & LABORATORY FINDINGS: Temperature, 36°C; blood pressure, 130/70 mmHg. Lethargic, chronic, morbid facies; moon-shaped face and buffalo back. Passive posture. No jaundice. No enlarged superficial lymph nodes. Head normal. Chest flat, expansion in the fourth intercostal space was 2.5 cm. Heart and lung negative. Abdomen soft, liver and spleen not palpable. Loss of physiological spine curvature with arch-shaped deformation and limited movement. Internal and external rotation of both iliac joints limited. Movement of the extremities passive. Right ankle swollen, no callus but tender.

Cervical (C1-C7) X-ray showed calcification of the lower cervical paravertebral ligament without changes in the intervertebral space and the physiological curvature. Thoracolumbar (T7-L3) X-ray showed calcification of the paravertebral ligaments and a bamboo-shaped spinal column. The physiological curvature flattened with blurring of the intervertebral facets. Osteoporotic changes of the vertebrae. Pelvic X-ray showed fusion of both the sacroiliac joint spaces with small transparent areas in the sacrum.

RBC, 4.07M/mm^3; hemoglobin, 13.3 gm%; WBC, 11,300/mm^3; neutrophils, 84%; lymphocytes, 16%. ESR, 60 mm/hr, RF, (-). Immunoglobulin normal. ECG normal. HLA-B27 (+).

INSPECTION OF TONGUE: Enlarged and dark tongue with white, thin coating.

PULSE CONDITION: Deep and fine.

MODERN MEDICINE DIAGNOSIS: Ankylosing Spondylitis.

TRADITIONAL CHINESE MEDICINE DIAGNOSIS: Wan Bi (Stubborn Arthralgia).

Symptom-complex differentiation: Insufficiency of Kidney Essence; stagnation of Phlegm and Blood.

THERAPEUTIC PRINCIPLES: Replenish Essence to tonify Kidney, relieve pain by dissolving Phlegm and remove Blood stasis and obstruction of the Channels.

PRESCRIPTION: Rhizoma cibotii, 30 gm; Semen cuscutae, 45 gm; Radix dipsacii, 45 gm; Rhizoma drynariae, 30 gm; Radix rehmanniae praeparatae, 60 gm; Radix paeoniae alba, 30 gm; Radix paeoniae rubra, 30 gm; Radix angelicae sinensis, 45 gm; Olibanum, 30 gm; Resina commiphorae myrrhae, 30 gm; Agkistrodon, 30 gm; Squama manitis, 30 gm; Spina gleditsiae, 45 gm; Semen sinapis alba, 30 gm; Hirudo, 30 gm; Scolopendra, 20 pieces; Colla cornus cervi, 30 gm; Colla plastri testudinis, 30 gm; and appropriate amount of pig spinal cord. Ground ingredients into powder and mixed with honey; made into 10 gm pellets. One pellet twice a day. Maintained the dosage of dexamethasone. The patient was asked to follow this therapeutic regimen for two months.

FOLLOW-UP/COURSE OF TREATMENT:

Second consultation on September 17, 1986: Marked improvement was observed with amelioration of pain and increasing freedom of spinal movement. Stiffness and soreness in the mid-section still present. ESR, 18 mm/hr. Dosage of dexamethasone was 0.75 mg × 4 daily and was reduced progressively. Tripterygium hypoglaucum discontinued.

Third consultation on January 11, 1987: Further improvement observed. Pellets were continued. Dexamethasone was on its maintenance dose (0.75 mg daily). No pain or other discomfort was noticed. Spinal movement tended to be normal. The patient was able to move actively. Swelling and tenderness had disappeared from his right ankle. Signs of moon-shaped face and buffalo back were remitting. The patient was vigorous and had a good appetite and enjoyed normal sleep. He was able to go back to work.

Fourth consultation on May 24, 1987: Disappearance of moon-shaped face and buffalo back and absence of discomfort made him a healthy person again. Mild soreness along the spinal column felt only during weather changes. X-ray film of the spinal column showed no deterioration from previous examination. ESR, 15 mm/hr. The patient was advised to take the pellets for another two months, then discontinue dexamethasone.

Follow-up on March, 1988: Medications discontinued. The patient was able to work without any discomfort.

DISCUSSION: Ankylosing spondylitis is a chronic progressive disease of the joints involving mainly the spinal column. It manifests clinically as pain and deformation of the spine. The involved joints tend to develop stiffness. It was categorized into arthralgia in traditional Chinese medicine and is closely related to the Bone and Kidney according to TCM teachings.

The Kidney stores the essence of life and dominates the bones. Kidney essence is of highest importance in promoting growth and development. If the bones are filled and nourished by marrow produced and supplied by the Kidney, then the functional activity of the bones and muscles can be well maintained.

The onset of this disease is usually characterized by lumbosacral pain and stiffness. As the disease progresses, it advances in a cephalad direction to the thoracic and cervical vertebrae. Movement of the back becomes limited. The waist is the residence of the Kidney and the Du Channel passes along the spine upward to the top of the head. Insufficiency of Kidney essence leads to emptiness of the Du Channel. Pain in the spinal cord caused by obstruction of the Channels is often associated with invading exogenous evils, trauma and fatigue. Wind, Cold and noxious Dampness prevail while body resistance weakens. Joints, muscles and bones are compromised because the stagnation prevents them from being nourished properly, i.e., Blood and Phlegm in the Channels. TCM theory believes that "emaciated patients must be treated with Qi-tonifying herbs to promote digestion; patients with deficiency of essence should be treated with animal or plant food or herbs rich in nutrients." Using "flesh and blood" food to nourish the body and "insect and ant" medications to search out the evil in the body, we treated the case with medications which strengthen the body resistance and dredge the stagnated Channels.

During the course of treatment, Radix rehmanniae praeparatae, Colla plastri testudinis, Rhizoma cibotii, Semen cuscutae, Radix dipsaciae and Rhizoma drynariae were used to tonify the Liver and Kidney and strengthen the muscles and bones; Radix paeoniae, Radix rehmanniae praeparatae and Radix angelicae sinensis to enrich the Blood; and Agkistrodon, Squama manitis, Scolopendra and Hirudo to dispel Blood stasis and promote the Channels. In addition, pig spinal cord was used to supplement the marrow and nourish the Kidney essence. Colla cornus cervi not only nourished the Kidney essence but also tonified the Du Channel.

Genetic factors, infection and auto-immunity are thought to be contributory to the pathogenesis of ankylosing spondylitis. Ankylosing spondylitis is a chronic inflammatory disease involving primarily the sacroiliac and apophyseal joints, intervertebral ligaments and tendovaginae. Adjacent cartilages and bones might also be destroyed with the formation of new bones. To date, there is no treatment of choice in modern medicine to effectively control the disease. Non-steroid, anti-inflammatory drugs are the drugs of choice to relieve pain. In unresponsive cases, analgesia can be afforded by corticosteroids, which, however, often cause severe and adverse side effects.

Chinese herbal medicine is of great importance in treating this disease. Herbs for replenishing Kidney essence can raise body resistance, promote metabolism, regulate the immune system and correct the adverse reactions to corticosteroids. Radix angelicae sinensis, Radix paeoniae, Hirudo, Scolopendra and Agkistrodon promote Blood circulation and disperse inflammation. Colla cornus cervi, which contains a large amount of ossein and Ca^{++}, plays an important role in preventing bone destruction. Therefore, this comprehensive approach consisting of replenishing Kidney essence, regulating the Du Channel and relieving pain by dispelling Blood stasis and Channel obstruction was obviously an effective therapeutic regimen.

8.17 OSTEOMYELITIS OF THE LEFT PHALANGES AND METATARSAL
(FU GU JU, ACCUMULATION OF DAMP-HEAT AND BLOOD STASIS)

Guo Saishan

Department of Traditional Chinese Medicine, Peking Union
Medical College Hospital, Beijing

Li Changfu, 24, male, Han nationality, single, worker. Medical record number: C-372400. Date of first consultation: March 11, 1987.

CHIEF COMPLAINT: Redness, swelling and pain on the left index and middle fingers and the left first toe, accompanied by fever for two months.

HISTORY OF PRESENT ILLNESS: About two months prior to consultation, the patient's left index finger was injured by a big hammer. Without special care, the injured finger seemed recovered when the patient had high fever abruptly, with body temperature ranging from 39.6°C-40°C, and peripheral WBC count of 14,100-18,900/mm³, PMN, 90%. Redness, swelling, hot sensation and pain radiated from the left index and middle fingers to the dorsum of the left hand, wrist and forearm and even to the first toe of the left foot. He was diagnosed as having skin inflammation and was treated with TMPco, penicillin, gentamycin and Medemycin for one month and physical therapy for half a month. Body temperature was decreased to 37.5°C, and swelling of the forearm had disappeared. X-ray examination on March 5, 1987, indicated osteomyelitis.

PERTINENT PHYSICAL EXAMINATION & LABORATORY FINDINGS: Redness, swelling, calor and pain on the left index and middle fingers, metacarpophalangeal joints, dorsum of the left hand and left first toe and the metatarsophalangeal joint. There was limitation of joint movements. The patient lost appetite and had dry stools. X-ray examinations of the left hand and left foot were done on February 25 and March 5. Result: irregular blurring shape of the second and third distal phalanges. Sequestrum was seen. Soft tissues with fusiform swelling. The distal part of the first metatarsal of the left foot had regional bony lesions penetrating the metatarsophalangeal joint and medial cortex. There was periosteal proliferation. Soft tissue swollen.

INSPECTION OF TONGUE: Dark red tongue with yellowish, greasy fur.

PULSE CONDITION: String-like and slippery.

MODERN MEDICINE DIAGNOSIS: Osteomyelitis of the Second and Third Distal Phalanges of the Left Hand; Osteomyelitis on the First Metatarsal of the Left Foot.

TRADITIONAL CHINESE MEDICINE DIAGNOSIS: Fu Gu Ju (Pyogenic Infection of the Bone); Accumulation of Damp-Heat and Blood Stasis.

THERAPEUTIC PRINCIPLES: Remove Heat and toxic materials, remove Dampness and invigorate the Spleen, remove Blood stasis and clear Heat from the Blood.

PRESCRIPTION: Flos lonicerae, 15 gm; Fructus forsythiae, 12 gm; Radix scutellariae, 10 gm; Rhizoma polygoni cuspidati, 30 gm; Rhizoma atractylodis, 10 gm; Cortex phellodendri, 10 gm; Semen coicis, 30 gm; Rhizoma pinellinae, 10 gm; Cortex moutan radicis, 10 gm; Radix paeoniae rubra, 15 gm; Semen persicae, 10 gm; Flos carthami, 10 gm; Scorpio, 4 gm; Ramulus mori, 30 gm; Radix achyranthis bidentatae, 10 gm; and Rhizoma corydalis, 10 gm. Twelve doses.

FOLLOW-UP/COURSE OF TREATMENT:

Second consultation: After twelve doses, the swelling on the dorsum of the left hand had disappeared. There was atrophy of the intermetacarpal muscles. Appetite was getting better. Regular urination and bowel movement. Red tongue tip, and small, string-like pulse. Continued the first prescription adding Radix astragali, 25 gm, and Endothelium corneum gigeriae galli, 10 gm; 20 to 40 doses.

Third consultation and X-ray follow-up on May 13, 1987: After two months and administration of 40 doses, the swelling on the left index and middle fingers and the left first metatarsophalangeal joint had disappeared. Slight tenderness and partial limitation of interphalangeal joint movement had remained. Appetite getting better. Regular urination and bowel movement. X-ray follow-up: Marked repair of bony lesions, especially on the distal phalanges of the left hand, with thin and regular-shaped cortex. Sequestrum and soft tissue swelling had disappeared. Bony lesion on the first metatarsal of the left foot diminishing. Red tongue tip with thin whitish fur. Continued taking the prescription.

Follow-up on August 20, 1987: After three months and administration of 60 doses, the patient's condition was getting better. There was no limitation of movement. Feeling of slight pain in the left hand. X-ray examination: Osteomyelitis of the second and third phalanges of the left hand had completely recovered. No marked change on the first metatarsal bone of the left foot. Red tongue tip with whitish, greasy fur and string-like, slippery pulse. Continued the prescription adding Semen cuscutae, 15 gm, Fructus ligustri lucidi, 15 gm, and Ramulus taxilli, 30 gm. The patient was required to exercise his finger joints.

Follow-up on December 17, 1987: Another three months and 60 doses administered. No limitation of movement. No pain in the left hand but slight pain in the left foot. General condition was good. X-ray examination: marked repair of lesion on the cortex of the first metatarsal cortex. Dark red tongue with thin, yellowish, greasy fur. Pulse string-like and slippery, sunken and small on the left side. Continued the prescription adding Fructus lycii, 15 gm, and changed the dosage of Radix astragali from 25 gm to 15 gm. Pulverized eight recipes together, mixed with honey and made into 10 gm pills; two to three pills per day.

By May 10, 1988, the patient had been taking the prescription for five months. There was no limitation of movement, no swelling and no pain on the index and middle fingers of the left hand and the first toe of the left foot. X-ray examination: Cortex complete with increased and identical bony density, trabecula reconstructed though the blurred line on the margin of the medulla and cortex remained. Repair of the bony lesion and reconstruction of the cortex on the first metatarsal of the left foot almost completed. Red tongue with thin, whitish, fur. Slippery pulse. Continued the same treatment. Pulverized four recipes together, mixed with honey and made into 10-gm pills; two to three pills per day.

DISCUSSION: According to TCM teachings, the characteristics of Fu Gu Ju (pyogenic infection of the bone) represent an invasion of exogenous toxic pathogens of Damp-Heat during injury and accumulation of Wind-Cold-Dampness in tendons and bones. There are two kinds of Fu Gu Ju, one involves injury by Damp-Heat, the other by Wind-Cold-Dampness evil.

Our case was one of hand injury attacked by toxic evil. The toxic Heat evil invaded the interior of the body and stayed on in the tendons and bones causing obstruction of the Channels, stagnation of the Vital Energy, stasis of Blood and accumulation of Damp-Heat evils which eventually led to erosion of the tendons and bones. Clinically, this condition manifested itself as bony lesions and formation of sequestrum on the second and third phalanges of the left hand and the first metatarsal of the left foot and soft tissue swelling. The patient had symptoms of redness, swelling, calor, pain and limitation of movement. The tongue was dark red with yellowish, greasy fur. Stagnation of Damp-Heat evil in the gastrointestinal tract caused loss of appetite and dry bowels. Symptom-complex differentiation indicated Fu Gu Ju (osteomyelitis) and accumulation of Damp-Heat and Blood stasis. The principle of treatment was to remove Heat and toxic materials, remove Dampness and invigorate the Spleen and remove Blood stasis and Heat from the Blood. In the prescription given, Flos lonicerae, Cortex phellodendri, Fructus forsythiae, Radix scutellariae and Rhizoma polygoni supidati removed Heat and toxic materials, removed Dampness with herbs bitter in taste and cold in nature and removed Blood stasis and dredged the Channels; Rhizoma atractylodis, Rhizoma pinellinae and Semen coicis were used as supplements in removing Dampness and together with herbs bitter in taste and warm in nature invigorated the Spleen and promoted diuresis to reduce fluid retention and edema. In addition, Semen persicae, Flos carthami, Scorpio, Cortex moutan radicis, Radix paeoniae rubra, Ramulus mori and Rhizoma corydalis were used to remove Blood stasis and Heat from the Blood, to dredge the Channels and to reduce edema. This prescription assembles a powerful spectrum of antibiotic herbs like Flos lonicerae, Fructus forsythiae, Rhizoma polygoni cuspidati, Radix scutellariae, Cortex phellodendri, Cortex moutan radicis and Radix paeoniae rubra. Among them, Radix scutellariae is very effective against penicillin-resistant staphylococci. This could be the key ingredient of the prescription.

Furthermore, some of the herbs are capable of removing Blood stasis, dredging the Channels, reducing edema and promoting tissue regeneration. They play a role in improving blood circulation of the bones and soft tissue, nourishing the bone tissue, promoting the repair of bony lesions and resolving the sequestrum, as well as reducing edema and alleviating pain. When evil Heat and toxic pathogens were removed, Radix astragali and Endothelium corneum gigeriae galli were added to supplement the Vital Energy and to invigorate the Spleen, accompanied by other herbs to activate Blood circulation, strengthen bones and tendons, support the healthy energy and eliminate the evil factors. It was only after two months of treatment that X-ray examination showed a marked repair of bony lesions and disappearance of sequestrum. Such a clinical course was considered too slow for the repair of the left first metatarsal. Since the Kidney controls the bone and nourishes the bone marrow as well as controls the Lower Burner, Semen cuscutae, Fructus ligustri lucidi and Ramulus tacilli were added to tonify the Kidney and strengthen the bones. This was followed by a remarkable repair of the first toe of the left foot.

8.18 THROMBOANGIITIS OBLITERANS (TUO ZHU, GANGRENE)

Zhao Runlai, Zhen Xuejun and Wei Beihai
Beijing Traditional Chinese Medicine Hospital, Beijing

Xu, male, single, peasant. First consultation on May 14, 1984.

CHIEF COMPLAINT: Necrotic ulcer of the right big toe with severe pain for the past 40 days.

HISTORY OF PRESENT ILLNESS: This condition began in winter of 1979. The patient felt cold and tense in the left lower extremity, sometimes with spasms. Intermittent claudication was noted. Tachogram showed that he suffered from thromboangiitis obliterans. The condition was essentially put under control after treatment. Last winter, similar condition was detected on the right lower extremity. Tip of toes became purple with intermittent claudication. He failed to respond to medical treatment and condition worsened abruptly 40 days ago. On examination, his right foot was swollen, dark purplish in colour with a black, festered big toe. Because of severe pain, he groaned a lot. He was not able to take any gainful sleep. The patient smoked 15 to 20 cigarettes a day for the past nine years and was exposed to prolonged cold two years ago.

PERTINENT PHYSICAL EXAMINATION & LABORATORY FINDINGS: Sallow complexion, emaciated with agonizing expression and restless. Tongue red with normal coating. Pulse rapid and fine. No enlarged lymph nodes. Chest and abdomen findings negative. He walked with the aid of two walking sticks.

Local Signs:

	LEFT SIDE	RIGHT SIDE
Leg circumference	29 cm	27.5 cm
Skin colour	White toe tip	Purple dorsum and toe tip
Trophic condition	Dry skin, scanty capillary hair	Loose calf, dry and rough skin, loss of hair
Toe nail	Hypertrophy, uneven	Hypertrophy with ridge
Dorsal pulse	(++) weak	(-) not palpable
Post pulse	(+) very weak	(-) not palpable
Gangrene	(-)	Gangrene of big toe with fetid, dirty secretion, exposed toe and tendon, sinus formation, six live maggots were picked out
Postural test of extremities	(±)	(±)
Time of reddening on dependency	30"	60"
Engorgement time of toe venous plexus by pressing	3"	5"
Tachogram	Lowered elasticity and insufficiency	= 0.26" = 0.25 D lost Difference of amplitude 65%

MODERN MEDICINE DIAGNOSIS: Thromboangiitis Obliterans with Gangrene; Left Leg: Stage II; Right Leg: Stage III.

TRADITIONAL CHINESE MEDICINE DIAGNOSIS: Tao Zhu (Gangrene).

Symptom-complex differentiation: Long-standing vascular obliteration, interior Heat produced by stagnation, extreme noxious Heat consuming the essence and damaging the vessels and bone.

THERAPEUTIC PRINCIPLES: Nourish the Vital Essence, strengthen the Vital Energy and clear away noxious Heat to lessen pathogenic inflammation.

PRESCRIPTION: Flos lonicerae, 30 gm; Fructus forsythiae, 20 gm; Radix scrophulariae, 30 gm; Radix paeoniae rubra, 15 gm; Radix achyranthis, 12 gm; Hirudo, 8 gm; Herba dendrobii, 30 gm; Pericarpium papaveris, 12 gm; Herba leonuri, 30 gm; and Pollen typhae, 12 gm. One dose per day. Lesions cleaned locally with H_2O_2 solution and granulation-promoting ointment applied. Changed dressing every other day.

FOLLOW-UP/COURSE OF TREATMENT:

Second consultation on June 2, 1984: After taking the above prescription, swelling of the foot and pain had receded. The patient had two hours of sleep each night. Pulsation of anterior and posterior tibial arteries not palpable. Tongue red, pulse rapid and fine. Astragalus root added to promote circulation.

Fifth consultation on June 24, 1986: The patient's condition improved markedly and pain gone. Twinge felt occasionally in his right leg. Able to sleep peacefully. Purple colour faded and swelling disappeared; foot and toe moist due to mild sweating. Scarring of ulcerated area. Pulsation felt on the right post-tibial artery. Toenail tended to be normal. Dark red tongue coated with white, thin fur. All these findings showed that the noxious Heat had receded, though stagnation of Qi and Blood was still evident. The aim of treatment then was to tonify Qi and warm the Meridian in order to promote circulation. Prescription: Ramulus cinnamomi, 15 gm; Radix astragali, 30 gm; Caulis akebiae, 6 gm; Flos lonicerae, 30 gm; Fructus forsythiae, 20 gm; Herba dendrobii, 30 gm; Radix paeoniae alba et rubra, 10 gm each; Pericarpium papaveris, 10 gm; Radix achyranthis, 12 gm; Herba leonuri, 30 gm; Pollen typhae, 12 gm; and Hirudo, 8 gm. One dose per day. Dressing for necrotic lesion applied.

Ninth consultation on July 23, 1984: Further improvement noted. Skin temperature had returned to normal. Pulsation palpable on the right post-tibial artery and evident on dorsal artery. Postural test of the right leg (+). The time of reddening on dependency, ‹ 30". Engorgement time of toe venous plexus by pressing, 3". Trophic condition of leg skin improved with appearance of capillary hair. The patient began to walk without the aid of a cane. Treatment should be that of promoting blood circulation by warming the Meridian. Some fruits were no longer used. Peach semen added instead.

Eleventh consultation on August 9, 1984: Normal skin and evident pulsation of dorsal and post-tibial arteries on the left leg. Swelling of the right foot had disappeared. Pulsation positive. Growth of new toenail had dislodged the old, thick one. A demarcation between normal tissue and the sequester was seen. The black end of the right big toe exposed. Sequester was then removed under local anesthesia and embedded with normal tissue. Wound sutured. Prescription: Ramulus cinnamomi, 15 gm; Radix astragali, 30 gm; Radix achyranthis, 12 gm; Radix pseudostellariae, 20 gm; Radix angelicae, 30 gm; Poria, 10 gm; Rhizoma atractylodis macrocephalae, 10 gm; Radix salviae, 30 gm; Radix paeoniae rubra et alba, 10 gm each; Cauli spatholobi, 30 gm; and Flos carthami, 10 gm.

Thirteenth consultation: Walking canes were discarded one week later. The patient was in good condition and able to take care of himself. He began to engage in light labour and got married in 1986.

DISCUSSION: Thromboangiitis obliterans (Burger's disease) is a common chronic vascular disease. It is seen most commonly in young men. Because of necrotic loss of the toe (or finger) caused by vascular ischemia, the disease was called Tao Zhu (gangrene) in traditional Chinese medicine and was first described in *Canon of Medicine* 2,000 years ago. An even more detailed description was found in medicine books of the Qing Dynasty. The Decoction of Four Wonderful Drugs for Quick Restoration of Health was introduced to treat gangrene of the extremities of the Toxic-Heat type. Gangrene has been considered a stubborn disease since ancient times. The exact cause of thromboangiitis obliterans is unknown. Tobacco sensitivity and exposure to cold in a Kidney deficiency person have been incriminated. Blood stasis due to pathogenicy Cold leads to stagnation of Qi and Blood and obstruction of vessels. Noxious Heat in the interior produced by long-standing stagnation destroys vessels and bones. There are three stages as categorized by traditional Chinese medicine.

The early stage is equivalent to the vasospasm stage. The blood vessel is stagnated by accumulating pathogenic Cold. Warming up the Meridian to promote circulation is the treatment of choice at this stage. The second stage coincides with the distrophic stage and is characterized by Qi and Blood stasis. The treatment is to promote circulation by strengthening the Qi. The third stage coincides with the gangrene stage. Symptoms are those of noxious Heat, Fire invasion and tissue necrosis. The therapy should be to nourish the Vital Essence and dispel noxious Heat and Fire from the Blood. The clinical picture of our case belonged to the third stage.

For our case, the course of treatment using traditional Chinese medicine was again divided into three stages. During the initial stage (first to fourth consultations), noxious Heat symptoms predominated. Thus, the patient was given large doses of Flos lonicerae, Fructus forsythiae, Herba dendrobii and Radix scrophulariae to remove toxic Heat and nourish the Vital Essence. Radix paeoniae rubra, Herba leonuri, Pollen typhae and Pericarpium papaveris were used to relieve pain by promoting Blood circulation, and raw Hirudo powder was used to remove Blood stasis.

The patient's condition was stable during the period from the fifth to the tenth consultations. Symptoms of toxic Heat in the Blood vessels had receded. The cause of disease, obstruction, was managed by promoting circulation and warming the Channels. Large doses of Radix astragali were used to strengthen his resistance by reinforcing Qi and promoting Blood circulation. During the succeeding stage (after the eleventh consultation), the symptoms subsided. Collateral circulation was established and affected vessels recanalized. Qi and Blood, excessively exhausted due to the long-standing disease, needed to be tonified and replenished next.

Under the guidance of TCM theories, the choice of medications were based on four key points:

1) Radix astragali which strengthens cardiac contraction, increases cardiac output, elevates arterial blood pressure and promotes blood circulation, was administered in large dosages.

2) Herbs which nourish the Vital Essence and dispel Heat, such as Herba dendrobii, Radix scrophulariae and Flos lonicerae, dilute the blood and decrease its viscosity, exerting and action similar to that of low molecular dextran.

3) Yang-warming and Channel-promoting herbs, such as Ramulus cinnamomi and Pericarpium papaveris, dilate the vessels and relieve pain by relaxing vasospasms.

4) Circulation-enhancing herbs, such as Radix salviae, Herba leonuri and Hirudo, have anticoagulant and thrombolytic actions. Radix salviae decreases viscosity and abates blood cell aggregating. It also activates the fibrinolytic system and degrades fibrins into FDP. The latter inhibits platelet aggregation, accelerates blood circulation and improves microcirculation. Hirudo impedes the process of clot formation and dilates the capillaries. Since it is thermolabile and liable to destruction by ethanol, it is better to use it in raw-powder form.

9. ORAL AND ENT DISEASES

9.1 BECHET'S DISEASE
(HU-HUO SYNDROME)

Guo Yungen, Wu Dehui and Chen Zeying
Emergency Clinic and Medical Department of the Fujian People's
Hospital and the Affiliated Hospital of the Fujian College of
Traditional Chinese Medicine, Fuzhou

Li, 21, male, single, worker. Medical record number: 6931. Date of admission: October 1, 1987.

CHIEF COMPLAINT: Fever and chills accompanied by joint and abdominal pain of several days duration.

HISTORY OF PRESENT ILLNESS: The patient consulted in one of the hospitals in Fuzhou City in February 1987, with the complaint of common cold and fever of several days duration. This was followed by congestion and pain of the eyes, markedly impaired vision and discharge from the right ear. In the same hospital, he was diagnosed as having iridocyclitis and acute otitis media. Treatment was given in the form of large doses of antibiotics and corticosteroids. Symptoms relieved and vision recovered. However, the symptoms relapsed soon after. In June of the same year, the patient experienced irregular bouts of shivering and fever with multiple, painful ulcerations on the oral mucosa and scrotum. In addition, there were numerous maculopapulae scattered on the skin over the trunk and extremities. Movement of the extremities was limited as finger and knee joints were swollen and painful. He also had intermittent abdominal pain and diarrhea with passage of three to four watery stools each day. His appetite declined markedly. Biopsy of the skin lesions disclosed acute and chronic inflammatory changes. A working diagnosis of Bechet's disease was entertained at this juncture in view of the clinical manifestations.

After being treated with large doses of prednisone for a month, the patient's condition seemed notably improved, and he was discharged with continued administration of corticosteroids. However, he withdrew the prednisone abruptly at the beginning of September. Soon after, he once again developed fever, shivers, joint pain, abdominal pain, ulcerations on the scrotum and a large number of rashes. Despite re-administration of large doses of corticosteroids, his condition remained unresponsive, and he was subsequently admitted to our hospital.

PAST AND FAMILY HISTORY: Non-contributory.

PERTINENT PHYSICAL EXAMINATION & LABORATORY FINDINGS: Temperature, 38°C; pulse rate, 110/min; respiratory rate, 18/min; blood pressure, 135/70 mmHg. Medium build and undernourished. Chronic illness facies, thin and frail with embarrassed gait. No jaundice and edema. Mild capillary congestion of both eyes. Throat not congested. Presence of nodules, 1.0-1.5 cm in diameter, moderate in texture, slightly tender and pruritic, some with accompanying hair follicle infection. No enlargement of superficial lymph nodes. Neck and thyroid normal. Bilateral breath sounded normal. Heart borders normal, cardiac rhythm regular with grade II systolic murmurs appreciated over the pulmonary area. Abdomen soft, liver and spleen not palpable. The joints of both forefingers and ring fingers swollen and slightly fusiform in shape. Spinal column normal. No pathological reflexes elicited. Hemoglobin, 8 gm%; WBC, 6,800/mm^3; PMN, 74%, eosinophils, 4%; lymphocytes, 22%; and ESR, 80 mm/hr. Urinalysis negative. Serum IgG, 1,900 mg/dl; IgA, 600 mg/dl; IgM, 200 mg/dl; lymphoblast transformation rate, 37%; E-rosette formation rate, 4%; LE cell (-); ANA (-); rheumatoid factor (+); serum mucoprotein 7.2 mg/dl (modified Harris method).

INSPECTION OF TONGUE: Tongue substance pink with thin, white and dry fur. Four small ulcers noted along the left side of the tongue.

PULSE CONDITION: Thready.

MODERN MEDICINE DIAGNOSIS: Bechet's Disease.

TRADITIONAL CHINESE MEDICINE DIAGNOSIS: Hu-huo Disease; Wetness-Heat of the Liver and Spleen.

Symptom-complex differentiation: In this case, attack of seasonal evil factors and internal stasis of Wind and Heat resulted in transformation of pathogens to Heat and Virulence. This Virulence advanced to the Upper Orifices manifested as reddened eyes; permeated outward to the skin as macules and sank down to the external genitalia producing ulceration and pustules. Persistence of exogenous evils resulted in damage of Blood and consumption of Vital Energy. As a result, healthy energy was deficient and evil factors overwhelming as evidenced by the presence of a red tongue with thin coating and rapid, small and weak pulse.

THERAPEUTIC PRINCIPLES: Eliminate the Damp and toxic pathogens, supplement the Vital Energy, nourish the Blood and calm the Wind.

PRESCRIPTION: Cornu bubali, 30 gm (decocted first); Radix rehmanniae, 24 gm; Cortex moutan radicis, 6 gm; Radix paeoniae alba, 12 gm; Rhizoma coptidis, 9 gm; Radix scrophulariae, 15 gm; Flos lonicerae, 15 gm; Radix codonopsis, 15 gm; Radix astragali, 30 gm; and Radix glycyrrhizae, 3 gm. One dose daily for three days.

The patient had been taking large doses of prednisone (more than 60 mg/day) for a prolonged period of time. Attempt to withdraw its administration was followed soon after by rebound of the symptoms. Since then, this large dosage of prednisone had not been able to control the symptoms. The patient was noted to have developed signs of steroid administration side effects, such as general consumption, diminished hypodermic fat and depletion of muscle mass. To avoid iatrogenic adrenocortical hypofunction, it was decided to prescribe prednisone at a relatively smaller dosage of 30 mg/day.

FOLLOW-UP/COURSE OF TREATMENT:

Second consultation on October 4, 1987: The patient complained of stomach discomfort with mild abdominal pain. He passed three to four loose stools every day and experienced tenesmus. Pink tongue substance with several ulcers on the sides, tongue fur slightly yellow. Continued the prescription with modifications. Cornu bubali, 60 gm (decocted first); Radix rehmanniae, 15 gm; Radix paeoniae alba, 12 gm; Rhizoma coptidis, 6 gm; Cortex phellodendri, 9 gm; Radix isatidis, 15 gm; Caulis lonicerae, 24 gm; Pollen taraxaci, 9 gm; and Radix glycyrrhizae, 3 gm. One dose daily for three days.

Third consultation on October 7, 1987: The patient had developed occasional fever of 38°C. Abdominal pain remained with passage of loose stool several times a day. Ulcers on the sides of the tongue had healed. Gingivitis present. The patient complained of left shoulder joint pain. Tongue substance pink with grimy fur. Pulse string-like and slippery. Prescription to clear away Heat and toxic pathogens together with intestinal astringent: Flos lonicerae, 9 gm; Cortex lycii radicis, 15 gm; Herba violae, 15 gm; Radix scutellariae, 6 gm; Radix paeoniae alba, 9 gm; Cortex phellodendri, 9 gm; Rhizoma coptidis, 9 gm; Radix pulsatillae, 9 gm; Radix pueratiae, 9 gm; Cortex fraxini, 9 gm; and Rhizoma drynariae, 9 gm. Three doses.

Fourth consultation on October 10, 1987: Abdominal pain and diarrhea had ceased. The patient complained of generalized arthralgia and tinnitus. Pink tongue substance with grimy fur. Pulse string-like and slippery. Continued the measures to clear away pathogenic Heat from the Blood, eliminate the Wind and excrete the Dampness. Caulis lonicerae, 24 gm; Radix achyranthis, 9 gm; Fructus chaenomelis, 9 gm; Radix paeoniae rubra, 15 gm; Fructus forsythiae, 9 gm; Radix rehmanniae, 15 gm; Semen phaseoli, 15 gm; Herba artemisiae scopariae, 15 gm; Cortex erythrinae, 15 gm; and Radix stephaniae tetrandrae, 9 gm. One dose daily.

Fifth consultation on October 13, 1987: The symptoms had been alleviated. There were more than 10 pruritic nodules over the extremities and forehead. Continued the same prescription adding Flos lonicerae, 15 gm. Reduced the dosage of prednisone by half to 15 mg/day.

Sixth consultation on October 17, 1987: Skin rashes had intensified and maculopapules appeared flushed and infected with small pustules in the centres. Lesions itchy and painful. The patient complained of dryness of the mouth, constipation and yellowish discolouration of urine. Tongue substance red with thin fur, pulse wiry and slippery. Administered the following prescription for 10 days: Flos lonicerae, 15 gm; Radix rehmanniae, 15 gm; Rhizoma smilacis glabrae, 15 gm; Fructus kochiae, 15 gm; Cortex dictami radicis, 15 gm; Radix scutellariae, 6 gm; Herba violae, 15 gm; Herba taraxaci, 15 gm; Fructus tribuli, 15 gm; Fructus cnidii, 9 gm; and Radix glycyrrhizae, 4.5 gm.

Seventh consultation on October 28, 1987: Skin lesions were alleviated gradually. Condition of the tongue and pulse remained the same as before. Repeated the prescription for 10 days.

Eighth consultation on November 7, 1987: Skin rashes had disappeared. The patient's physical activity had improved markedly. There was no difficulty in getting about. He experienced mild pain in the muscles and joints of the extremities. Tongue substance red with white fur and pulse small and wiry. Modified the prescription to eliminate the Wind and Dampness: Cortex erythiae, 15 gm; Semen phaseoli, 15 gm; Radix rehmanniae, 15 gm; Herba artemisiae capillaris, 15 gm; Radix paeoniae rubra,

9 gm; Fructus chaenomelis, 9 gm; Caulis lonicerae, 20 gm; and Radix stephaniae tetrandrae, 9 gm.

Ninth consultation on November 16, 1987: All symptoms relieved. Condition of the tongue and pulse remained the same as before. Modified the prescription to dispel the pathogenic Heat from the Blood and clear away the Virulence: Fructus gardeniae, 9 gm; Radix scutellariae, 6 gm; Radix gentianae, 9 gm; Caulis akebiae, 4.5 gm; Herba artemisiae capillaris, 15 gm; Semen phaseoli, 15 gm; Rhizoma smilacis glabrae, 15 gm; Herba oldenlandiae diffusae, 15 gm; and Herba lophatheri, 9 gm.

The last prescription was to be modified according to the clinical manifestations. After taking 12 doses, joint and skin symptoms were relieved completely in succession, but there was still dull abdominal pain. For this reason, the prescription was modified by the removal of Caulis akebiae and Fructus gardeniae and the addition of Radix codonopsis, Pollen typhae and Fructus aurantii to be administered for four days. The patient recovered fully after administration and was discharged from hospital in good condition. Follow-up after six months revealed no relapse of the symptoms, and his condition was stable and good.

DISCUSSION: This case was characterized by the presence of a prolonged irregular fever, typical eye manifestations and ulceration of the oral cavity and external genitalia. It is also known as eye-oral-external genital syndrome. In addition, there were subcutaneous nodules, hair follicular papules, joint pain and GI tract symptoms, such as abdominal pain, diarrhea and others. In short, this was a disease involving multiple systems. Laboratory examinations showed increased level of serum immunoglobulin, decreased rate of lymphoblast transformation and E-rosette formation. Also evident were increased ESR and serum mucoprotein. LE cell detection was negative. Based on these clinical observations and clinical findings, a definitive diagnosis of Bechet's disease was reached.

Bechet's disease is a modern medicine nomenclature. As recorded in the TCM classic *Synopsis of the Golden Chamber* by Zhang Zhongjing of the Han Dynasty, it was known as Hu-huo disease. Zhang Zhongjing states that "the signs and symptoms of Hu-huo disease are similar to those of exogenous febrile disease; the pathogenic ulcerations attack the throat or external genitalia. When ulcers develop, the patient loses appetite and feels nauseated upon ingestion of food ... and has flushed face or diminished and somber complexion now and then. Development of ulcers on the upper part of the respiratory tract will lead to hoarseness of the voice." Zhang also advised that Gan Cao Xie Xin Tang be the prescription of choice for treatment and recommended Ku Shen Decoction as a gargling solution to alleviate dryness of the throat when the lower part of the throat is involved, as well as Sophora flavescens Art. solution to fumigate the ulcerative lesions on the anus. Manifestations described by Zhang agree rather with those of Bechet's disease. Since then, Zhang's description of the disease has been quoted in works by other noted traditional medicine practitioners, such as *A Handbook of Prescription for Emergencies* by Ge Hong and *Sphygmology* by Wang Shuhe of the Jin Dynasty; *General Treatise on the Etiology and Symptomology of Diseases* by Chao Yuanfang of the Sui Dynasty; and *Medical Secrets of an Official* by Wang Tao of the Tang Dynasty.

Wei Nianting of the Qing Dynasty states that Hu-huo disease results from Yin deficiency and Blood Heat. According to TCM theory, it is believed that Hu-huo disease is caused by invasion of certain infectious factors or accumulation of Dampness and Heat and should be treated mainly by clearing the Heat, excreting the Dampness and eliminating the Virulence. Recently, Hu-huo disease has been classified into three clinical types: (1) Wetness-Heat of the Liver and Spleen, treated by clearing the Heat, eliminating the Dampness and removing Virulence. Prescription based on Long Dan Xie Gan Tang and Xie Huang San; (2) Accumulation of Dampness due to deficiency of the Spleen, treated by strengthening the Spleen, supplementing the Vital Energy, elevating the Yang, eliminating Wetness and clearing away Virulence. Prescription based on Bu Zhong Yi Qi Tang; and (3) Endogenous Heat syndrome caused by Yin deficiency, treated by nourishing the Yin and the Liver and clearing away the Heat with Yi Guan Jian, Er Zhi Wan and Liu Wei Di Huang Wan.

Our case belongs most likely to the first type. Treatment by clearing away the Heat and eliminating and removing Virulence has brought about a satisfactory outcome.

This case had multiple organ involvement with complex and severe clinical conditions. It was further complicated by unresponsiveness to corticosteroids and presence of rebound symptoms upon withdrawal of the drug.

On admission, Xi Jiao Di Huang Tang was first prescribed in order to purge the Heat, clear away the Virulence and consolidate the Yin. After administration of three doses, the patient still complained of diarrhea and abdominal pain. Prescription was modified by adding herbs effective in regulating the Intestines and Qi. For the next one week, the patient's condition improved markedly. As soon as gastrointestinal tract symptoms were put under control, the patient was given prescriptions to dispel pathogenic Heat from the Blood together with herbs to eliminate the Wind and excrete Dampness. On October 13, in view of the relapse of skin rashes, emphasis was put on clearing away the Virulence and dispelling the Heat from the Blood. Subcutaneous nodules and skin rashes faded away in about 20 days, and thereafter the prescription was administered with necessary modifications according to the clinical conditions.

By this mode of application, successful withdrawal of corticosteroids and alleviation of clinical symptoms were achieved and sustained for a long period of time.

9.2 BECHET'S DISEASE
(HU-HUO SYNDROME)

Bian Tianyu and Liu Shiming
Dermatological Institute of Integrated Traditional Chinese
and Western Medicine, Tianjin Changzheng Hospital, Tianjin

Yue, 51, male, Han nationality, married, farmer. Medical record number: 26. Date of first consultation: May, 1969.
CHIEF COMPLAINT: Recurrent ulcerations of the mouth and scrotum with eye

pain for three years.

HISTORY OF PRESENT ILLNESS: At the onset of the disease, the patient was noted to have ulceration of the mouth and scrotum. Erythematous nodular lesions were also noted on the lower extremities. There were accompanying fever and chills during episodes of attack. A few months later, pain was experienced in both eyes, which appeared congested. Gradually, visual acuity was noted to be deteriorating with eyes sensitive to light exposure. Isomorphine reaction (+). He also complained of arthralgia. At the time of consultation, ulceration of the mouth and scrotum had been present for 10 days with chills and fever, arthralgia, especially prominent on the ankle joints, pallor, general weakness and lumbago.

PAST HISTORY: Positive history of cigarette smoking.

PERTINENT PHYSICAL EXAMINATION & LABORATORY FINDINGS: Chronic disease facies; moderate development and nutrition status. Two bean-sized ulcers on the inner aspect of the lower lip and one on the scrotum measuring 0.5 cm in diameter. Papules of follicular inflammation scattered over the extremities, chest and back. Presence of erythematous nodules on the lower extremities with tenderness. Left ankle joint slightly swollen and tender. Ophthalmological examination: adhesion of iris to cornea; pupil pin point in size with flaccid response; O.D., 0.2; O.S., light sensitive. Hemoglobin, 10 gm%; RBC, 3M/mm^3; WBC, 7,000/mm^3; ESR, 7 mm/hr. Chest X-ray findings negative.

INSPECTION OF TONGUE: Scanty amount of white coating.

PULSE CONDITION: Slippery and weak.

MODERN MEDICINE DIAGNOSIS: Bechet's Disease.

TRADITIONAL CHINESE MEDICINE DIAGNOSIS: Hu-huo Syndrome.

THERAPEUTIC PRINCIPLES: Tonify the Spleen and Kidney, promote Blood circulation to remove stasis.

PRESCRIPTION: Rhizoma rehmanniae praeparatae, 9 gm; Cortex cinnamomi, 9 gm; Rhizoma pinelliae, 9 gm; Radix salviae, 9 gm; Rhizoma atractylodis macrocephalae, 9 gm; Poria, 9 gm; Rhizoma sparganii, 9 gm; Rhizoma zedoariae, 9 gm; Radix angelicae, 9 gm; Radix paeoniae, 9 gm; Flos carthami, 9 gm; and Fructus forsythiae, 6 gm.

FOLLOW-UP/COURSE OF TREATMENT:

Second consultation on May 30, 1969: The patient had taken eight doses of the prescription over the past two weeks. Ulcers of the mouth and scrotum cleared up. Symptoms of chills and fever, arthralgia and general weakness alleviated markedly.

For the next two to three months, the prescription was taken at a dosage of one dose per two to three days. Joint swelling, lumbago and other symptoms disappeared and vision did not deteriorate any further. The patient was back to work on the farm.

Followed up 10 years later by mail, the patient reported that there had been sporadic episodes of ulceration of the mouth and scrotum during the spring and autumn which could usually be cleared up by about 10 doses of the same prescription. Condition of the eyes and vision had not deteriorated.

DISCUSSION: Ulceration of the mouth and scrotum in this case had been relapsing for three years. Though slightly tender, these ulcers were usually not accompanied by significant swelling or erythema. By symptom-complex differentiation, this was a case of

Blood stasis with the ulcers classified as "Cold ulcers." Satisfactory outcome was obtained by pursuing the principle of tonifying the Spleen and Kidney. It should be pointed out here that this mode of treatment is markedly different from that for "Heat ulcers." In treating cases of "Heat ulcer," the therapeutic principle to be applied is to clear away the Heat and to detoxicate. Ulcer, by TCM symptom-complex differentiation, is divided into two types, and each merits its own appropriate therapeutic regimen.

9.3 RECURRENT ULCERATIVE STOMATITIS (ORAL ULCER)

Xu Zhihong

School of Stomatology, Beijing Medical University, Beijing

Wang Zhenhong, 38, male, Han nationality, married, engineer. Date of first consultation: October 6, 1974.

CHIEF COMPLAINT: Recurrent oral ulcers for more than 10 years.

HISTORY OF PRESENT ILLNESS: The patient had been suffering from recurrent oral ulcers for more than 10 years. The ulcers usually appeared at labial, buccal and lingual mucosa. During the last year, severity and frequency of the attacks occurred progressively almost without interval of remission. Healing time was prolonged from a week to a month. The number of ulcers increased during each attack. The patient was noted to have taken a large quantity of water. Urination and defecation were normal.

PAST HISTORY: Positive history of pulmonary tuberculosis and digestive disturbance.

PERTINENT PHYSICAL EXAMINATION & LABORATORY FINDINGS: 0.3 × 0.5 cm ulcers on tip of tongue and inner aspect of upper lip mucosa; borders distinct, hyperemic and swollen. Ulcer cicatrication on margins of tongue also present.

INSPECTION OF TONGUE: Tongue substance red with thin, yellowish fur.

PULSE CONDITION: Taut, slippery and rapid.

MODERN MEDICINE DIAGNOSIS: Recurrent Ulcerative Stomatitis.

TRADITIONAL CHINESE MEDICINE DIAGNOSIS: Oral Ulcer.

THERAPEUTIC PRINCIPLES: Replenish Yin and remove Heat.

PRESCRIPTION: Radix rehmanniae, 20 gm; Radix scrophulariae, 15 gm; Radix paeoniae alba, 12 gm; Radix paeoniae rubra, 12 gm; Radix asparagi, 15 gm; Radix ophiopogonis, 12 gm; Herba dendrobii, 15 gm; Radix scutellariae, 10 gm; Fructus schisandrae, 6 gm; Caulis spatholobi, 15 gm; Radix achyranthis, 10 gm; Radix platycodi, 10 gm; Caulis akebiae, 6 gm; and Powder of Cortex cinnamomi, 1 gm (prepared by pouring liquid on it).

Local application: Yangyinshenzhi San, 0.1% Rivanal mouth rinse solution.

FOLLOW-UP/COURSE OF TREATMENT:

Second consultation: Symptoms subsiding, pain alleviated and the patient's general condition was getting better. Ulcerative lesions healing. Prescription: Radix astragali, 15 gm; Rhizoma atractylodis, 15 gm; Rhizoma rehmanniae praeparatae, 15 gm; Rhizoma anemarrhenae, 10 gm; Rhizoma dioscoreae yam, 12 gm; Radix scutellariae, 10 gm; Herba dendrobii, 12 gm; Radix achyranthis, 10 gm; and Poria, 15 gm.

Third consultation: Ulcer on the tip of the tongue had been healed though the area was still a little tender as if the ulcers were about to recur. The lips were red in colour. Tongue substance slightly red with thin, white and dry coating. Modified the previous prescription by removing Cortex cinnamomi, Fructus schisandrae, Caulis akebiae and Caulis spatholobi and adding Gypsum, 30 gm, and Rhizoma rehmanniae praeparatae, 15 gm.

Fourth consultation: All the ulcers were healed and there was no recurrence. The patient complained of thirst and drank a lot of water. His urine became yellow.

After a treatment course of one and a half months, oral ulcers were essentially under control. Although there was a tendency for the condition to relapse, the situation was mild and could be controlled rapidly. General condition of the patient was good.

During the next 12 years of follow-up, the patient's condition was stable.

DISCUSSION: The authors applied the Four Methods of Diagnosis in traditional Chinese medicine to gather the relevant clinical information. Based on the result of symptom-complex differentiation analysis, this case was judged to be of ulcer and Fire symptoms caused by consumption of Yin leading to a flaring up of Evil Fire. The patient's face and lips were flushed and tongue proper was also red. Pulse fine and slightly rapid. Colour of urine yellow and stool dry. The patient also complained of insomnia, irritability and dryness of the mouth and tongue. These clinical manifestations indicated accumulation of internal body Heat secondary to deficiency of the Vital Energy. Deficiency of the vital function and vital essence of the Kidney was evidenced by positive history of tuberculosis, weak constitution, pallor, weak and fine pulse and aching on the back and legs. The therapeutic principle applied in this case was to clear away the Heat and nourish the Yin. Oral ulcers were contained within three months time and did not recur within six months after the course of treatment. The patient's condition was stable during the next three years with occasional recurrence of the ulcers, which tended to be difficult to control at the onset. Full recovery was finally obtained when, using traditional Chinese medications, the balance of the patient's viceral and bowel functions were restored and his resistance to pathogens enhanced.

9.4 INFECTIOUS STOMATITIS (ORAL EROSION)

Xu Zhihong

School of Stomatology, Beijing Medical University, Beijing

Song Wen, 60, male, Han nationality, married, cadre. Medical record number: 105290. Date of first consultation: October 15, 1985.

CHIEF COMPLAINT: Mucosal eruption of the palate for three weeks.

HISTORY OF PRESENT ILLNESS: Three weeks ago, eruption of the mucosa was noted at the centre of the palate. Several antibiotics had been administered including spiramycin, penicillin and prednisone, but none afforded any relief. Lesion was neither painful nor pruritic.

PAST HISTORY: Non-contributory.

PERTINENT PHYSICAL EXAMINATION & LABORATORY FINDINGS: An ulcer, 2.0 × 2.5 cm in size, situated at the centre of the soft palate; fundus smooth with yellowish exudate; border distinct and slightly elevated. Area around the ulcer hyperemic and congested. Routine peripheral blood examination finding normal.

INSPECTION OF TONGUE: Yellow coating.

PULSE CONDITION: Fine and taut.

MODERN MEDICINE DIAGNOSIS: Infectious Stomatitis.

TRADITIONAL CHINESE MEDICINE DIAGNOSIS: Oral Erosion.

THERAPEUTIC PRINCIPLES: Nourish Yin and remove evil Heat.

PRESCRIPTION: Radix rehmanniae, 15 gm; Radix rehmanniae praeparatae, 15 gm; Radix paeoniae alba, 12 gm; Radix scrophulariae, 15 gm; Radix cimicifugae, 9 gm; Cortex moutan, 10 gm; Red sage root, 15 gm; Radix scutellariae, 10 gm; Herba violae, 15 gm; Os draconis, 30 gm; Concha ostreae, 30 gm; Radix astragali, 20 gm; Radix glycyrrhizae, 10 gm; and Catecha, 12 gm.

Local application: Yang-yin Shen-zi San and E-Hou Ning, 0.05% Chlorexidine solution for mouth wash.

FOLLOW-UP/COURSE OF TREATMENT:

Second consultation: Symptoms and pain of the lesion alleviated and size of ulcer reduced. Ulcer crater became shallower and amount of exudate reduced as well. Area of hyperemia diminishing. Tongue fur thin and white at the tip but slimy and greasy at the back.

Third consultation: The patient's condition continued to improve. Size of ulcer reduced to 0.2 × 0.6 cm, surrounding hyperemia minimal. Swelling reduced.

Fourth consultation: Ulcer was healed and all swelling and hyperemia eliminated.

DISCUSSION: A ruptured mass was present at the centre of the palate and was suspected to be a carcinoma initially. Pathological diagnosis was suspected eosinophilic granuloma. There was no history of recurrent attacks or trauma. Laboratory examination was negative. The patient's general condition was good. Examination revealed a palatal ulcer surrounded by a wide zone of congestion. Surface of the ulcer was covered by secretions of intense yellow colour. In traditional Chinese medicine, oral ulcer is caused by Fire, so this case was treated with the methods of clearing away Heat, alleviating Fire and cooling and invigorating the Blood. In addition, diseases of the oral mucous membrane are usually accompanied by Yin insufficiency of varying degrees, thus herbs which can nourish the Yin and clear away the Heat should be used, such as Radix rehmanniae, Radix scrophulariae, Cortex moutan, Rhizoma anemarrhenae and Radix paeoniae. On second consultation, the inflammation was remitting and herbs effective in reinforcing the Spleen and drying up the moisture were added. These herbs could improve the processes of epithelialization and wound healing. On the third consultation, herbs astringent in nature and capable of promoting granulation were added. The patient's condition had recovered completely when last seen. Such a rapid recovery indicates that appropriate modifications of the prescription based on clinical manifestations were necessary in treating this kind of disease.

9.5 RECURRENT ULCERATIVE STOMATITIS (ORAL ULCER)

Xu Zhihong

School of Stomatology, Beijing Medical University, Beijing

Luo Moutang, 38, male, engineer. Medical record number: 16657. Date of first consultation: April 4, 1972.

CHIEF COMPLAINT: Recurrent oral ulcer for more than 20 years; frequency of attack had increased in recent years.

HISTORY OF PRESENT ILLNESS: Recurrent bouts of oral ulcer for more than 20 years. Recently, symptoms exacerbated with lesion involving the pharynx. Each course of the disease lasted for several months. In the last three months attack was continuous without intermission. The patient also had history of ulcers on the genitals. Eyes normal. Various treatment in the past using antibiotics, vitamins, steroids, tissue therapy, smallpox vaccine inoculation and placental globulin injection did not afford relief from the condition.

PAST HISTORY: Positive history of chronic enteritis, colitis, drug rashes (sulfanilamide anaphylactic reaction), tracheitis and rhinitis. Often complained of insomnia, tinnitus and sticky, loose stool.

PERTINENT PHYSICAL EXAMINATION & LABORATORY FINDINGS: Ulcers present on right upper lip and right lingual margin measuring 0.4 × 0.6 cm in size with another large and deep ulcer present on retropharyngeal mucosa; margins irregular accompanied by grayish yellow exudates. Surrounding area hyperemia and swelling prominent.

INSPECTION OF TONGUE: Presence of thin, yellow coating.

PULSE CONDITION: Fine, taut and moderate.

MODERN MEDICINE DIAGNOSIS: Periadenitis Mucosal Necrotica Recurrens.

TRADITIONAL CHINESE MEDICINE DIAGNOSIS: Oral Ulcer.

THERAPEUTIC PRINCIPLES: Replenish Qi, invigorate Spleen function and remove Heat.

PRESCRIPTION: Radix astragali, 20 gm; Poria, 12 gm; Radix paeoniae, 12 gm; Radix asparagi, 10 gm; Radix ophiopogonis, 10 gm; Radix scutellariae, 10 gm; Cortex moutan, 10 gm; Radix trichosanthis, 12 gm; Rhizoma polygonati, 12 gm; Rhizoma polygonati odorati, 15 gm; Semen cassiae, 15 gm; and Radix platycodi, 12 gm.

Local application: 0.1% Rivanal solution to rinse mouth.

FOLLOW-UP/COURSE OF TREATMENT:

Second consultation: Ulcer of the tongue healed. Size of buccal mucosa ulcer reduced. Retropharyngeal and upper labial ulcerative exudate diminished. The patient still passed sticky and loose stool. Principle of treatment: strengthen the Kidney by way of reinforcing the functions of the Spleen.

Third consultation: Size of retropharyngeal ulcer reduced. Swelling and hyperemia still noted. The patient complained of common cold and cough with pharyngalgia. Prescription: Tong Xuan Li Fei Pills and Decoction of Lonicerae and Forsythiae.

Fourth consultation: Symptoms of common cold and cough alleviated. Size of retropharyngeal ulcer continued to be reduced and was becoming shallower. No occurrence of new ulcer. Tongue with yellow coating. Prescription: Pills of Six Drugs with Rehmanniae and modified Bu Zhong Yi Qi Pills.

Retropharyngeal ulcer healed completely after one and a half months of treatment. The lesion recurred once but was healed rapidly. The patient continued the treatment for another six months. His condition had been stable during the succeeding 15 years of follow-up. There was occasional recurrence of ulcer which was mild in severity and usually healed rapidly.

DISCUSSION: This was a case of ulcer caused by Fire secondary to consumption of Vital Essence. This diagnosis was made based on the patient's clinical manifestations, the application of the Four Methods of Diagnosis and TCM symptom-complex differentiation. Traditional Chinese medicine believes that skin abscess or sores with pain, inflammation and pruritus are due to excessive Heat (Fire) in the Heart and Blood. It regards ulcers and many other types of sores as caused by or related to accumulation of visceral Heat which is subsequently transformed into Fire. Excessive Fire syndrome can further be classified as due to consumption or due to excessive pathogenic factors.

The patient in this case manifested deficiency or inadequacy of the Heart, Spleen, Vital Energy and Blood. This was due to disharmony of the Spleen and Stomach, which are the source of Blood and Vital Energy. Disturbed digestive functions in this case were evidenced by a history of chronic enteritis and colitis, fatigue and intolerance to cold, susceptibility to catching colds, rhinitis, dreamful sleep, irritability and restlessness. The therapeutic principles of strengthening and reinforcing the Heart and Spleen, nourishing Yin and removing Heat were applied in this case to rectify the patient's condition. The resulting short course of treatment served to regulate the patient's health and was also effective in putting the ulcerative lesions under control. Also effectively remedied by this treatment course were Spleen deficiency, diarrhea, chronic enteritis and others. The patient's physical condition was also improved. These results show that traditional Chinese medicine, by using symptom-complex differentiation to treat the body as a whole, is of advantage in regulating a patient's health and controlling the course of his or her disease.

9.6 ORAL LICHEN PLANUS
(ORAL EROSION, ORAL MUSHROOM)

Xu Zhihong
School of Stomatology, Beijing Medical University, Beijing

Xie Benglian, 60, female, Han nationality, teacher. Medical record number: 124589. Date of first consultation: November 20, 1986.

CHIEF COMPLAINT: Erosive lesion of buccal mucosa of five years duration.

HISTORY OF PRESENT ILLNESS: Recurrent attack of erosive lesions in the buccal mucosa for the past five years. Condition worsened progressively and had not been in remission for the past three months. Vitamins were taken as treatment but without evident effects.

PAST HISTORY: Positive history of diabetes mellitus, neurodermatitis and hypertension.

PERTINENT PHYSICAL EXAMINATION & LABORATORY FINDINGS: Grayish white, reticular and fine striae on both sides of buccal mucosa with evident hyperemia and erythema. Multiple erythema papula, effusion and scab with obsolete pigmentation spots on skin of extremities.

INSPECTION OF TONGUE: Tongue substance slightly red in colour with yellow and slimy fur.

PULSE CONDITION: Fine, taut and slippery.

MODERN MEDICINE DIAGNOSIS: Lichen Planus.

TRADITIONAL CHINESE MEDICINE DIAGNOSIS: Oral Erosion.

THERAPEUTIC PRINCIPLES: Replenish Yin and nourish Blood, dispel external Wind, remove Heat, quench Liver Fire and dispel Heat from Blood.

PRESCRIPTION: Cortex moutan, 12 gm; Fructus kochiae, 30 gm; Radix paeoniae, 12 gm; Radix rehmanniae, 20 gm; Radix scutellariae, 12 gm; Herba lophatheri, 12 gm; Cortex dictamni, 12 gm; Radix scrophulariae, 12 gm; Semen coicis, 20 gm; Fructus cridii, 12 gm; Concha haliotidis, 30 gm; and Fructus gardeniae, 10 gm.

Long Dan Xie Gan Pills (per os).

Vit. Bco and Oryzanol (per os).

Local application: Acetonidi unguentum acetatis fluocinoloni.

FOLLOW-UP/COURSE OF TREATMENT:

Second consultation: The patient reported alleviation of most of the symptoms. Progress of the lesions controlled with the disappearance of erosion. No new lesion had occurred on the skin. Broom cypress fruit, 3 gm; Cortex moutan, 10 gm; Radix rehmanniae, 15 gm; Radix paeoniae, 12 gm; Radix scutellariae, 12 gm; Fructus forsythiae, 15 gm; Semen coicis, 15 gm; Herba violae, 15 gm; Herba portulacae, 15 gm; Fructus cridii 10 gm; Fructus aurantii, 10 gm; and Poria, 12 gm. Also administered Fang Feng Tong Shen Pills, Vit. B6 and Vit. Bco (per os).

Third consultation: The patient's condition continued to improve. Most areas of congestion had disappeared and no new lesions were noted. Herba artemisiae, 15 gm;

Radix scutellariae, 12 gm; Herba lophatheri, 10 gm; Poria, 12 gm; Fructus kochiae, 20 gm; Radix spirodelae, 12 gm; Herba portulacae, 12 gm; and Semen coicis, 15 gm. Fang Feng Tong Shen Pills, Vit. B$_6$ and Vit. Bco (per os).

Fourth consultation: Most of the original lesions had subsided and mucosa was normal. Only vague striae remained. Most of the buccal lesions had disappeared. Continued the previous prescription.

Fifth consultation: Disappearance of grayish-white striae from the buccal mucosa.

Oral and skin lesions improved steadily during the two-month course of treatment. The patient's condition was stable during the ensuing six months of follow-up.

DISCUSSION: This was a case of typical oral lichen planus accompanied by neurodermatitis, hypertension and diabetes mellitus. The patient's clinical manifestations indicated internal infiltration by Wind-Evil which accumulated in the skin and muscles, resulting in insufficiency of Yin and Blood. Such a condition led to production of Heat and Wind, stagnation of the Blood causing Heat, Blood insufficiency and Wind Dryness. Clinically, these were manifested as lesions in the muscles, skin and mucosa. Pruritus was evident with congestion and erythema of the mucosa. Pathogenic factors of Wind, Wetness and Heat were transformed to Dryness first then to Fire leading to consumption of Blood and damage of the Yin. Nutritional insufficiency of the muscles, skin and mucosa secondary to this condition was evidenced by keratinized striae on the buccal mucosa with rupture, exudation and erosion. The treatment was to nourish the Yin and Blood, dredge the Wind, clear away the Heat, clear the Liver, cool the Blood, regulate the flow of Vital Energy and invigorate the circulation of the Blood.

This case is a good illustration of the correct approaches, both locally and systemically, for treating diseases with this particular symptom-complex.

9.7 IDIOPATHIC DEAFNESS
(DEAFNESS CAUSED BY EXOGENOUS WIND-EVIL)

Wang Dongxi and Wang Xiaohui
Fujian Provincial Hospital, Fuzhou
People's Hospital, Fujian College of Traditional Chinese Medicine, Fuzhou

Chen Zigui, 20, male, Han nationality, single, student. Medical record number: 5603.

CHIEF COMPLAINT: Impairment of hearing and tinnitus on the left side for seven days.

PRESENT SYMPTOMS: The patient complained that his hearing on the left side was impaired suddenly on May 9, 1988. He did not pay much attention to it in the beginning. The same night, tinnitus of varying tones was experienced in the same ear. Tinnitus was described as continuous and got louder when the surroundings were noisy. He was dizzy but did not experience rotatory sensation. Impairment of hearing was noted to have aggravated progressively. He consulted the Provincial Hospital, and an audiometry was performed, results of which indicated that his appreciation of the 1,000 Hz pitch was reduced to 90-100 dB. He was diagnosed as having sudden deafness and received an injection, the name of the medication he could not recall. Hearing did not improve and tinnitus worsened after the medications. The patient consulted our clinic and was subsequently admitted on May 16.

PAST HISTORY: Bilateral ptosis of eyelids since childhood.

PERTINENT PHYSICAL EXAMINATION & LABORATORY FINDINGS: Conscious and under strain. Of moderate nutritional status. Skull normal. Inspection of both external auditory canals normal. No hyperemia or perforation seen on drumheads; light cones intact. Tuning fork test revealed air conduction of the low pitch (C128) of the left ear was normal but the high pitch (C2048) range reduced severely. Rinne's test negative. Right ear normal. No spontaneous nystagmus appreciated. Head position test normal. Romberg's sign and finger-nose test negative. Caloric test to follow. Nasal septum deviated to the left with slightly congested mucosa. Pharynx and larynx essentially normal. Neck supple. No superficial lymph nodes palpated. Thyroid not enlarged. Heart and lung findings normal. Abdomen flat and soft, liver and spleen not palpated. No pathological reflexes elicited.

INSPECTION OF TONGUE: Bright red tongue substance with thin and yellowish fur.

PULSE CONDITION: String-like (wiry) and slippery.

MODERN MEDICINE DIAGNOSIS: Sudden Deafness, Left Ear; Blood Vessel Disorder (?).

TRADITIONAL CHINESE MEDICINE DIAGNOSIS: Deafness and Tinnitus of the Left Ear.

Symptom-complex differentiation: The cause and pathogenesis of this disease are due to flaring up of the dominant liver Fire, stagnation of Vital Energy and Blood stasis.

THERAPEUTIC PRINCIPLES: Clear the Liver and purge the sthenic Liver Fire.

PRESCRIPTION: Modified Longdan Xiegan Tang and Taohong Siwu Tang. Radix gentianae, 6 gm; Fructus gardeniae, 9 gm; Radix scutellariae, 9 gm; Radix bupleuri, 9 gm; Radix rehmanniae, 15 gm; Rhizoma alismatis, 9 gm; Semen persiae, 9 gm; Flos carthami, 6 gm; Rhizoma ligustici Chuanxiong, 6 gm; Radix paeoniae alba and rubra, 15 gm each; Radix salviae miltiorrhizae, 20 gm; and Radix angelcae sinensis, 6 gm. Placed in water for 15 minutes, then decocted for 30 minutes. One decoction per day in three divided doses.

Other management: Avoid food which is Dryness-Fire and acrid-peppery in nature. Salviae Compound for injection, 2.0 ml, IV drip, q.d.; Low monocular dextran, 500 ml, IV drip, q.d.; Vitamin B1, 100 ml, IM, q.d.

FOLLOW-UP/COURSE OF TREATMENT:

Second consultation on May 16: After taking the prescription, the patient's general condition was better. Blood pressure, 134/90 mmHg. Tinnitus generally alleviated in the morning but tended to be aggravated in afternoons. Routine peripheral counts showed WBC, 5,800/m³; neutrophiles, 40%; eosinophiles, 1% and lymphocytes, 53%.

Viral infection was considered the cause of the condition in view of elevated lympho-cyte count. Oral Moroxydinum prescribed.

Third consultation on May 18: The patient reported that symptoms of deafness and tinnitus remained the same. He experienced sore throat. It was evident at this point that he was suffering from invasion by exogenous Wind-Evil. Discontinued the previous medications and applied the therapeutic principles of expelling the Wind-Evil and eliminating the evil factors. Qu Feng Yin was prescribed made up of Flos lonicerae, 9 gm; Folium isatidis, 9 gm; Lasiosphaera seu calvatia, 3 gm; Fructus arctii, 9 gm, and Radix glycyrrhizae, 3 gm. Prepared in the same way as the prescription above. One dose per day.

Fourth consultation on May 19: Tinnitus alleviated but deafness remained. Liver function tests normal. HBsAg test negative.

The results of caloric test were:

	Left 2'10"		Left 2'10"
30°C		44°C	
	Right 2'		Right 2'10"

Fifth consultation on May 22: The patient reported that tinnitus had disappeared, though deafness remained the same. He slept well and dryness of the mouth was relieved. This prescription, based on the principles of expelling Wind-Evil and elimi-nating the evil factors, had been effective in achieving the desired result and now the emphasis was put on removing Blood stasis. Prescription: Herba ephedrae, 3 gm; Ramulus cinnamomi, 3 gm; Radix astragali seu Hedysari, 9 gm; Radix paeoniae, 6 gm; Radix angelicae, 6 gm; Radix codonopsis pilosulae, 9 gm; Radix ophiopogonis, 9 gm; Fructus schisandrae, 3 gm; and Radix glycyrrhizae, 3 gm. One dose per day.

Sixth consultation on May 25: The patient reported significant improvement in hearing. The high pitch of tinnitus had disappeared; only a low-pitch, machine-like sound remained. Dizziness had disappeared. Chest X-ray findings normal. Continued the treatment.

Seventh consultation on June 1: The patient reported distinct recovery of his hearing and further alleviation of tinnitus. On audiometry, auditory acuity over the 1,000 Hz - 6,000 Hz range was significantly enhanced.

The patient was discharged on June 3 after a total admission period of 20 days.

DISCUSSION: The patient was admitted due to sudden unilateral hearing loss followed by tinnitus. In view of absence of systemic disorder and definitive precipitat-ing factors, the cause of the condition was considered to be depression resulting in disability of the Liver to clear and disperse. This stagnant Liver energy was trans-formed subsequently into Fire-Evil which disturbed the lucid orifices and led to stagnation of Vital Energy and Blood. Accordingly, the initial therapeutic principles to adopt were those of dispersing the depressed Liver energy and purging the sthenic Fire as well as those of promoting Vital Energy and removing Blood stasis. Modern medications were also used to improve microcirculation and nourish the nervous system. Later on, the patient reported a sore throat with a CBC picture of leukopenia and lymphocytosis which was likely caused by Wind-Evil-virus infection. Since the patient belongs to the age group which is unlikely to be suffering from vascular disease, the therapeutic principle adopted was then shifted to that of eliminating the viral infection.

In the Qu Feng Yin prescription, Folium isatidis is effective as an antiviral agent, while Flos lonicerae, Lasiosphaera seu catvatia and Fructus arctii are effective as antibacterials. The combination of these herbs can eliminate viral infection of the upper respiratory tract and accompanying bacterial infection.

One week after admission, the patient reported alleviation of the symptoms. Leukocyte count was elevated and lymphocyte count down. This indicated that Wind-Evil had been controlled. It was necessary at this point to emphasize removal of Blood stasis to improve Blood circulation. Ma Hui Tang was prescribed in addition to administration of dextran. In this prescription, several herbs were effective in promoting the circulation of Vital Energy and Blood. Theoretically, they could dilate the blood vessels and improve local circulation in order to facilitate nerve ending healing. In such a way, hearing could recover.

Although the definite diagnosis had been established for seven days, the patient only received therapy in the outpatient department. From previous experience, should treatment for sudden deafness be delayed for more than three days, the damage could be irreversible. In our case, application of a full spectrum combination of traditional Chinese and modern medications and timely modifications of the prescriptions based on adjustment of therapeutic principles enabled the course of treatment to achieve a successful outcome.

9.8 PERITONSILLAR ABSCESS (ABSCESS OF THE THROAT)

Wang Dongxi and Wang Xiaohui
Fujian Provincial Hospital, Fuzhou
People's Hospital, Fujian College of Traditional Chinese Medicine, Fuzhou

Wang Wenyu, 19, female, Han nationality, single, waitress. Medical record number: 7525. Date of admission: November 24, 1987.

CHIEF COMPLAINT: Sore throat for seven days complicated by fever and difficulty in swallowing for three days.

HISTORY OF PRESENT ILLNESS: One week prior to admission, the patient experienced a sore throat. She self-medicated with Huo Xian Pian which relieved the symptom temporarily. Three days prior to admission, the sore throat aggravated, and she was given oral erythromycin in the Provincial Hospital; it afforded no relief. The ailment was noted to have remained and localized to the right side. One day prior to admission, the patient experienced nasal congestion with a scanty amount of discharge and blood. She consulted our clinic and was diagnosed as having "Ru-E" (milky moth, or acute lacunar tonsillitis complicated with peritonsillar abscess, and was subsequently admitted.

PAST HISTORY: Non-contributory.

FAMILY HISTORY: Both parents living and well.

PERTINENT PHYSICAL EXAMINATION & LABORATORY FINDINGS:
Conscious and of normal nutritional status. Voice low and sunken with nasal twang.
Gross inspection of external auditory canals normal. No hyperemia nor perforation of
the tympanic membrane on otoscopic examination. Light cones intact. No impairment
of hearing. No deviation of the nasal septum. A bleeding lesion on the antero-inferior
portion of the left side. Nasal mucosa slightly congested with smooth and moist
surface. Right inferior turbinate red and swollen slightly. No enlargement of the
middle turbinate. Purulent discharge noted on the right common meatus. Trismus
evident with the gap between upper and lower rows of teeth only one and a half fingers
broad. Red and congested mucous membranes of fauces and oropharynx. Both faucial
tonsils were red and swollen (second degree). There were multiple pus thrombi in the
lacunae of both tonsils. The right anterior palatine arch was markedly red and swollen
and protruding anteriorly. Uvula deviated to the left. Submaxillary nodes on the right
side swollen and tender. Heart and lung findings negative. Abdomen flat and soft, liver
and spleen not palpable. Neurological examinations normal. Routine blood examination: hemoglobin, 8.8 gm%; WBC, 17,000/mm³; neutrophils, 81%; lymphocytes, 18%;
and monocytes, 1%. Liver function tests normal. HBsAg negative. Urine and stool
examination normal. Chest X-ray findings negative.

INSPECTION OF TONGUE: Bright red tongue substance with thick and turbid
fur.

PULSE CONDITION: String-like (wiry).

MODERN MEDICINE DIAGNOSIS: Acute Lacunar Tonsillitis Complicated with
Peritonsillar Abscess.

TRADITIONAL CHINESE MEDICINE DIAGNOSIS: "Ru-E" (Milk moth) Secondary to Heat-Wind Evil Complicated with Abscess of the Throat, Right Side.

THERAPEUTIC PRINCIPLES: Clear away the Heat and toxic materials, expel
the Wind and promote sweating to remove exogenous evil from the body surface.

PRESCRIPTION: Qu Feng Yin Formula. Flos lonicerae, 9 gm; Folium isatidis, 15
gm; Radix isatidis, 9 gm; Lasiosphaera seu calvatia, 3 gm; Fructus arctii, 9 gm; and
Radix glycyrrhizae, 3 gm. Placed ingredients in water for 15 minutes and decocted for
30 minutes. One decoction daily in three divided doses.

Fluid diet with avoidance of food of Dryness-Fire and acrid-peppery natures.

FOLLOW-UP/COURSE OF TREATMENT:

Second consultation on November 25: After admission, the patient reported
exacerbation of a sore throat and difficulty in swallowing. Food ingestion was minimal
and disturbed. Intravenous administration of 50% glucose was instituted. Trismus
slightly alleviated. Pharynx still red and swollen. Right anterior palatine arch bulging.
Puncture was done under 1% Xylocaine local anesthesia but no pus was aspirated.
Continued the medication.

Third consultation on November 26: The patient reported significant alleviation
of sore throat. Temperature lowered to normal. Trismus had disappeared. Food
ingestion had increased and constipation was relieved. Signs of recovery noted on

pharynx, tonsils, right anterior palatine arch and uvula. Tongue with thick and yellowish fur, pulse wiry. Findings of routine blood examination and urinalysis were normal.

Fourth consultation on November 27: Sore throat had disappeared. Food ingestion had increased and the patient could sleep well. Redness and swelling of tonsils reduced. Palatine arches remained slightly red and swollen. Thick tongue fur began to go down. Continued the medication.

Fifth consultation on November 28: Sore throat gone completely. Redness and swelling of throat reduced. Submaxillary lymph nodes still palpable and slightly tender. Chest X-ray findings normal.

Sixth consultation on November 30: The patient reported feeling better. Tongue coating slightly yellowish in colour with red tongue tip. Pulse remained wiry. In addition to the previous prescription, Radix scrophulariae, 15 gm; Radix rehmanniae, 15 gm; and Radix glehniae, 10 gm, were added for two days.

Seventh consultation on December 1: Repeated CBC showed WBC, $9,900/mm^3$; neutrophils, 75%; eosinophils, 3%; and lymphocytes, 22%.

The patient was discharged from hospital after 10 days of admission.

DISCUSSION: Peritonsillar abscess generally develops rapidly when the patient's condition is serious. Most of the cases are complicated by acute lacunar tonsillitis. At the beginning, it is the acute inflammation in the peritonsillar fossa which progresses to suppurative change and abscess formation. Clinically, the terms "peritonsillitis" and "peritonsillar abscess" actually denote the same thing. It means that almost every case of peritonsillitis results in suppuration and abscess formation. In our experience, if a case could be treated by traditional Chinese medicine promptly, suppurative changes could be prevented.

In modern medicine, it is considered that this disease is caused by suppurative bacteria. Thus, antibiotics or sulphonamides are usually prescribed. Since these agents are only bacteriostatic, not bactericidic, in effect, suppuration will result in most cases.

As understood by traditional Chinese medicine, this disease entity is caused by poor personal hygiene or unhealthy living habits as well as unchecked or excessive and irregular intake of food and beverages. In such circumstances, the weakened body constitution will be vulnerable to invasion by Heat-Evil which damages the tissues and leads to abscess formation. The principle of treatment is essentially that of clearing away the Heat and toxic material supplemented by that of expelling the Wind and promoting sweating to remove exogenous evils from the body surface. In the prescription used, the six herbs are all bactericidic in effect, which is the reason behind the successful outcome. These effective herbs not only shortened the course of treatment but also prevented further suppuration.

10. INFECTIOUS DISEASES

10.1 FEVER RELEVANT TO INTERNAL INJURY (FAMILIAL MEDITERRANEAN FEVER, FMF)

Kuang Ankun

Shanghai Second Medical University

Shao Zuze, 38, male, Han nationality, married, official. Medical record number: 85856. Admitted to Ruijin Hospital, Shanghai, on April 15, 1964.

CHIEF COMPLAINT: Periodic fever.

HISTORY OF PRESENT ILLNESS: In August 1958 the patient was afflicted with periodic fever of unknown cause. There was about one high fever period per month; the body temperature could be over 40°C for 3 to 4 days or 6 to 7 days, or even 15 to 20 days. He felt chill and pain all over the body, and had shortness of breath. He was listless and somnolent. Besides, he complained of vexation and palpitation. Defervescence was accompanied by diaphoresis. He suffered also from hemorrhoid and later it was complicated by prolapsus ani. From August 1958 to July 1959, he was treated as common cold without success. From July 1959 to March 1964, he was treated with TCM and Western medicine in different hospitals of the town where he worked and was hospitalized more than 10 times in those hospitals under excellent care. The following examinations were done: Leucocyte count, urine and feces examination, ESR, Aso, sternal puncture, liver puncture, radiographic examination of the lungs, gastro-intestinal system and gallbladder, biopsy of lymphatic nodes in the neck, axilla, inguinal-femoral and other regions, OT, search of germs and parasites and exploratory laparotomy, etc. All the above investigations, which were repeated many times, were negative except OT (+) and leukocyte count occasionally › 10,000. Antituberculosis treatment was used; then amygdalectomy and appendicectomy were done because amygdalitis and chronic appendicitis were found. Antibiotics and other drugs were given. During the six years of his sickness, he was treated by many TCM physicians. All the treatments were unsatisfactory. As the illness was getting worse, the patient was referred to the department of medicine of Shanghai's Ruijin Hospital by a hospital in his town. Asked about his life in the countryside, he told us that he had worked very. hard from December 1957 to January 1959. According to TCM, overstrain and overfatigue cause fever due to internal injury which manifests as lassitude, listlessness, shortness of breath, fever and spontaneous sweating. This clinical picture matched well the case of our patient and we believed that it had something to do with his illness.

PERTINENT PHYSICAL EXAMINATION & LABORATORY FINDINGS:

Body temperature, 37.6°C; pulse rate, 76/min; respiratory rate, 20/min; and blood pressure, 105/60 mmHg. His mind was clear, he was rather thin, and he had a chronic illness facies. He was found to have painless, movable, enlarged lymphatic nodes in the neck, axilla, inguinal-femoral and other regions. The lower border of the liver was palpable 2 cm below the right costal margin and the spleen was just palpable below the left costal margin. No other physical abnormalities were noted.

PAST AND FAMILY HISTORY: In August 1958, he had dysentery. All the members of his family were healthy.

INSPECTION OF TONGUE: White, greasy and enlarged.

PULSE CONDITION: Taut and soft pulse.

MODERN MEDICINE DIAGNOSIS: Familial Mediterranean Fever (FMF).

TRADITIONAL CHINESE MEDICINE DIAGNOSIS: Fever Relevant to Internal Injury.

THERAPEUTIC PRINCIPLES: We followed the fundamental strategic concept of the famous TCM physician Li Gao (1180-1251), known also as Li Donghuan, using sweet and warm medicaments to treat fever relevant to internal injury in order to invigorate the spleen and stomach, promote the Vital Energy, dispel the Dampness and quench the Fire. We made a combination of Buzhong Yiqi Tang (Decoction for Reinforcing Middle-Jiao and Replenishing Qi) and Si Jun Zi Tang (Decoction of Four Noble Drugs for Qi Deficiency), etc.

PRESCRIPTION: (1) standard dosage (SD): Pilose asiabell root, 9 gm; Astragalus root, 9 gm; White atractylodes rhizome, 6 gm; Porio with horsewood, 12 gm; Licorice root, 3 gm; Polygala root, 4.5 gm; Spiny jujube seed, 12 gm; Chinese angelica root, 9 gm; Costus root, 3 gm; Bamboo shavings, 6 gm; Waxgourd seed, 18 gm; Coix seed, 18 gm; Tangerine peel, 4.5 gm; Magnolia bark, 3 gm. (2) Moderate dosage (MD): Pilose asiabell root (PAR), 15 gm; and Astragalus root (AR), 15 gm. (3) Big dosage (BD): PAR, 30 gm, and AR, 30 gm. In MD and BD, the dosages for the other drugs are the same as in SD. We used SD in the interval period, MD in moderate fever and BD for obstinate high fever. SD and MD: one dose per day, divided in two decoctions; BD: one dose per day, divided in two decoctions; two doses per day, devided in four decoctions, and three doses per day, in six decoctions.

FOLLOW-UP/COURSE OF TREATMENT:

First high fever period: six days after admission, April 20, 1964, 8 pm, 38.2°C. No treatment was given. April 21, 4 pm, the patient felt cold in the lower extremities. One MD was given at 5 pm, and two hours afterwards, the lower extremities became warm, the soles of the feet were sweating and the temperature began to decline. April 22, one BD was given, the temperature became normal and the patient took one SD per day.

Second high fever period: May 11, 1964, midnight, 37.7°C. No treatment was given. May 12, after two BD were given, temperature became normal.

Third high fever period, July 19, 1964, midnight, 38.2°C. No treatment was given. July 20, 4 pm, 39.4°C. The fever declined spontaneously. No treatment was given. July 22 and July 23, 38°C in the afternoon, one SD each day. July 24, two BD were given. The temperature became normal the following day.

Fourth high fever period: August 17, 1964, 8 pm, 38.2°C. Two BD that day. August

18, also two BD that day. August 19, 12 am, 39.4°C. Three BD were given and the fever declined sharply.

Fifth high fever period: September 26-28, 1964, three days of high fever. September 27, 4 pm, 39.4°C. Three BD were given for two days (26 and 27) and two BD the third day, and the temperature became normal.

From September 29, 1964, to December 21, 1964, the day of the patient left our hospital, there was no more periodic fever. He went back to his hometown, where he resumed work and enjoyed good health for nearly nine years. Between 1969 and 1973 during the "cultural revolution," he was forced again to do hard work and in 1973 the periodic fever recurred. He was treated by old TCM physician Wei Longxiang, with Chaihu Guizhi Tang (Bupleurum root-Cinnamon Twig Decoction), but he used also high dosage of Pilose asiabell root (60 gm) per day and Astragalus (30 gm per day). The patient recovered and since then he has enjoyed good health.

DISCUSSION: The patient was sick for six years. His illness being related to hard work, we treated him with sweet and warm Chinese drugs. He regained his health and resumed work for nearly nine years, but the same disease relapsed due to the same reason and he was recovered by similar treatment. Fever is frequently induced by spleen injury relevant to overstrain. High fever injures Yin and causes deficiency of the Vital Energy. When Fever-Yin is mounting the Yang Qi declines instead of elevating. The clinical picture with lassitude, listlessness, etc, coincided with that of our patient. The type of pulse was also coincidental.

Buzhong Yiqi Tang composed of sweet and warm Chinese drugs, was specially invented by Li Gao for fever due to internal injury. The prescription slightly modified by us was very successful for our patient.

The patient, who was weak from protracted sickness, wouldn't be able to tolerate high dosages of medicament; on the other hand, the disease was so obstinate that regular dosage wouldn't work, so we decided to use the progressive-regressive method. During his hospitalization, we prescribed MD for moderate fever; SD for the intervals between high fever periods and rarely for obstinate high fever, for which we were forced to prescribe two or three BD per day. On those occasions I often stood by to watch the patient closely, until he was completely recovered. If overstrain is the unique aetiology of fever induced by internal injury, such periodic fever should be a common disease, but it was very rare in our country. Western medicine has widely studied periodic fevers among which is FMF, which is very common among patients of Sephardic Jewish, Armenian and Arabic ancestry. However the disease has been seen among people of Italian and Anglo-Saxon descent as well as others. Nevertheless approximately 50 percent of the patients give no family history of the disease. There are about 25 percent of FMF patients in Israel who are known to have amyloidosis and this complication leads to death. Up to now, there is no satisfactory treatment for FMF. Our patient looked like having been afflicted with concealed FMF factor as well as internal injury. Buzhong Yiqi Tang modified by us was very successful in our case. Could it be also successful in proved FMF cases? This question can be answered only when the drug is tried out in countries where FMF is common.

10.2 AIDS
(WARM TOXIC DISEASE)

Jean Yu and Chen Keji
Santa Barbara College of Oriental Medicine, California, U.S.A.
Xiyuan Hospital, China Academy of Traditional Chinese Medicine, Beijing

In the spring of 1981, the Centre for Disease Control (CDC) was informed of the first case of acquired immunodeficiency syndrome (AIDS). Of 41,735 cases reported as of September 7, 1987, 24,019 have died. Thus, AIDS has become a major health concern. So far, the only approved drug for human use, AZT (Azidothymidine), has shown the serious side effect of bone marrow suppression. Consequently, AIDS victims have been searching for alternative therapies in order to increase life expectancy and to ameliorate symptoms. Chinese medicine has become one of those choices.

Modern Chinese and Japanese researchers have shown that Chinese herbs can enhance both humoral and cellular immunity. It is believed that treatment with Chinese herbal medicine can prolong life expectancy and considerably ameliorate the symptoms of AIDS patients. Therefore, from May 1986 to September 1987, we prescribed herbal medicine in a diagnosed AIDS case with very encouraging results.

Case No. 335: A 38-year-old white male. First visit: May, 1986. The patient's chief complaints were chronic diarrhea of eight to nine months duration, profound malaise and lethargy and a viral-like syndrome with swollen lymph nodes for three to four years. The initial site of enlarged lymph nodes noted by the patient was in the head and neck region, where the nodes varied in location and size. The patient lacked appetite, suffered nausea and experienced weight loss and distention in the epigastric area. The stool was very loose, often watery, foul-smelling and contained undigested food. Additional symptoms include recurrent and distressing sinus congestion, pharyngitis, thrush and herpes zoster.

The patient tested positive for presence of the putative AIDS agent, HIV-III, in May and June of 1984. Because of elevated serum SGPT and SGOT, he was informed that he had type-B hepatitis and AIDS, but at this time there was nothing available for the treatment of his condition. Faced with this devastating disease and rejection by the public, the patient lost interest in life, became depressed and withdrew from human contact.

The patient's history included a 10-year period, from 1974 to 1984, of active homosexual relationships with about 25 apparently healthy men, aged 25 to 28. He was particularly active between 1981 and 1984 while working as a bartender in the Hollywood area of Los Angeles. In 1982, his homosexual contacts developed insidious symptoms of adenopathy, weakness, and chronic fatigue. As of September 1987, all of his contacts had died of opportunistic infections.

PERTINENT PHYSICAL EXAMINATION & LABORATORY FINDINGS: The patient was emaciated and spiritless, with a very pale complexion. Findings were otherwise unremarkable with the exception of the lymphoreticular system. The patient had a congested throat with non-streptococcal pharyngitis. Unilateral lymph nodes were found to have been enlarged to about $3 \times 4 \times 2$ cm in the axillary, inguinal and posterior cervical areas. They were non-tender, non-indurated and of various sizes. Splenic enlargement was palpated under the left hypochondria and a hepatic enlargement was palpated 2 cm under the right hypochondria. No tenderness or blunt edges were present.

The patient had a normal whole blood count. Blood chemistry studies showed primarily hepatocellular dysfunction reflected by elevations of SGOT to 136 IU/L and SGPT to 268 IU/L. Serum albumin was 4.2 gm/dL and $\gamma\mu$-globulin was 2.8 gm /dL. A/GM 1.5, prothrombin time 15.2 sec. (normal value = 11-13 sec) and activity 43% (normal value 70%).

INSPECTION OF TONGUE: Red body delicate with a longitudinal crack; tip and edge exhibited red spots; a thin, yellowish, greasy coating; thickness towards the root and invitro culture revealed candida.

PULSE CONDITION: Rapid (over 90/min), wiry and slippery.

According to TCM theory, the patient's condition was diagnosed as a Warm-Toxic conformation with deficiencies of the Kidney, Spleen and Heart. It was located in both Qi and Blood portions.

The treatment has been classified into the following three stages:

Stage 1 (May-August, 1986): The purpose of treatment in this stage was to clear away the Heat, cool the Blood, eliminate the Damness and detoxify. The main formula was modified Gan Lu Xiao Du Yin (Antiphlogistic Decoction of Dew), with added Scutellariae barbata, Oldenlandia diffusa, Lonicerae japonica, Forsythiae suspensa, Isatis tinctoria, Radix isatis, Paeoniae suffruticosa and Gardeniae jasminoides. Hordeum vulgare and Cretaegus cuneatas were added for improving digestion and decreasing flatulence, and for the purpose of clearing away Heat and detoxification. The above formula was prescribed at four to five doses a week.

Stage 2 (September 1986-May 1987): By September 1986, the patient exhibited subjective signs of improvement, with less fatigue and an uplifting of spirits. His digestive functions had also improved as evidenced by an increased appetite and more consistency to the form of his stools. But he continued to display anxiety and depression which manifested as a reactive psychiatric disturbance resulting from the death of his previous sexual partners. Due to encouraging signs of improvement, the patient began to work on a part-time basis.

The tongue picture altered with the tongue body changing from red to pale-pink in colour. The tongue shape was puffy with tooth marks and wet overall. The pulse was wiry and slippery at a normal rate (64-72 beats/min). On October 15, 1986, laboratory findings revealed SGOT and SGPT reduced to 91 IU/L and 162 IU/L respectively.

According to TCM theories, in this second stage (October 1986 to March 1987) the Warm-Toxic symptom complex was less predominant. The herbs had cleared most of the Dampness and Turbidity out of the body system, but the Qi and Yin were still deficient. Therefore, the goal of treatment in this stage was to replenish the Qi and Yin. The formula used was modified Shen Mai Yin (Pulse-producing Decoction) with added Scrophulariae radix, Rehmanneae radix, Ligustrum lucidum and Eclipta alba for the purposes of nourishing Yin and promoting the secretion of body fluids.

On March 4, 1987, laboratory findings showed that SGOT and SGPT had been reduced to 73 IU/L and 169 IU/L respectively. Serum albumin was 4.5 gm/dL and γ-globulin was 2.5 gm/dL. A/GM 1.8, triglyceride reduced from 146 mg/dL to 91 mg/dL, VLDL from 28 mg/dL to 18 mg/dL.

On May 5, 1987, the patient suffered a repeated attack of herpes zoster. The lesions, which were lateral along the T12-L1 neural pathway, consisted of grouped, tense, deep-seated vesicles with intensive pain after medication with Heat- and toxin-dispelling herbs, such as Coptis chinensis, Amebia eucroma, Baphicacanthis folium and Moutan radicis cortex.

Two weeks later (on May 19), the eruption was gone and the pain relieved without post zoster neuralgia. After June 1987, the patient's subjective feelings were much improved and his diarrhea was relieved. The sore throat was no longer a main complaint and adenopathy was reduced. The patient began working part-time and attended a vocational school. At this period of time the tongue picture showed it was pale, puffy and wet. Pulses were deep and thready. The patient's main complaint was palpitation and a feeling of dizziness.

From the TCM point of view, the patient was suffering from a Kidney and Spleen Qi deficiency symptom-complex. Modified Gui Pi Tang (Decoction to Strengthen the Spleen and Heat) was applied through large dosages of Radix astragali and with the addition of Kidney-tonifying herbs such as Cuscuta chinensis, Epimedium saggitatum and Lingustrum lucidum for replenishing the Yang and Yin of the Heart, Spleen and Kidney.

At the end of September, the patient's condition was stable. He was satisfied with his subjective energy level and had not caught a cold or flu for several months. Recently, he was checked for his T-helper cells. The result was 91/mm^3 and has since remained low.

DISCUSSION: According to recent literature, 93% of those who are infected with AIDS are male; 72% of AIDS patients are homosexual or bisexual men; 90% of whom are under 35 years of age. The racial distribution is 59% whites, 26% blacks and 14% Hispanics. Homosexual AIDS patients are primarily white. Those people at risk for AIDS may demonstrate early nonspecific findings, including chronic generalized lymphadenopathy, unexplained weight loss, fever, profound malaise and lethargy, idiopathic thrombocytopenia and leukopenia in addition to immunologic abnormalities. With currently available tests, 100% of lymphadenopathy patients show evidence of past infection with AIDS retrovirus.

Although the patient reported on this study did not suffer from Kaposi's sarcoma and/or pneumocystis carnii pneumonia, AIDS diagnosis was confirmed through case history, symptoms and signs and positive result of the HIV-III test.

In accordance with the manifestations of this case and TCM theories, AIDS is diagnosed as a Warm Toxic symptom-complex. The deficiencies of both Spleen and

Kidney Yang are primary causes (Ben) while the invasions of Warm Toxic and Turbid Dampness pathogens are secondary factors (Biao). The therapeutic regimen for this AIDS patient was initially to clear away Heat, deoxify, eliminate Dampness, cool the Blood and tonify the Kidney, Spleen and Heart. The clinical results demonstrate that this therapeutic regimen had a certain efficacy in this case. However, it is necessary to make further observations and identify the effectiveness of this course of treament for retrovirus before drawing final conclusions.

Chinese clinical and immunological researchers have found that Chinese herbs have enhancing effects on humoral and cellular immunity. These herbs include Radix astragali, Ginseng, Lucidum ligustrum, Codonopsis pilosula, Eleuthero ginseng, Curculigo orchioides, Cuscuta chinensis, Cornus officinalis, Oldenlandia diffusa and Coix lachryma jobi. Astragali radix can increase the interferon production of human cells dramatically. Curculigo orchioides, Cuscuta chinensis and Cynomorium songaricum can promote the formation of antibodies.

Herbs for tonifying Yang and nourishing Yin, which clear away Heat, dispel toxins and promote circulation of Blood also enhance cellular immunity by promoting macrophage phagocytosis. The compound Dan Gui Bu Xue Tang has the same effect.

Polygonatum sibiricum, Ganoderma lucidum and Tremella polysaccharide increase the T-cell ratio. There has been some progress in the study of the active ingredients of those herbs which influence the immune system. It is currently believed that AIDS patients lose the delicate balance of the T-suppressor cell ratio. The T-suppressor cell ratio of AIDS patients may be reduced from a normal value of about 1.8 to 1.1 or less. The T-helper cell count may drop from a normal value of over $400/mm^3$ to below 50 or $20/mm^3$. It will be very encouraging if Chinese herbal medicine is effective in this respect.

It is known that free radicals can damage cells, produce genetic changes and cause Kaposi's sarcoma, which is one of the most common causes of death for AIDS patients. Therefore, the treatment of AIDS requires the continued study of free radical scavengers. Recently, American physicians have applied massive doses of Vitamin C (60-170 gm/24 hrs) as scavengers for AIDS patients. Chinese researchers have found that some compound prescriptions and single herbs possess antioxidant action and some Kidney-tonifying formulas can reduce plasma lipidperoxide levels in elderly persons. It may be possible that Chinese herbs are an effective choice in clinical practice for the treatment of AIDS.

So far, the only approved drug available to AIDS patients is AZT. The expense of such treatment ranges from RMB¥ 7,000 to RMB¥ 10,000 a year, excluding costs for blood transfusions for the anemia caused by bone marrow suppression. We have applied Chinese herbal medicine in the treatment of AIDS and demonstrated that it is effective, safe, economical and acceptable. Efforts should be made to treat additional cases and to increase the efficacy through further clinical and experimental studies.

10.3 EPIDEMIC HEMORRHAGIC FEVER (WIND-FEBRILE SYNDROME)

Hong Yongshen and Cheng Jianyong
Hangzhou Red Cross Hospital, Hangzhou

Qi Gui'er, 43, female, Han nationality, married, farmer. Medical record number: 75453. Admitted on April 3, 1986.

CHIEF COMPLAINT: Fever and lumbago for 10 days, oliguria for four days.

HISTORY OF PRESENT ILLNESS: The patient had abdominal distention and pain in the lower back and around the orbital cavities accompanied by headache, slight chills and fever (temperature not recorded) 10 days ago when she was working in the field. The temperature stood at 39.6°C during the night three days later. She was restless and thirsty so she drank a lot of water, but the amount of urine decreased progressively. The average amount of urine in 24 hours was 500 ml for four days, and it was yellowish or reddish in colour. The patient had a flushed appearance as if drunk. The pain in the lower back and both calves became worse. She received chloromycetin and dexamethasone in a local clinic but to no avail. The night before admission, she visited this clinic complaining of restlessness, thirst, aversion to fluids and scanty urine. Laboratory tests showed WBC, 11,000/mm³; neutrophils, 80%; abnormal lymphocytes, 12%, urine protein, (++); RBC, (+); and granular cast, (+++). She was admitted as a case of epidemic hemorrhagic fever.

The patient did not complain of sore throat, cough, chest pain, stiff neck, frequent and urgent urination, abdominal pain or diarrhea, but she experienced loss of appetite and constipation for three days.

PAST HISTORY: Non-contributory.

PERTINENT PHYSICAL EXAMINATION & LABORATORY FINDINGS: Temperature, 38.5°C; pulse rate, 104/min; respiratory rate, 22/min; and blood pressure, 100/70 mmHg. Conscious and cooperative; of normal nutritional status. Bleeding spots on both the upper palate and axilla. Lymph nodes not enlarged. Slight puffiness of the eyelids. Bulbar conjunctival congestion; pupils isochoric with normal light reflex. No deformity nor discharge from external auditory canals. Mastoid processes not tender. Slight congestion of the throat; first-degree enlargement of the tonsils. Neck supple; no distention of the jugular vein. Thyroid gland not enlarged. Heart and lung findings negative. Pain on percussion on the kidney area. Abdomen soft, flat, non-tender, no mass palpable; liver and spleen not palpable. Positive shifting dullness. Slight tenderness on costal-spinal areas. No edema of the lower extremities. Neurological examination negative. WBC, 11,000/mm³; neutrophiles, 80%; and abnormal lymphocytes, 12%. Epidemic hemorrhagic fever antibody detection positive. Urine protein, (++); RBC, (+); WBC, few; and granular cast, (+++).

INSPECTION OF TONGUE: Red tongue substance with dry and yellowish fur.

PULSE CONDITION: Overflowing and rapid.

MODERN MEDICINE DIAGNOSIS: Epidemic Hemorrhagic Fever.

TRADITIONAL CHINESE MEDICINE DIAGNOSIS: Wind Febrile Syndrome (Excessive Heat on Qi-Fen and Ying-Fen).

THERAPEUTIC PRINCIPLES: Clear away Heat from Ying-Fen.

PRESCRIPTION: Modified Shigao Dihuang Formula and Qing Ying Tang. Gypsum fibrosum, 30 gm; Rhizoma anemarrhenae, 12 gm; Radix rehmanniae, 12 gm; Radix ophiopogonis, 10 gm; Radix scrophulariae, 10 gm; Leaf buds of Herba lophatheri, 3 gm; Flos lonicerae, 15 gm; Fructus forsythiae, 12 gm; Rhizoma coptidis, 9 gm; and Radix salviae, 12 gm. Decocted in 500 ml of water with appropriate intensity of fire for 30 minutes to obtain a resultant decoction of 200 ml. Taken orally in two equal proportions. Three doses. One dose a day.

Other management: Rest in bed, semi-liquid, high-calorie diet rich in vitamins; 1,500 ml of normal saline infusion daily. Monitor fluid input and output as well as acid-base balance.

FOLLOW-UP/COURSE OF TREATMENT:

Second consultation: Number of bleeding spots did not increase after taking the prescription, but high fever, restlessness and thirst remained. The amount of urine was 700 ml per day, yellowish or reddish in colour. The patient experienced difficulty in moving her bowels because of the dryness of stool. Sensation of distention experienced on the lower abdomen. Blood pressure, 100/60 mmHg. Tongue substance bright red with dry, yellowish coating, pulse rapid. WBC, 15,000/mm^3; abnormal lymphocytes, 10%; urine protein, (++); and RBC, (++).

Modified the previous prescription by removing Flos lonicerae and Fructus forsythiae and adding Radix et rhizoma rhei, 12 gm; Fructus aurantii immaturus, 10 gm; and Cortex magnoliae officinalis, 10 gm. When the herbs had been boiled for 85 minutes, placed Rhei in it and boiled for another 5 minutes. Two doses. One dose daily in two divided portions.

Amount of urine had increased day by day after treatment. Lower abdomen distention had disappeared. Body temperature 37.6°C. Tongue substance red with yellowish coating, pulse weak and rapid.

Third consultation: Continued the previous prescription with modifications. Removed trifoliate orange, Cortex magnoliae officinalis and Rhei and added Radix rehmanniae, 15 gm; Radix scrophulariae, 15 gm; Radix ophiopogonis, 15 gm; and Rhizoma anemarrhenae, 15 gm. Five doses.

In addition, 15 gm of Herba dendrobii and 30 gm of Rhizoma rehmanniae were boiled to drink ad libitum.

The amount of urine at this point was about 1,500 ml daily and bleeding had stopped. All of the symptoms were gone. Body temperature had returned to normal. The patient's appetite was getting better. Tongue reddish and moist with thin, yellowish coating.

Fourth consultation: Continued the previous prescription with modifications. Radix rehmanniae, 12 gm; Radix scrophulariae, 12 gm; Rhizoma anemarrhenae, 12 gm; Rhizoma coptidis, 6 gm; Radix salviae, 15 gm; Rhizoma polygonati odorati, 10 gm; Rhizoma polygonati, 15 gm; and Radix glycyrrhizae, 4.5 gm. Seven doses. One dose daily.

Thirty gm of fresh common reed rhizoma and 6 gm of leaf buds of Herba lophatheri were boiled to drink ad libitum. The patient had recovered completely after seventeen doses of the prescription. All symptoms had disappeared. The patient's appetite was normal. Urination and bowel movements were normal as well. Urine protein detection negative and there was no abnormal lymphocytes in the blood.

DISCUSSION: This case had the following clinical features:

1) The disease developed in the springtime. The patient had fever, chills, headache and pain around orbital cavities.

2) The patient had high fever, especially at night, restlessness, thirst, craving for drinks, oliguria with yellowish or reddish discolouration of urine, flushed appearance, poor appetite and dry stool before treatment.

3) Tongue substance was red with dry and yellowish coating. Pulse overflowing and rapid.

This disorder is classified as "seasonal febrile disease." The etiologic factor is invasion of the Febrile-Evil. Lungs were involved first since the Lung controls the skin and hair and the Wei-Energy goes through the Lung. Should the measures to expel the evils be applied at this time, the evils in the Lung-Wei would have been driven out. Unfortunately, the patient did not receive any treatment at this stage. Yang evils of Wind and Heat invaded the body and together they produced Fire which penetrated the Ying-Fen and Blood-Fen easily. Subsequent appearance of high fever, thirst, restlessness and red rashes on the skin indicated presence of evils in the Qi-Fen and Ying-Fen. Therapeutic principles applied at this point were clearly stated in TCM literature: "If evil is in Wei-Fen, seating method should be used; if evil is in Qi-Fen, clear away the turbid Qi; if evil is in Ying-Fen, remove the Heat; and if the evil is in the Blood-Fen, cool the Blood and promote its circulation."

Accordingly, measures to clear away the Ying-Fen and expel Heat-Evil were used at the time of first consultation. Though the Febrile-Evil did not involve the Blood-Fen (the bleeding stopped without an increase in the number of lesions), it dwelled in the Ying-Fen. This was evidenced by Yangming excess syndrome manifested in the form of high fever, restlessness, abdominal fullness and dry stool. The principles of clearing away the Ying-Fen and expelling Heat-Evil alone at this point were inadequate to achieve the desired effect. Radix et rhizoma rhei, which is bitter in flavour and cool in nature, was used as the main ingredient in the second prescription. Rhei is effective in dredging the Nine Orifices, increasing urine excretion and bowel movement and clearing away Heat-Evils in the organs. Fructus aurantii immaturus, which is also bitter in flavour and cool in nature, was used to relieve Qi stasis and to eliminate abdominal fullness and distention. Cortex magnoliae officinalis was effective in regulating the functions of the Stomach and Spleen and promoting Qi circulation in the Middle Burner. Diseases caused by Febrile-Evil usually damage the body fluid, and in order to avoid further damage in this regard, Mild Purgative Decoction was omitted on the third consultation. Emphasis was placed on replenishing the body fluid and nourishing the Yin. Herba dendrobii and Rhizoma phragmitis nourished the Yin and promoted production of body fluid and were boiled to be taken as daily drinks. As body fluid was being replenished, the amount of urine increased without loss of body fluid. The tongue picture turned red and moist. The prescription on the fourth consultation was designed to further enhance these effects. The patient's condition returned to normal consequently.

It is important to mention here that modern medicine also played a significant part in this treatment course as 1,500-2,000 ml of normal saline was given by slow IV infusion each day to maintain the electrolyte and acid-base balance.

10.4 CHOLESTASIS OF ACUTE VIRAL HEPATITIS (DISTURBANCE OF THE SPLEEN DUE TO COLD-DAMPNESS, BLOOD STASIS AND HEAT)

Wang Chenbai

Department of Traditional Chinese and Western Medicine, No. 302 Hospital of the People's Liberation Army, Beijing

Du Xinping, 29, male, Han nationality, married, worker. Medical record number: 101589. Date of admission: June 12, 1984.

CHIEF COMPLAINT: Progressively deepened jaundice and pruritus of two months duration.

HISTORY OF PRESENT ILLNESS: The patient first experienced fever on April 15, 1984, and was diagnosed as having acute tonsillitis. His urine was noted to be yellow and his stool was light-coloured two days later, and his appetite was getting worse. Xanthochromia of the skin and sclera was evident and bilirubin test positive four days after the onset of fever. He was admitted to a hospital in Beijing on April 29 where the treatment received consisted of phenobarbital, energy-sustaining mixtures, Qing Gan Ning (Pills for Removing Heat from Liver), albumin, pancreatic glucagon-insulin, branched amino acids chain and Injection 6912 (compound prescription of Heat-clearing and detoxifying Chinese herbs). Adrenocortical hormones were added to the regimen when his bilirubin level was elevated to 16.8 mg% on May 8. The hormone's dose was reduced two weeks later because his jaundice persisted and the rate of elevation of the bilirubin level became faster than before. The patient was subsequently transferred to our hospital. On admission, he was noted to have pruritus, thirst but with no desire for drinks, chest fullness, dyschesia (twice a day), yellow-coloured urine and decreased appetite.

PAST HISTORY: Non-specific.

PERTINENT PHYSICAL EXAMINATION & LABORATORY FINDINGS: Severe jaundice of the skin and sclera; scratch marks on the lower extremities with no petechiae nor ecchymoses. Heart and lungs normal. Liver palpable 2 cm below the right costal margin, soft and non-tender. Spleen likewise palpable. HBsAg, anti-HBs, anti-HBcIgM, anti-HAV IgM detection negative, while the values of bilirubin, GPT, AKP, 5-NT, Y-GT and LP-X were 37.5 mg%, 240 units, 6.8 units, 28 units and 21.2 mg%, respectively. First limulus test was found to be (q) at peak time of jaundice, strikingly positive at the time when bilirubin reduced to 2.8 mg%, (+++) by the end of 30 minutes and (++++) by the end of 24 hours. Serum endotoxin quantitation was greater than 10 µg% and negative in the control group. TXB_2 was 470 pg/dL (normal value, 120q27 pg/dL). Liver bipsy findings: cord-like liver tissues with intact hepatic lobules occasionally seen, disarrangement of cord-like liver tissues, occlusion of hepatic sinusoid, loose cytoplasm, mild retrograde and acidophilic degenerations, eosinophilic bodies, focal necrosis, cholestasis in the liver cells, bile thrombosis, intrahepatic diffuse infiltration of inflammatory cells and moderate reactions of Kupffer's cells.

INSPECTION OF TONGUE: Dark to purplish tongue substance with thin and white fur.

PULSE CONDITION: Taut and slippery.

MODERN MEDICINE DIAGNOSIS: Cholestasis of Acute Viral Hepatitis.

TRADITIONAL CHINESE MEDICINE DIAGNOSIS: Infiltration of Damp-Heat into the Three Burners; Disturbance of the Spleen due to Cold-Dampness; Blood Stasis and Heat Accumulation.

THERAPEUTIC PRINCIPLES: Invigorate the Three Burners and eliminate Damp-Heat.

PRESCRIPTION: Modified Decoction of Three Kinds of Kernels and Sweet Dew Detoxification Drink. Semen armeniacae amarum, 15 gm; Semen coicis, 18 gm; Talum, 30 gm; Semen amomi cardsmomi, 15 gm; Rhizoma pinelliae, 15 gm; Radix salviae, 30 gm; medulla terapanacis, 10 gm; Herba artemisiae scopariae, 15 gm; Fructus forsythiae, 18 gm; Radix paeoniae rubra, 80 gm; Flos lonicerae, 20 gm; Radix rubiae, 30 gm; Radix puerariae, 30 gm; Radix notoginseng, 1.5 gm; and Cornu bubali, 15 gm. Decocted and taken at a dosage of twice a day. In addition, oral vitamins and glucurolactone, IV infusion of 10% glucose (500 ml) and vitamins C and K_1 were also prescribed. Course of treatment discontinued when the patient's GI tract symptoms were relieved.

FOLLOW-UP/COURSE OF TREATMENT:

Second examination and consultation on June 25, 1984: On examination, the following signs and symptoms were seen: intolerance of cold without chills, thirst and preference to hot drinks, distention and fullness in epigastrium that could be relieved by pressure and warmth, loose stools (twice a day), dark-coloured urine, restlessness at night, dark rims of orbits, splashing sound in the stomach and scratch marks and ecchymoses on the skin. Tongue substance was dark or purplish with white to yellowish, greasy fur. These signs and symptoms supported the diagnosis of disturbance of Spleen functions due to Cold and Dampness, and Blood stasis and Heat which should be treated by warming the Middle Burner and removing Dampness with Blood-cooling and detoxifying herbs. Prescription: Ramulus cinnamomi, 15 gm; Poria, 30 gm; Rhizoma zingiberis, 15 gm; Rhizoma ligustici, 15 gm; Gypsum fibrosum, 30 gm; Flos carthami, 15 gm; Rhizoma alpiniae officinarum, 15 gm; Radix rubiae, 30 gm; Fructus forsythiae, 15 gm; Flos lonicerae, 15 gm;

Radix puerariae, 30 gm; Radix paeoniae rubra, 8 gm; Radix notoginseng, 15 gm; and Cornu bubali, 15 gm.

DISCUSSION: It was difficult to determine the etiology of this case since both virus antigens and antibodies of hepatitis A and B were negative, and indices of non-A and non-B hepatitis were also not detected. The diagnosis of cholestasis of acute viral hepatitis was confirmed by case history, biochemical indices and liver biopsy. There were four possible causes to progressive elevation of jaundice:

1) Endotoxemia. Cholestasis could have given rise to endotoxemia which might have been a result of liver disease, but limulus test at peak time of jaundice could only provide an index of suspicion which was probably associated with the inhibiting effect of severe bilirubinemia on the limulus test. The strikingly positive reaction of the limulus test when the level of jaundice had reduced to normal on the whole showed that the patient was suffering from endotoxemia, but it was not the direct cause of jaundice elevation;

2) Cholestatic factor. Cholestasis due to various causes could have induced lymphokine production which would lead to jaundice elevation. As it was not assayed in this case, it was difficult to confirm its actual effect;

3) Increased TXB_2. TXB_2 value assayed at peak time of jaundice and at the time when the patient was seen the first time was four times greater than its normal value. It decreased along with the decrease of bilirubin during the course of treatment. As TXB_2 is a powerful cholecystokinetic agent, it might have also been the cause of jaundice elevation; and

4) Prolonged administration of hormones. Clinical and animal studies have shown that administration of hormones can result in an elevated level of jaundice. Sasaki also discovered that jaundice level increases when hormones are used and decreases when hormones are discontinued. Application of large doses of hormones in this case might be one of the important causes for the rapid elevation and decrease of jaundice, though the bilirubin level continued its increase when hormones were discontinued.

The patient responded very poorly to various treatments using Chinese herbs and modern medications, but noticeable therapeutic effect was achieved by administration of Bian Zhen Lun Zhi. By symptom-complex differentiation, the patient was diagnosed initially as having Damp-Heat infiltration of the Three Burners, and as such he had a poor response to the compound prescription of Decoction of Three Kinds of Kernels and Sweet Dew Detoxication. Once correctly diagnosed on the next consultation, symptoms and signs disappeared rapidly after treatment, demonstrating that an accurate symptom-complex differentiation is indispensable in order to obtain a favour-able clinical outcome.

On the other hand, this case also manifested Blood stasis and Heat accumulation as well as disturbance of the Spleen due to Cold and Dampness. Traditional Chinese medicine considers Damp-Heat the cause of acute hepatitis. Though Damp-Heat of hepatitis accumulates in the Liver and Spleen, it could eventually lead to pathological lesions in the Heart and Kidney. Invasion of Qi at the onset of hepatitis and its gradual progression into the Blood could lead to the manifestations of a blood system syndrome. Zhang Zhongjing, a renowned traditional medicine practitioner, states in his classics that "jaundice is mostly a result of Damp-Heat, but prolonged illness of the Channels would certainly give rise to Blood stasis," "Blood stasis of hepatitis is in the Liver" and "if Blood stasis exists in the body, persistent evil heat would give rise to jaundice." Symptoms and signs of Blood stasis and heat were found when the patient was examined on the second visit. Increased TBX_2 level is a new index for the diagnosis of Blood stasis syndrome. In order to normalize the function of the Gallbladder and to cure jaundice, Blood-cooling and detoxifying herbs such as Radix salviae, Radix paeoniae rubra and Flos carthami were selected, while TBX2-inhibiting and bile duct-dilating herbs were also used in the prescription.

A sound described as splashing was appreciated in the stomach in this case, which was an indication of fluid retention in the epigastrium. This showed that there was fluid retention in the stomach since it was situated in the epigastrium. Sputum and fluid are derived from the same source, and Phlegm retention is due to Spleen deficiency. It was pointed out in *Standards of Diagnosis and Treatment* that "since presence of sputum is due to deficiency of Spleen Qi, it should be treated by reinforcing the Spleen so that once the Spleen function is restored, sputum will be resolved.... Priority should be to give Decoction of Poria, Radix atractylodis macrocephalae, Cinnamom and Radix glycyrrhizae when fluid retention is found in the epigastrium." As Phlegm results from Yin deficiency, Decoction of Poria, Radix atractylodis macrocephalae, Cinnamom and Radix glycyrrhizae was given to suppress its Yang. Radix atractylodis macrocephalae was used to strengthen and activate the Yang and to open the Channels by regulating the nutrient system so that spontaneous micturition could be achieved when Yang Qi was relieved; Poria was used in large doses to remove fluid retention, as it is sweet in taste and neutral in nature. Though Rhizoma atractylodis macrocephalae, Glycyrrhizae and Poria all exhibit similar properties in strengthening the Spleen and relieving distention, the former two take priority in the treatment of hepatitis complicated with abdominal distention because they are more powerful than Poria in relieving distention.

To reinforce the effects of Rhizoma atractylodis macrocephalae and Poria in removing Dampness, Rhizoma alpiniae officinarum and Rhizoma zingiberis were added to the prescription to warm the Middle Burner and to dispel the Cold. Rhizoma ligustici was effective in promoting Blood flow, removing Blood stasis and invigorating the flow of Qi. It was added to the prescription to facilitate the removal of fluid retention, as a healthy flow of Qi would render a normal Blood flow which in turn would lead to normal transportation of fluid. Heat-removing and detoxifying herbs such as Flos lonicerae and Fructus forsythiae were used to relieve endotoxemia and occasional low-grade fever.

This prescription has been successful in treating the apparent contradiction of Blood stasis due to Heat syndrome and disturbance of the Spleen due to Cold and Dampness. It is formulated by bearing in mind the possible causes of jaundice and as such has achieved satisfactory therapeutic effects in reducing jaundice in the short term and in preventing its recurrence in the long run.

10.5 SEVERE ICTERIC AND CHOLESTATIC ACUTE HEPATITIS-B COMPLICATED WITH COMBINED CRYOGLOBULINEMIA (JAUNDICE DUE TO STAGNANT HEAT)

Wang Chenbai

Department of Traditional Chinese and Western Medicine, No. 302 Hospital of the People's Liberation Army, Beijing

Zhang Chunhua, 26, female, Han nationality, married, worker. Medical record number: 94528. Date of admission: November 15, 1981.

CHIEF COMPLAINT: Asthenia, poor appetite, vomiting and yellow-coloured urine for more than 20 days.

HISTORY OF PRESENT ILLNESS: About a month prior to admission, the patient experienced generalized weakness, aversion to greasy food, vomiting one to several times a day and dark-yellow to strong, tea-like urine. Jaundiced sclera, grayish-coloured stools, generalized pruritus and epistaxis were found 10 days later. Laboratory tests performed on November 15 in our hospital showed GPT greater than 200 units, TTT and serum bilirubin 15 units and 7.15 mg%, respectively.

When first seen in our clinic on December 12, 1981, the patient presented signs and symptoms such as severe pruritus which interfered with his sleep, nausea and vomiting, poor appetite, grayish-coloured stools, absence of thirst and desire to drink, severe jaundice of the skin, multiple scratch marks, bloody crusts and massive ecchymoses of the lower extremities with tenderness. His jaundice increased (bilirubin level 22.8 mg%), area of ecchymoses was enlarging and pruritus worsened after treatment by Heat-clearing and detoxifying herbs and adrenocortical hormones in our hospital.

PAST HISTORY: History of gastroenteritis and gastroptosis in 1974.

PERTINENT PHYSICAL EXAMINATION & LABORATORY FINDINGS: Blood pressure, 132/190 mmHg. Conscious and cooperative. Skin and sclera moderately jaundiced with sporadic ecchymoses of the lower extremities. Heart and lung findings negative. Liver palpable 2.0 cm below the right costal margin on midclavicular line, 4.0 cm palpable under the xiphoid process, soft in consistency and tender on percussion; spleen not palpable. Pitting edema of the lower extremities positive. GPT, 824 units; serum total bilirubin/direct bilirubin and prothrombin time/activity was 11.05/8.6 mg% and 12 seconds/1005; 5'NT, r-GT and AKP, 12 m, 23 units and 3.18 units, respectively. Total cholesterol/cholesterol ester, 180/650 mg% (the patient's maximum value being 245 mg% during hospitalization), while sedimentation rate was 9 mm/hr. CH_{50}, C_3, HBsAg and anti-HBc were 38 μ/mL, 1652.5 mg/mL, 1:16 and 1:10, respectively. Serum cryoglobulin 165 μgm/mL (normal value ‹14 μgm/mL). Anti-mitochondrion antibodies and anti-smooth muscle antibodies were negative. No immunocomplex sedimentation was found in biopsies of the skin at the site of ecchymoses.

Liver biopsy: Liver cords found to be arranged in order, hepatic sinusoid stenosed and hepatic cytoplasm loose with ballooning degeneration occasionally found. Proliferation of Kupffer's cells, focal necrosis and infiltration of lymphocytes were also found with sporadic thrombosis in bile capillaries and cholestasis in liver cells.

INSPECTION OF TONGUE: Dark-red to purplish tongue with petechiae, ecchymoses and thin, whitish coating.

PULSE CONDITION: Taut.

MODERN MEDICINE DIAGNOSIS: Severe Icteric and Cholestatic Acute Hepatitis-B complicated with Combined Cryoglobulinemia.

TRADITIONAL CHINESE MEDICINE DIAGNOSIS: Jaundice due to Stagnant Heat.

THERAPEUTIC PRINCIPLES: Cool the Blood, invigorate the circulation, dispel the Wind and arrest the itchiness.

PRESCRIPTION: Radix paeoniae rubra, 60 gm; Radix puerariae, 30 gm; Radix rehmanniae, 18 gm; Radix salviae, 18 gm; Radix scutellariae, 15 gm; Cortex moutan radicis, 15 gm; Herba artemisiae capillaris, 15 gm; and Radix ledebouriellae, 15 gm.

FOLLOW-UP/COURSE OF TREATMENT:

Second consultation on December 15, 1981: After taking two doses of the prescription, grayish-coloured stool turned yellow, while pruritus was relieved and ecchymotic areas reduced, though one to two new ecchymotic areas were noted. Because of vomiting (which could have been due to withdrawal of hormones), the herbal prescription was withdrawn, but grayish-coloured stool returned and jaundice deepened a day later. Bilirubin level was 35.6 mg% and no change was found in the condition of the tongue and pulse. Modified the prescription to contain Fructus trichosanthis, 30 gm; Rhizoma pinelliae, 15 gm; Herba plantaginis, 15 gm; Radix thalictribaicalensis, 15 gm; Radix paeoniae rubra, 80 gm; Herba leonuri, 15 gm; Radix puerariae, 30 gm; Radix lidebouriellae, 15 gm; Radix salviae, 15 gm; Cortex moutan radicis, 15 gm; Fructus kochiae, 15 gm; Rhizoma ligustici, 15 gm; and Rhizoma imperatae, 18 gm.

Third consultation on December 22, 1981: After taking four doses of the modified prescription, the patient reported only mild pruritus with disappearance of ecchymoses and epigastric distention. He had bowel movement three times a day with right interphalangeal arthralgia. Jaundice was reduced with bilirubin level lowered to 23.5 mg%. Continued the same prescription.

Fourth consultation on January 7, 1982: The patient complained of mild pruritus, nausea, soft stools, symmetrical arthralgia and local pachylosis with a sensation of numbness. The patient was referred to a specialist and was diagnosed as having allergic arthritis due to hepatitis infection. Tongue substance was dark-red to purplish with white, greasy fur and pulse was taut. Modified the prescription to contain Radix gentianae macrophyllae, 15 gm; Radix paeoniae rubra, 60 gm; Radix paeoniae alba, 18 gm; Radix scutellariae, 15 gm; Radix salviae, 15 gm; Rhizoma ligustici, 15 gm; Radix glycyrrhizae, 6 gm; Rhizoma pinelliae, 15 gm; Radix lidebouriellae, 6 gm; Radix puerariae, 30 gm; and herba siegesbechiae, 15 gm.

Fifth consultation on February 6, 1982: GPT, 130 units; bilirubin, 2.15 mg%;

anti-HBc, 1:10 with negative HBsAg and no complaint of discomfort. After discharge from the hospital, the patient continued to take the prescription and had no relapse during the succeeding year of follow-up.

DISCUSSION: The diagnosis of acute and cholestatic hepatitis-B was established in this case based on clinical signs and symptoms, biochemical tests findings and liver biopsy. The patient had the characteristic trilogy of symptoms of fatigue, purpura and arthralgia accompanied by cryoglobulinemia. The incidence of its occurrence in acute hepatitis-B could be as high as 70% and is common in young female patients suffering from hepatitis. The condition is characterized by damage of the skin and small renal vessels. The common manifestation is purpura which is often localized on the lower extremities with a tendency to develop concentric diffusion; 72.5% of the patients we have treated had multiple symmetrical arthralgia of hands and knees, but generally there was no deformity. The diagnosis was made definite by detection of cryoglobulin in the blood. It is seldom effective to treat the disease using adrenocortical hormones, cytotoxic drugs (such as butyric nitrogen mustard), cyclophosphamide, agathiopurine, penicillamine, splenectomy or plasma exchange.

Signs and symptoms important to TCM symptom-complex differentiation are jaundice, ecchymoses and arthralgia. The cause of jaundice is associated with Warm and Heat pathogens. The Spleen is the vicera primarily involved. According to TCM literature the "Spleen will inevitably become yellow in colour if stagnant Heat is present." The pathogenesis of jaundice as documented in *Si Shen Xin Yuan* is "Damp-Earth and ultimately results from Wind and Wood." This indicates that jaundice causes injury to both the Spleen and Liver. Sun Simiao points out that "severe jaundice of seasonal febrile diseases, such as virus hepatitis, is probably due to endogenous stagnant Heat." The rapid onset of the disease could be attributed to internal invasion of epidemic pathogens and toxic Heat. A sharp increase in the jaundice level is due to bile being forced out of the bile ducts by epidemic pathogens of toxic Heat, while ecchymosis results from invasion of the skin by the same pathogen. Traditional Chinese medicine holds that "jaundice complicated by hemorrhage is due to pathogenic Fire in the Spleen and Stomach, Heat injuries to the Heart which governs the Blood circulation and excessive Heat." It was evident that jaundice secondary to stagnant Heat was the etiology and pathogenesis in our case. Arthralgia was associated with excessive internal Heat, which is a Yang pathogen interacting with the Blood and Qi; spasms of the muscles were due to the invasion and obstruction of the Channels which led to intolerable pain. Excessive Heat damaging the Blood circulation and Blood deficiency secondary to endopathic Wind resulted in pruritus.

Though the patient displayed signs of excessive toxic Heat as the dominant pathogen, his Vital Energy could still resist it. Since the pathogenic invasion was not that severe, it could be treated by applying the principles of cooling the Blood and invigorating the circulation with attention also paid to the nourishment of Yin. The prescription to achieve these goals was made up of Radix paeoniae rubra, Radix puerariae, Radix salviae, Radix rehmanniae, Cortex moutan radicis, Rhizoma ligustici, Flos carthami, Radix scutellariae, Herba artemisiae scopariae, Rhizoma imperatae itchin, Radix ledebouriellae, Cortex Illicii broom and Cypress fruit with Cortex dictamni radicus added to dispel Wind and arrest the pruritus. Since the prominent manifestation of this case in the later stage was arthralgia, which is believed to be caused by Heat, Radix gentianae macrophyllae and Herba siegesbechiae were added to regulate the Blood, remove the Heat and relieve the arthralgia. In addition, Radix glycyrrhizae and Radix paeoniae alba were used to relieve spasms and pain.

Administration of this prescription led to a rapid turn for the better in the patient's condition. Jaundice, ecchymosis and arthralgia had disappeared, and he was discharged from hospital fully recovered.

10.6 CHRONIC ACTIVE HEPATITIS-B, DECOMPENSATED HEPATOCIRRHOSIS, ENDOTOXEMIA (BLOOD STASIS AND BLOOD DEFICIENCY, NOXIOUS HEAT AND INTENSE FIRE)

Wang Chenbai

Department of Traditional Chinese and Western Medicine, No. 302 Hospital of the People's Liberation Army, Beijing

Wang Xiangtong, 15, male, Han nationality, single, student. Medical record number: 101547. Date of admission: June 6, 1984.

CHIEF COMPLAINT: Nausea and asthenia for more than a year; edema of the lower extremities for one and a half months.

HISTORY OF PRESENT ILLNESS: One year prior to admission, the patient experienced nausea, poor appetite, aversion to fatty food, generalized weakness, jaundice and yellow-coloured urine. Blood examination showed levels of GPT, TTT and STB to be 644 units, 13 units and 4.4 mg% , respectively. Jaundice disappeared when TTT level was reduced to 9 units and GPT to 628 units after six weeks of treatment using medications such as Yi Gan Ling in a hospital. He continued to take the medication after discharge from hospital. GPT level was 500 units when re-examined in June of the same year and fluctuated between 600 and 700 units thereafter. Jiang Mei Ling was given to treat the condition. Four months later, GPT and TTT levels were detected to be 680 and 20 units, respectively, with serum HBsAg positive. He was admitted to the same hospital as a case of chronic active hepatitis. Taking diphenyl diester for six months, his GPT and TTT were reduced to 180 and 128 units, respectively, and he was discharged. The patient continued to take the medication, but edema of the lower extremities was noted in April of 1984 with STB level detected to be 3.1 mg% in May of the same year. He was subsequently admitted to our hospital.

On admission, the patient complained of dizziness, generalized weakness, numbness of the right lower extremity, thirst but with no desire for drinks, afternoon fever (temperature around 38°C), edema of the lower extremities, abdominal distention (with presence of moderate ascites) and acne of the skin.

PAST HISTORY: Non-contributory.

PERTINENT PHYSICAL EXAMINATION & LABORATORY FINDINGS: Blood pressure, 100/60 mmHg; conscious and cooperative; non-icteric. Spider nervi, liver palm, acne, scattering petechiae, ecchymotic areas on the lower extremities, icteric sclera and abdominal distention were evident. Heart and lung findings negative. Positive shifting dullness with tenderness on percussion of the liver region. Liver and spleen not palpable. Hemoglobin, 7 gm%; RBC, 1.79 M/mm^3; WBC, 2,800/mm^3; neutrophils, 61%; lymphocytes, 36%; monocytes, 2%; eosinophils, 1%; and platelet count, 42,000/mm^3. Urinalysis revealed WBC, 3-4/hpf and RBC, 0-1/hpf. Serum total bilirubin/combined bilirubin, 5.0/2.8 mg%; TTT, 15 units; GPT, 130 units and albumin/globulin, 2.6/2.4 gm%, prothrombin time/activity, 33 sec/15.6%; and aFP, 1:00 (+). IgM, IgA and IgG levels were 5.01 mg/mL, 5.88 mg/L and 25.08/mL, respectively. Protein electrophoresis showed albumin, 53.6%; γμ-globulin, 30.8%; ESR, 16 mm/hr; HBsAg, 1:64; inhibiting rate for anti-HBc, 91%; anti-HBcIgM, 4.5; HBeAg, positive; anti-HBs and anti-HBe negative. Limulus test positive.

INSPECTION OF TONGUE: The tongue was slightly enlarged and reddish in colour with rhagades and thin, whitish fur.

PULSE CONDITION: String-like.

MODERN MEDICINE DIAGNOSIS: Chronic Active Hepatitis-B; Decompensated Hepatocirrhosis; Endotoxemia.

TRADITIONAL CHINESE MEDICINE DIAGNOSIS: Blood Stasis and Blood Deficiency; Presence of Noxious Heat and Intense Fire.

THERAPEUTIC PRINCIPLES: Cool the Blood, invigorate the circulation and clear away Heat and toxic materials.

PRESCRIPTION: Radix paeoniae rubra, 60 gm; Radix puerariae, 30 gm; Flos lonicerae, 30 gm; Fructus forsythiae, 30 gm; Rhizoma cimicifugae, 6 gm; Radix angelicae, 15 gm; Cortex moutan radicis, 15 gm; Rhizoma alismatis, 60 gm; Rhizoma imperatae, 15 gm; Herba agrimoniae, 15 gm; Radix rubiae, 15 gm; Radix notoginseng, 1.5 gm; and Cornu bubali, 1.5 gm. Twice a day.

Other management: hydrochlorothiazide, 25 mg/day; antisterone, 20 mg/day; IV infusion of vitamin K1, 10 mg/day and transfusion of 1,000 ml of blood and 35 ml of prothrombin complex. A total of 380 gm of albumin was also transfused over five occasions.

FOLLOW-UP/COURSE OF TREATMENT:

The patient ran a persistent, low-grade fever and intermittent high fever every four to eight days which persisted two to three days each time (10 times in all) after he was admitted to our hospital. Eight days of treatment using gentamicin (240,000 units a day) failed to lower his temperature. Fever had not occurred since November 13, 1984.

Second consultation on June 18, 1984: Levels of bilirubin, GPT, TTT, A/G ratio and Pt/Pa were 9.3/3.9 mg%, 216 units, 16 units, 2.5/3.4 gm% and 33 seconds/15.6% (maximum value being 8.9%), respectively. Edema of the lower extremities had disappeared, while he had thirst and taste of blood in his mouth with no change in the picture of the tongue and pulse condition. The patient went on taking the prescription modified by increasing the dose of Bai Mo Gen (Cogongrass rhizome) to 30 gm.

Third consultation on September 27, 1984: Bilirubin, 5.5/2.2 mg%; GPT, 334 units; GOT, 304 units; Pt/Pa, 1 second/23.8%; and A/G, 2.38/3.16%. Limulus test (+) at 0 time, (+++) by the end of 30 minutes and (++++) by the end of 24 hours. Quantitative endotoxin was greater than or equal to 10 mg%. Tongue substance red with rhagades and yellowish fur. Pulse rapid and string-like. Modified the prescription to contain Radix paeoniae rubra, 80 gm; Herba taraxaci, 15 gm; Rhizoma zedoariae, 15 gm; Radix puerariae, 30 gm; Radix scrophulariae, 15 gm; Fructus crataegi, 30 gm; Rhizoma sparganii, 15 gm; Flos lonicerae, 15 gm; Fructus forsythiae, 15 gm; Radix astragali, 15 gm; Radix achyranthis, 15 gm; Radix rehmanniae, 15 gm; Carapax trionycis, 15 gm; Plastrum testudinis, 15 gm; Squama manitis, 15 gm; Radix notoginseng, 1.5 gm; and Cornu bubali, 1.5 gm. Taken twice daily.

Fourth consultation on April 18, 1985: Bilirubin, 2.3/1.0 mg%; TTT, 5 units; GPT, 130 units; A/G, 3.27/1.85%; and Pt/Pa, 24 seconds/28.1%. The patient reported no specific discomfort and the signs of ascites had disappeared. Tongue substance remained red with rhagades. Modified the prescription to contain Radix paeoniae rubra, 30 gm; Radix puerariae, 30 gm; Rhizoma cimicifugae, 30 gm; Fructus crataegi, 30 gm; Rhizoma zedoariae, 15 gm; Rhizoma sparganii, 15 gm; Fructus forsythiae, 15 gm; Radix astragali, 15 gm; Radix achyranthis, 15 gm; Plastrum testudinis, 15 gm; and Squama manitis, 15 gm.

Fifth consultation on August 4, 1985: SGPT, GOT and TT levels all normal; A/G, 3.38/2.55 gm%, bilirubin, 2.5/1.4 mg%; and Pt/Pa, 24 seconds/28.1%; HBsAg, 1:64; inhibiting rate for anti-HBc, 99% and hematochrome, 10.5%; HBeAg and anti-HBcIgM negative. The patient continued to take the prescription up to the time of discharge from hospital. Prescription was then changed to honeyed-pill form which the patient took for another year after various biochemical indices returned to normal.

When last seen in early 1988, the patient was in good health.

DISCUSSION: The diagnosis of chronic active hepatitis-B with decompensated hepatocirrhosis was established based on the medical history of chronic hepatitis, severe deterioration of liver functions, marked reduction of serum albumin, hypersplenia, ascites, edema and positive indices of hepatitis-B virus.

The chief characteristic of this disease is severe endotoxemia. Hepatocirrhosis causes intestinal wall edema and portal hypertension which in turn enhances intestinal absorption of endotoxins. Endotoxins pass into systemic circulation directly through collateral pathways leading to an increased level in blood and positive limulus test. Antibiotics have little effect in treating intermittent fever due to endotoxemia. Damage to the inner walls of blood vessels by endotoxins cause platelet aggregation leading to reduction in the number of platelets. Impaired prothrombin activity is due to endotoxin-induced chronic-disseminated intravascular coagulopathy resulting in consumption of coagulation factor II. The lowest prothrombin activity level of this case was 8.9%.

Though drugs such as lactulase and antibiotics resistant to intestinal absorption can be used in the treatment of endotoxemia, none of them so far has had a satisfactory therapeutic effect. The author believes that a combined treatment employing traditional Chinese and modern medicine can achieve good therapeutic effects in this respect. The patient was finally cured by traditional Chinese medicine together with a large amount of albumin transfusion.

According to traditional Chinese medicine, this case should be treated by relieving the abdominal distention and clearing away the noxious Heat. Traditional medicine believes that abdominal distention is due to ascites secondary to hepatocirrhosis. Its etiology and pathogenesis are very complicated. As stated in *Principles and Prohibitions for Medical Profession: Abdominal Distention,* "Without exception, abdominal distention is a result of fluid retention, Qi stagnation and Blood stasis." Our case was complicated with jaundice, which is usually secondary to accumulation of Damp-Heat. In due course of time, Damp-Heat led to injury of the Spleen and loss of Qi in the Middle Burner, disturbance in regulatory functions, retention of water within the body and loss of Liver Qi. Liver, Spleen and Kidney dysfunctions were the key pathogenesis of abdominal distention. Liver Qi stagnation and Blood stasis gave rise to obstruction of the Channels, which was the fundamental cause of abdominal distention.

Abdominal distention should be treated first of all by differentiating between the symptom-complex of deficiency and excess. It is pointed out in *Complete Works of Jing Yue: Abdominal Distention* that those who have red and yellow complexion and puffing and blowing breath are probably suffering from excess syndrome, while those who appear thin and pallid with short breath suffer from deficiency syndrome. Those who are young and vigorous and have airway obstruction probably suffer from excess syndrome, while those who have insufficiency of the Middle Burner and look tired with stagnation of Qi probably suffer from deficiency syndrome. Our patient was a young man and it is likely that he suffered from both deficiency and excess syndromes because he had Blood stasis and Blood Heat complicated with Blood deficiency according to our comprehensive analysis.

This case also had an irregular and persistent fever and a prolonged, lingering course of the disease was complicated by subcutaneous hemorrhage and ecchymosis. Heat dwelled in the Yin Blood, and the condition was further complicated by Yin injury. The appropriate principles of treatment were to clear away the Heat, cool the Blood and nourish the Yin.

Taking into consideration the etiology and pathogenesis, the patient was treated in accordance with the principles of cooling the Blood, invigorating the circulation and clearing away the Heat and toxic materials. In the prescription, Radix paeoniae rubra, Radix puerariae, Plastrum testudinis and Radix notoginseng were used to cool the Blood and invigorate the circulation; Cornu bubali to clear away Heat and toxic materials; Radix astragali to supplement the Qi; and Rhizoma sparganii, Rhizoma zedoariae, Squama manitis and Carapax trionycis to eliminate Blood stasis, soften hard masses and remove obstruction of the Channels. Rhizoma alismatis was added to promote micturition.

This case involved severe jaundice (bilirubin level of 9.3 mg%) which was due to Blood stasis and Blood Heat. Satisfactory therapeutic effects were achieved in reducing and eliminating jaundice by using Blood-cooling and circulation-invigorating herbs instead of oriental wormwood. These prescriptions are better than others in clearing away heat and toxic materials and in invigorating Blood circulation and removing Blood stasis.

10.7 CHRONIC PERSISTENT HEPATITIS (MELANCHOLIA)

Gao Chiyan, Liu Qingxiang and Wu Weiwei
Xiamen Traditional Chinese Medicine Hospital, Xiamen

The patient is a 63-year-old male of Han nationality, married, retired worker. Medical record number: 63139. Date of first consultation: May 7, 1986.

CHIEF COMPLAINT: Chest and hypochondria distention, lassitude, decreased appetite for about one year. Pain on the right upper abdomen. Loose stools for more than one month.

HISTORY OF PRESENT ILLNESS: The patient went to hospital about a year ago because of pain in the right hypochondrium, decreased appetite and lassitude. He was treated as "Chest Bi" for several months without effect. Other symptoms he complained of were epigastric distention, indigestion and loss of appetite, vertigo, lassitude, irritability with bitter taste in the mouth and dry throat, restlessness, sleep with frequent dreams, scanty, dark urine and loose stools two to three times a day.

PAST HISTORY: History of dysentery in 1964.

Personal History: A widower, the patient is a smoker, a light drinker and fond of spicy food.

PERTINENT PHYSICAL EXAMINATION & LABORATORY FINDINGS: Temperature, 36.3°C; pulse rate, 76/min; respiratory rate, 20/min; blood pressure, 130/80 mmHg; conscious, with lustreless complexion, emaciated. Non-icteric sclera, skin normal; red palm (liver palm), no nevus arachnoideus. No enlargement of superficial lymph nodes. Heart and lungs normal. Abdomen soft, upper limit of the liver on the fifth intercostal space and the lower limit 2.5 cm below right costal margin. Liver consistency moderate with tenderness on percussion. Spleen palpable, soft and without tenderness. No edema of the lower extremities. Nervous system examination negative. Hemoglobin, 11.5 gm%; WBC, 6,000/mm³; neutrophils, 52%; eosinophils, 3%; lymphocytes, 45%; platelet, 135,000/mm³; and ESR, 5 mm/hr. Liver function test: icterus index, 7 units; total protein, 7.4 gm; albumin, 4.0 gm; globulin, 3.5 gm; TTT, 20 units; TFT, (+++); ZnTT, 14 units; SGPT, 90 units (normal value 40 units); HBsAG, 1:64 positive; HBVM: HBsAG, (+); HBsAB, (-); HBeAG, (+); HBeAB, (+); HBcAB, 1:100 (+++). Urine test: bilirubin, (-); urobilinogen, (-); urobilin, (-). Routine stool examination negative.

INSPECTION OF TONGUE: Red tongue substance with yellowish and glossy fur.

PULSE CONDITION: String-like, faint and rapid.

MODERN MEDICINE DIAGNOSIS: Chronic Persistent Hepatitis (Type B).

TRADITIONAL CHINESE MEDICINE DIAGNOSIS: Melancholia; Depressed

Liver with Insufficient Spleen.

Symptom-complex differentiation: This was a case of consumed and weak Vital Energy. The patient was temperamental, irascible and depressed. There was presence of Liver Qi stasis. He has been treated for a long time but without satisfactory results. Liver was depressed and Spleen insufficient. Liver Qi affected the Spleen, which lost its normal transporting functions, leading to onset of the disease. The primary pathology was dysfunction of the dissipation and excretory functions and disorder of Qi. The patient complained of pain in the chest and liver region. Depression of Wood generated Fire, causing bitter taste and dry throat and red tongue substance with yellowish and glossy fur. Disturbance of the mind by pathogens caused restless sleep with frequent dreams. Accumulation of Dampness and Heat in urinary bladder was manifested by a scanty amount of dark urine. Indigestion and loss of appetite resulted from impairment of the Spleen's normal transporting functions. Deficiency of Vital Energy caused lack of Qi and Blood. Inadequate nutrition to the extremities and trunk was evidenced by lassitude and lustreless complexion. Physical sign of red (Liver) palms was due to stagnation of Blood.

THERAPEUTIC PRINCIPLES: Based on the teaching of "treating the Biao (secondary) aspect for emergency and the Ben (primary) aspect for chronicity," this case was treated by clearing the Liver, regulating the Qi and dissipating Heat and detoxification.

PRESCRIPTION: Modified Dan Zhi Xiao Yao Fang. Fructus gardeniae, 6 gm; Radix bupleuri, 9 gm; Radix paeoniae alba, 12 gm; Herba menthae, 3 gm; Radix angelicae sinensis, 6 gm; Rhizoma atractylodis macrocephalae, 9 gm; Radix curcumae, 9 gm; Herba hypericum, 15 gm; Herba arteaisai scopariae, 15 gm; and Medicated leaven, 10 gm. Five doses. The patient was advised to maintain a calm and relaxed way of life. Light meals and avoidance of greasy and spicy food as well as food of dry and heat nature were also recommended.

Second consultation on May 12, 1986: After taking the prescription, the pain on the chest and hypochondrium was alleviated slightly. The patient could sleep more peacefully, and he was more relaxed. He felt hungry in the morning and could eat two small bowls of porridge but still complained of bitter taste in the mouth and dry throat with occasional abdominal distention and vague pain in the right hypochondrium. Pulse was string-like and tongue had yellowish and glossy fur. These signs indicated that stagnation and Damp-Heat had not been dissipated. Removed Radix angelica and Radix curcumae from the previous prescription and added Fructus citri sarcodatylis, 9 gm, and Rhizoma coptidis, 6 gm. Seven doses.

Third consultation on May 19, 1986: At this visit, the patient was in a good mood and smiled a lot. He reported that after taking the prescription and following the doctor's advice, he could sense that his condition was improving. His appetite had returned to normal. Hypochondriac pain and abdominal distention occurred only occasionally. He slept had better now and did not experience bitter taste and dry throat. Body of tongue had changed from red to clear and yellowish fur disappeared. Pulse was slow and appeared string-like when pressed forcibly. These clinical manifestations indicated that the patient's condition had improved greatly, and it was likely that the pathogens and stagnation in the body had been successfully removed. Disappearance of pain and abdominal distention signified that pathogens no longer dwelled in the Channels. Now that depression of Wood had been dissipated and the Earth was at peace, it was necessary to readjust the therapeutic measures according to the new clinical condition. Attention was drawn to strengthening the Spleen to reinforce the patient's constitution. One must bear in mind that strengthening the body resistance and expelling the pathogens must be done simultaneously. The final goal of the treatment was to reach a state of "normal health with pathogens dissipated." The therapeutic principle at that point was to strengthen the Spleen and reinforce the Stomach.

Modified Xiang Sha Liu Jun Tang: Fructus amomi, 6 gm; Radix pseudostellaria heterophylla, 15 gm; Poria, 15 gm; Pericarpium citri reticulatae, 6 gm; Rhizoma atractylodis macrocephalae, 10 gm; Herba hyperieum, 15 gm; Radix smilax sinensis, 15 gm; Endothelium corneum gigeriae galli, 9 gm; Radix et Fructus gardeniae, 10 gm; and Radix glycyrrhizae, 3 gm. Ten doses.

Fourth consultation on May 26, 1986: After taking the prescription for three weeks, the patient appeared in good health. His complexion was lustrous, his voice deep and he moved around full of energy. At a glance, he did not appear to be a 60-year-old man. He reported passing loose stools twice a day, and he could engage in some light household chores. However, he still got tired and sweated easily. Tongue substance was light red in colour with clear fur and the pulse slow and weak. According to the teaching recorded in *Nei Jing (Canon of Internal Medicine)* "a healthy and strong interior prevents invasion by the pathogens," therefore, herbs effective in strengthening the Spleen and tonifying the Qi were added to the previous prescription.

Modified Si Jun Zi Tang: Radix astragali seu hedysari, 30 gm; Radix pseudostellaria heterophylla, 15 gm; Poria, 15 gm; Rhizoma atractylodis macrocephalae, 10 gm; Rhizoma dioscoreae, 15 gm; Fructus amomi, 6 gm; Endothelium corneum gigeriae galli, 9 gm; Radix smilax sinensis, 15 gm; Herba hypericum, 15 gm; and Radix glycyrrhizae, 3 gm. Fifteen doses.

Fifth consultation on June 10, 1986: The patient had no specific complaint. His diet was normal, and there was no epigastric and abdominal upset. Urination and bowel movements were normal. He slept well and appeared healthy. Pulse slow but strong.

Re-examination showed non-icteric sclera; normal heart and lungs. Abdomen soft, lower limit of the liver 1.5 cm below the right costal margin, soft and non-tender on percussion. Spleen not palpable. No edema of the lower extremities. Liver function test: total protein, 7.3 gm; Albumin, 4.4 gm; globulin, 2.9 gm; TTT, 6 units; TFT, (+); ZnTT, 8 units; SGPT, 40 units; HBsAG, 1:16 (+); HBVM; HBsAG, (+); HBsAB, (-); HBsAG, (+); HBeAB, (+); HBcAB, 1:100 (++).

From these findings, it was evident that the patient's Liver stasis had been dissipated essentially and the Spleen deficiency remedied. Because of the recovery of the primordial Qi, pathogens were now difficult to conceal in the body. The goal of "reinforcing the body resistance and eliminating pathogens" had basically been achieved. The patient was to take the following prescription to further consolidate the therapeutic effect. Radix astragali hedysari, 20 gm; Radix pseudostellaria heterophylla, 20 gm; Rhizoma atractylodis macrocephalae, 10 gm; Poria, 15 gm; Semen nulumnis,

15 gm; Radix smilax sinensis, 15 gm; and Rhizoma polygonati, 15 gm. One dose daily for 15 days.

Liver function tests were done on follow-up visit to our clinic on July 25, 1986. All findings were normal. HBsAG, (-).

DISCUSSION: This patient had suffered from hepatitis-B for about a year. Although treated in another hospital, the results were not satisfactory. Clinical symptoms such as lassitude, indigestion and loss of appetite, abdominal distention, diarrhea, distress and pain over the liver region remained. In addition, liver and spleen were swollen with liver functions abnormal. HBsAG detection was (+). These findings confirmed the diagnosis of chronic active hepatitis. Presently, modern medicine has no treatment of choice for this disease. The condition can be treated by using antiviral agents and immunotherapy, but no definite outcome can be expected. In this case, a course of treatment was mapped out based on TCM symptom-complex differentiation and a satisfactory result was obtained.

"Stasis" was the main pathology. The patient became a widower in his middle age, there was no one to take care of his daily life and, by traditional point of view, this led to stasis of the Mind. Stasis of the Mind resulted in Qi dysfunction and damage to the Liver. Depression of body Qi generated Fire with hepatic Qi running wild and unchecked. This deranged energy invaded the Spleen and Stomach resulting in a depressed liver and insufficient Spleen. Such a state was manifested by clinical signs and symptoms of chest and hypochondriac pain, irritability and excitability, bitter taste in the mouth and dry throat, red tongue and string-like pulse due to excessive liver Fire; and epigastric distention, indigestion, loss of appetite and loose stools attributed to Spleen deficiency. The coexistence of excess and deficient syndromes was thus evident in this case. Both the Liver and Spleen were in a disturbed state. *Jin Gui Yao Lue (Synopsis of the Golden Chamber)* states that "Liver ailment will inevitably transmit to the Spleen, so it is essential to strengthen the Spleen first." Clinical conditions of our case conformed with this teaching. The deranged internal condition and lowered body resistance caused by a prolonged course of disease was susceptible to invasion by external pathogens. *Nei Jing* states that "pathogens strike wherever there is insufficiency." Deficiency of Qi was the internal etiologic factor, while invasion by pathogens was the external etiologic factor.

In our case, it was advisable to expel first the pathogens which caused the stasis. However, if the measures to expel were applied indiscriminately, the Zhen Qi (Vital Energy) could be injured and rendered deficient and the pathogens could infiltrate from the exterior to the interior and to the Qi and blood, resulting in serious illness. The safe and appropriate measure was to simultaneously reinforce the body resistance and eliminate the pathogens. Emphasis on the initial stage was on strengthening the resistance rather than eliminating the pathogens, thus treating the disease slowly and allowing the patient to benefit fully from the treatment. It was prudent to follow the teaching of "slow treatment for chronic disease" in this case in order to achieve the final goal of full recovery.

The patient was diagnosed as having Liver depression with the presence of Fire at first consultation. Therapeutic principles applied were to clear the Liver and relieve the depression and eliminate the Fire and toxic materials. In line with the method of "facilitating the stagnant Wood" documented in *Nei Jing*, Dan Zhi Xiao Yao San with stasis-dissipating and toxin-eliminating herbs was prescribed to treat the patient in the hope that the Qi of solid and hollow viscerae would be cleared and the Channels would be opened, thus facilitating the dissipation of stagnant Qi and Fire. Having taken five doses of the prescription, the hypochondriac pain was alleviated, and the patient regained his appetite. This indicated a gradual restoration of the Qi function and dissipation of the pathogens. Wood Qi was smooth at the second visit because of "inhibition of Wood to restrain Earth," while there was no urgency in altering the "acquisition." Should the Spleen be given a considerable period of time to recover, its Qi would be vigorous, thus we could get twice the result with half the effort. The patient's tongue had a yellowish and glossy fur which indicated presence of residual Dampness and Heat in the Middle Burner. Accordingly, Fructus citri sacrodactylis was added to the prescription at the last visit to regulate Qi and eliminate stagnation and distention with Rhizoma coptidis added to eliminate retained Heat in the Middle Burner. By applying an uninterrupted course of treatment, pathogens were dissipated completely. The major feature of this therapy was a continuous harmonization of the Liver and Stomach and dissipation of the pathogens. After taking this prescription for more than one month, most of the symptoms disappeared. The patient reported that his condition had improved greatly and he was in a much better mood. Careful examination showed clear fur of the tongue and presence of a slow pulse. Such physical signs demonstrated complete removal of the pathogens and clearing away of the Dampness and Heat. It was then necessary to modify the treatment taking into consideration the new clinical circumstances. Appropriate therapeutic principles at this juncture were to strengthen the Spleen and mitigate the Stomach to achieve a vigorous Earth. The transport and digestion functions recovered and the goal of "normal health with pathogens dissipated" was achieved. Modified Xiang Sha Liu Jun Tang was prescribed to reinforce the Spleen and Stomach in order to strengthen the Yang, enhance the Spleen Qi and eventually lead to a rapid recovery. Should administration of pathogen-clearing herbs have continued in large doses when symptoms such as loose stool, lassitude and spontaneous sweating were still present, the Spleen and Stomach could have been damaged. Manifestation of these symptoms indicated the Spleen and Stomach functions had been compromised for a long time, their transport and digestion functions were impaired and general condition of the patient had just been brought under control. It was imperative that transport and digestion functions be reinforced. Si Jun Zi Tang was then prescribed to obtain this goal. Pathogen-clearing herbs were also administered concurrently, thus making the therapeutic measure one composed of both elimination and reinforcement properties, the same approach used to treat the coexistence of excess and deficiency syndromes.

Through the five visits, the patient took Chinese medicines for several months. His condition improved day by day. Findings from physical examination and liver function tests performed two months later were all normal with detection of HBsAG negative. It is evident from this experience that appropriate therapeutic measures are always based on sound symptom-complex differentiation. In this case, principles applied were clearing the Liver, regulating the Qi and strengthening and reinforcing the Spleen and Stomach. Together with the application of pathogen-clearing herbs, such as Qicunjin, Yinchen, Zhizigen and Baqi, satisfactory clinical results were obtained.

10.8 CHRONIC HEPATITIS-B
(HYPOCHONDRIAC PAIN,
SPLEEN AND STOMACH DEFICIENCY)

Wei Beihai and Wang Binfang
Beijing Traditional Chinese Medicine Hospital, Beijing

Wang Suzi, 53, female, Han nationality, married, worker. Medical record number: 4081. Date of first consultation: May 4, 1985.

CHIEF COMPLAINT: Left hypochondriac pain, weakness and poor appetite of more than one year's duration.

HISTORY OF PRESENT ILLNESS: For the past year prior to consultation, the patient suffered from hepatitis without icterus, accompanied by nausea, vomiting, fever, poor appetite, weakness and dizziness. Laboratory examination showed GPT level, 960 units; and III, 9 units. After treatment by a combination of modern and Chinese medicine, the liver functions recovered gradually, but her condition was not stable and HBsAG was positive. The patient had been under treatment for the whole year, yet the symptoms had not disappeared completely. She subsequently came to our clinic, and on the first visit she complained of dull pain in the liver region, fullness in the chest and hypochondrium, poor appetite, frequent sweating aggravated by physical activity, shortness of breath, weakness, restless sleep, diarrhea (watery, two to three times a day) and clear and long stream of urine.

PAST HISTORY: Non-contributory.

PERTINENT PHYSICAL EXAMINATION & LABORATORY FINDINGS: Yellowish face, white sclera. Heart and lungs negative. Abdomen distended; liver palpable 2 cm below right costal margin and 4 cm below xiphoid process; spleen not palpable; borborygmus significant. Liver function test: icteric index, 4 units; III normal; LDH, 480 units; R-GT, 46 units, SGOT and SGPT normal. Serum total protein, 6.96%; albumin, 4.35%; globulin, 2.61 gm%; cholesterol, 220 mg%; HBsAG, (1:32); anti-HBs, (-); HBeAG, (+); anti-HBc, (+); DNAp, (+); and E-rosette test, 46%.

INSPECTION OF TONGUE: Red tongue substance with ecchymotic areas; thin and white tongue fur.

PULSE CONDITION: Deep and weak.

MODERN MEDICINE DIAGNOSIS: Chronic, Persistent Hepatitis-B.

TRADITIONAL CHINESE MEDICINE DIAGNOSIS: Hypochondriac pain; Deficiency and Stagnation of Liver-Qi.

Symptom-complex differentiation: The depressed Liver, impaired by Dampness and Heat, gives rise to stagnation of Vital Energy leading to diminished function of the Spleen and Stomach.

THERAPEUTIC PRINCIPLES: Soothe the Liver, smooth the flow of Vital Energy, warm and tonify the Spleen and Stomach.

PRESCRIPTION: Radix astragali, 30 gm; Rhizoma atractylodis macrocephalae, 15 gm; Poria, 30 gm; Rhizoma dioscoreae, 20 gm; Radix glycyrrhizae, 10 gm; Radix angelicae, 15 gm; Radix paeoniae alba and rubra, 15 gm each; Os dranati and Concha ostreae, 30 gm each; and Charred triplet, 30 gm. Seven doses.

Method of preparation: Soak ingredients in water first for one to two hours, then boil for 30 minutes. Boil two times to obtain a resultant decoction of 300 ml; 150 ml per dose, twice a day at morning and evening.

Second consultation: After taking the decoction, dull pain in the liver region was lightened and appetite improved. Other symptoms remained the same. Continued the same prescription, 14 doses. Added Fu-Xiao-Mai, 30 gm per dose.

Third consultation: After taking 14 decoctions, the patient's body energy had improved, she did not complain of easy sweating, but diarrhea, occurring twice a day, still remained due to Spleen deficiency with accumulation of Dampness. Another 14 doses of the prescription with the addition of Galla chinensis, 15 gm, and Rhizoma atractylodis macrocephalae, 30 gm, were given.

Fourth consultation: The patient looked well. She did not complain of pain in the liver region; appetite good, but thirst appeared with thin, yellow tongue fur and fast pulse due to deficiency. Modified the previous prescription by removing Rhizoma corydalis and adding Radix astragali, 15 gm.

After another 50 decoctions, all symptoms had disappeared. Liver functions were normal, though HBsAG remained positive. In order to consolidate the therapeutic effect and to render HBsAG negative, the patient was asked to take extracts of the prescription for oral ingestion.

After four months of taking this preparation, HBsAG detection was negative and liver functions normal. The same findings were still true after relapse of another two months. The patient was advised to continue the medication for another two months, then discontinue. In June 1987, and February 1988, two follow-up examinations showed normal results and confirmed a clinical cure.

DISCUSSION: Most cases of chronic hepatitis-B result from acute viral hepatitis. Its mechanism, most experts believe, may be due to an inability to eliminate the virus completely. HBV-DNA or its fragments integrate with the genes of host cells resulting in depression of cellular immunity and endogenously induced interferon. However, the immune system still functions causing auto-immune reactions leading to injury of the immune system, which makes the disease difficult to treat.

The most important aspect of the treatment is elimination of the virus, but up to this date there is still no specific medicine for this purpose. Numerous measures have been proposed in the past. Attempts have been made to eliminate the virus by raising the immune function; the results have been encouraging. A number of modern medications can enhance the immune ability, but to patients with secondarily lowered immune function, the effects are not as good as traditional Chinese medications. Our case was treated by a combination of modern and traditional medicines, and a satisfactory outcome was obtained.

In this case, the patient suffered from chronic hepatitis, the liver functions were stable and there were no serious symptoms. However, HBsAg and DNAp were positive, which mean that the virus was being reproduced. The finding of 46% from the E-rosette test indicated low immune function. In view of the serious deficiency state, the priority of the treatment was to refresh the Vital Energy and strengthen the immune functions. Modern studies have shown that deficiency of Vital Energy can lead to compromised immune function. Pharmacological research confirms that Radix astragali, Rhizoma atractylodis, Herba epimedii and other herbs which were used in the prescriptions are effective in promoting immune ability. This prescription has been widely used in clinics, and comparatively good results have been obtained. The distending pain in the liver and the ecchymotic spots on the tongue were indications of Qi stagnation and Blood stasis resulting from Wet-Heat evil in the Liver Channel or stagnation of Liver Qi. It has been recorded that nail bed blood supply and microcirculation of the nail folds of hepatitis patients undergo pathological changes, more seriously in the patients with Qi and Blood stasis. Radix angelicae, Radix paeoniae alba and rubra and Radix salviae are effective in promoting Blood circulation and removing Blood stasis, and their application in chronic hepatitis can lead to satisfactory outcomes. Their efficacy in promoting circulation has been confirmed by pharmacological studies.

This case is one of many hepatitis patients treated in our clinic. With the application of modern medicine diagnosis and TCM symptom-complex differentiation, good clinical results have been achieved. The authors believe that further research on a simpler and easy-to-use therapeutic measure in treating cases of chronic hepatitis-B must be done.

10.9 CHRONIC DYSENTERY
(DIARRHEA DUE TO SPLEEN-ASTHENIA)

Ye Wangyun
Yongji Hospital, Tongji Medical University, Wuhan

Shen Xiaomao, 10 months old, female, Han nationality. Date of admission: June 28, 1973.

CHIEF COMPLAINT: Intractable diarrhea of six months duration; last bout occurred four days ago.

HISTORY OF PRESENT ILLNESS (history related by the patient's mother): Because of improper feeding, the baby had diarrhea four months after she was born and had been treated as "dyspepsia." However, the diarrhea was refractory to therapy. Exacerbation and remission occurred alternately. A month later, purulent, blood-streaked and mucous stool appeared and the temperature reached 39.8°C (rectal). Microscopically, a lot of pus cells were seen in the stool. Bacillary dysentery was diagnosed. Antimicrobial agents for treating dysentery, such as neomycin, kanamycin, furazolidon and berberine, were used which were only effective in controlling the diarrhea transiently. Diarrhea exacerbated soon after, and all of these drugs were ineffective. By means of elaborate treatment, careful nursing and diet control, pus and blood disappeared from feces, but the patient still passed watery or loose stools several times a day. Occasionally, mucous and jelly-like substances were noted in the stools. Symptoms waxed and waned during the six-month period prior to admission.

In the four days prior to admission, diarrhea worsened again with passage of five to six bowel movements of loose stool a day. The stool contained a large amount of mucous and jelly-like substances with a fetid smell. Pus and blood could not be seen grossly. Apart from lack of energy and loss of appetite, the baby had no other particular abnormality. She had not been given any therapy recently.

PAST HISTORY: Frequent diarrhea and occasional common cold.

PERTINENT PHYSICAL EXAMINATION & LABORATORY FINDINGS: Chronic illness appearance, emaciated, asthenic and languid. Non-pitting edema on the face and eyelids with a slightly distended abdomen. Microscopically, large number of pus cells found in the stool.

INSPECTION OF TONGUE: Pale tongue covered with white, thin fur and imbued with saliva.

PULSE CONDITION: Superficial venules on the index fingers of both hands were fine and pale and through the strategic Wind Gate (Feng Guan).

MODERN MEDICINE DIAGNOSIS: Chronic Dysentery.

TRADITIONAL CHINESE MEDICINE DIAGNOSIS: Diarrhea due to Spleen Asthenia.

THERAPEUTIC PRINCIPLES: Invigorate the Spleen and eliminate Wetness-Evil with astringent method.

PRESCRIPTION: Modified Shen Ling Bai Zhu Pulvis. Radix codonopsis pilosulae, 6 gm; Rhizoma atractylodis macrocephalae, 3 gm; Rhizoma dioscorae opposita, 9 gm; Semen dolichos lablab, 9 gm; Semen coicis, 9 gm; Semen nelumbinis, 9 gm; Fructus mume, 9 gm; Pericarpium granati, 9 gm; Flos lonicerae, 24 gm; Talcum, 10 gm; and Radix glycyrrhizae, 2 gm. Decoction for oral ingestion. Three doses, one dose per day.

FOLLOW-UP/COURSE OF TREATMENT:

Second consultation on July 6, 1973: The day after taking one dose of the prescription, stool was noted to be paste-like, and frequency of bowel movement reduced. After taking three doses, the patient passed formed stools, one to two times a day. Her appetite increased. She took in food eagerly and was becoming vigorous again. Two days ago the patient was given an egg, which caused an increased number of bowel movements with watery and undigested stool. Upon physical examination, it was shown that the patient was attentive, abdominal distention had increased and tongue coating was thick. Colour of the tongue and of superficial venules on the index fingers and other signs remained the same as during the first visit. Diagnosis by traditional Chinese medicine this time was Spleen asthenia with food retention. Principles of treatment were to invigorate the Spleen, remove food stagnation and promote digestion.

Modified the previous prescription to contain Radix codonopsis pilosulae, 6 gm; Rhizoma atractylodis macrocephalae, 3 gm; Rhizoma dioscorae opposita, 9 gm; Semen coicis, 9 gm; Semen nelumbinis, 9 gm; Poria, 9 gm; Pericarpium granati, 9 gm; Pericarpium citri reticulatae, 3 gm; Fructus crataegi, 6 gm; Medicated leaven, 6 gm; Fructus hordei germinatus, 9 gm; Fructus oryzae germinatus, 9 gm; and Radix glycyrrhizae, 1.5 gm. Decoction for oral ingestion. One dose per day for three consecutive days.

Follow-up on September 30, 1973: The patient's mother reported that after taking three doses of the second prescription, the baby passed formed stools again, once a day, and she was in good health, full of vigour and lively. She had rosy cheeks and was getting stronger. She could walk by herself (at that time she was 13 months old), and she had a good appetite. Besides breast feeding, the mother fed the child with cow's milk, noodles, congee and other supplementary food. For the past three months her bowel movement had been normal, with formed stool once a day. Occasionally she had soft stool because of improper feeding. Thereafter, she never experienced dyspepsia and dysentery again.

DISCUSSION: The patient had repeated diarrhea accompanied by fever. Her stools contained a large number of pus and blood. The diagnosis of dysentery was given by a pediatrician. Although the diagnosis was not confirmed by stool culture, other Gi disorders such as enteritis or infection of intestines could be ruled out based on clinical findings. Antibiotics were applied and proved to be effective at the early stage of the disease, suggesting that these medications were indicated for this disease. However, the same regimen was ineffective at the latter stage of the disease, ultimately indicating these drugs were not suitable for the treatment of this disease.

Therapeutic measures were adjusted regularly in accordance with the clinical manifestations. TCM theories believe that "Yang of children is not mature" and that "Yin of children is not sufficient" as well as that Zang (Solid Organs) and Fu (Hollow Organs) are delicate. Their conditions are extremely variable, easy to become asthenic or sthenic. TCM teachings believe that "treatment must aim at the root cause of the disease." A clear distinction must be drawn between asthenia-syndrome and sthenia-syndrome. "Treat the asthenia-syndrome by invigoration and the sthenia-syndrome by purgation"; these are the principal rules of traditional Chinese medicine. At the beginning of dysentery when Wetness and Heat evils are dominant, the illness is a sthenia syndrome and should be treated by purgation. To achieve this, traditional Chinese medicine always uses Heat-clearing and Wetness-drying, bitter-flavour and cold-nature herbs. Satisfactory results were thus achieved. Modern medicine uses chloromycetin, neomycin, kanamycin, furazolidon, berberine and others, and good outcomes can be reached as well since these agents are, in effect, purgative in nature. In our case, the patient ran a high fever during the course of the disease, with stools containing pus, blood and a large amount of mucous and jelly-like substances. The symptoms of Wetness and Heat evils were evident, and these herbs were effective in controlling the condition.

However, with numerous recurrent bouts of the same illness, the Spleen and

Stomach had been injured and healthy energy was insufficient. Evil had retreated but Spleen Qi was deficient and weak, water and cereals could not be transported and converted to energy. The patient's temperature had come down, stools had no pus and blood, but diarrhea remained. At this point, her condition had transformed from sthenic- to asthenic-syndrome and required treatment by invigoration. Had neomycin, kanamycin, furazolidon and berberine and others continued to be used to purge sthenia, the result would naturally have been unproductive.

Heat-clearing and Wetness-drying herbs used routinely for the treatment of dysentery, such as Rhizoma coptidis, Radix scutellariae, Cortex phellodendri, Cortex fraxini and Radix pulsatillae, were not part of the author's two prescriptions. Instead, the principle of invigoration was applied. Modified Shen Ling Bai Zhu Pulvis was used to invigorate the Spleen and supplement the Qi. The rationale was that asthenia-syndrome was prominent in the patient's condition as manifested by symptoms of pale complexion, emaciation, languidness, pale lips, mild edema of face and eyelids, slight abdominal distention, pale tongue substance, fine and pale superficial venules of the index fingers and loose and fetid stools containing mucous and jelly-like substances which were devoid of pus and blood. In addition, the patient had not the faintest signs of Heat and sthenia-syndrome. In the prescriptions, Radix codonopsis pilosulae, Rhizoma atractylodis macrocephalae, Poria, Rhizoma dioscorea, Semen dolichoris and Semen nelumbinis were used to invigorate the Spleen and supplement the Vital Energy and Semen dolicos lablab, Semen coicis and Talcum to dispel the Wetness. Furthermore, Fructus mume and Pericarpium granati were added as astringents; Flos lonicerae was added to clear away the remaining Heat-toxin. With functions of the Spleen recovered, water and cereals could be transported and converted to energy. As a result, stools became normal rapidly. During this course of treatment, improper diet, an egg, caused recurrence of diarrhea, and the patient's tongue coating turned thick. Fructus crataegi, medicated leaven, Fructus hordei germinatus and others were added to promote digestion and relieve stasis.

Throughout the course of treatment, the author applied the principle of invigoration as the primary therapeutic measure with stasis dispersing and heat clearing as adjuvant measures. Treating the primary and secondary aspects of the disease simultaneously yielded a very satisfactory result in this particular case. The symptoms were put under control quickly. This case of chronic dysentery of more than six months duration was cured by only six doses of herbal recipe within a period of about 10 days.

11. GYNECOLOGICAL DISEASES

11.1 MENOPAUSAL SYNDROME
(EXCESSIVE FIRE IN THE HEART AND LIVER)

Wang Dazeng

Longhua Hospital, Shanghai College of Traditional Chinese Medicine,
Shanghai

*Yan, 49, female, Han nationality, married, worker. Medical record number: 30.
Date of first consultation: October 8, 1987.*

CHIEF COMPLAINT: Generalized sensation of heat with sweating for two years.

HISTORY OF PRESENT ILLNESS: In the past two years prior to consultation, the patient frequently experienced heat with flushing of the face and sweating of the neck and face and crawling sensation of the skin. She got upset easily. Sleep had been disturbed, and she complained of dryness of the mouth. Urination and bowel movement were normal.

PAST HISTORY: Non-contributory.

PERSONAL HISTORY: Menopausal for four years.

PERTINENT PHYSICAL EXAMINATION & LABORATORY FINDINGS: Well-developed and well-nourished. Flushed appearance of the face. Blood pressure, 150/90 mmHg. Gynecological examination: external genitalia normal, cervix smooth and hyperemic, scanty amount of secretion, uterus normal in size and movable, lateral fornices negative. RIA serum hormone level detection: FSH, 198 IU/m; LH, 191, IU/ml; E_2, 18 pg/ml; T, 30 ng/dl.

INSPECTION OF TONGUE: Tongue substance plump; tip red with thin fur.

PULSE CONDITION: Thready and taut.

MODERN MEDICINE DIAGNOSIS: Menopausal Syndrome.

TRADITIONAL CHINESE MEDICINE DIAGNOSIS: Excessive Fire in the Heart and Liver.

THERAPEUTIC PRINCIPLES: Tonify the Vital Energy and nourish the Vital Essence; remove Fire from the Heart and subdue hyperactivity of the Liver.

PRESCRIPTION: Radix astragali, 15 gm; Radix codonopsis, 9 gm; Radix paeoniae alba, 9 gm; Radix ampelopsis, 9 gm; Rhizoma coptidis, 3 gm; Radix ophiopogonis, 9 gm; Radix salviae, 9 gm; Cortex moutan radicis, 9 gm; Radix achyranthis, 9 gm; and Os draconis, 15 gm.

FOLLOW-UP/COURSE OF TREATMENT:

Second consultation on October 15, 1987: Sensation of heat and sweating alleviated after taking the prescription, and crawling sensation of the skin had subsided. Sleep improved. Tongue and pulse manifestation remained the same as before. Continued the prescription for another seven days.

Third consultation on October 22, 1987: Since the first consultation, the patient had taken 14 doses of the prescription which was aimed at tonifying the Vital Energy, nourishing the Vital Essence, removing Fire from the Heart and subduing hyperactivity of the Liver. Sensation of heat experienced occasionally, sweating had disappeared and sleep was normal. Recently, abdominal fullness had developed. Tip of tongue was red and tongue thinly coated, pulse thready and taut. The therapeutic principles adopted were to remove Fire from the Heart, subdue the hyperactivity of the Liver and soothe and regulate the flow of gas. Modified the prescription by removing Radix astragali and adding Fructus aurantii, 9 gm, and Fructus citri sacrodactylis, 9 gm. Seven doses.

Fourth consultation on November 19, 1987: Sensation of heat and sweating had subsided and abdominal distention disappeared. Administration of the prescription had been discontinued for three weeks at the time of consultation. No new medication was prescribed.

DISCUSSION: Menopausal syndrome and its counterpart, climacteric syndrome in males, are complaints commonly encountered in clinical practice. The incidence of occurrence is higher in females because their physiological functions, such as menstruation, leukorrhea, pregnancy and parturition, are intimately related to the sex organs.

Canon of Internal Medicine states that "in women, deficiency of the Ren Channel (Conception Meridian), failure of the Chong Channel (Vital Channel) and exhaustion of Tiangui (Sex-Stimulating Essence) occur at the age of seven times seven." This teaching points out that occurrence of menopausal syndrome is related to deficiency of Kidney Qi. Therefore, the treatment of this syndrome should start with the Kidney.

The fundamental cause of this disease was in the Kidney. Physiological and psychological changes and clinical symptoms of the menopausal syndrome were due to the failure of Kidney Qi, but incidental manifestations were referred to the Heart, Liver and Spleen, especially the Heart and Liver.

Based on clinical manifestations of heat sensation, sweating, fidgetiness and irritability, insomnia and others, the condition was diagnosed as excessiveness of Fire of the Heart and Liver by TCM symptom-complex differentiation. Lassitude, fatigue and anorexia were due to Spleen deficiency. The Heart and Kidney are Fire and Water, respectively, and complement each other, while the Liver and Kidney (Yi and Gui) are from the same origin. The relation of the Spleen and Kidney represents the acquired and the congenital, respectively.

With deficiency of Kidney Yin, Water and Fire fail to complement each other. Water fails to provide proper nourishment for Wood (Liver) and syndromes of excess of Fire of the Heart and Liver ensue. Deficiency of Kidney Yang results in dysfunction of the Spleen in transporting and distributing the nutrients and water followed by deficiency syndrome of the Spleen. All of these show clearly the relationship between the Heart, Liver, Spleen and Kidney.

Emphasis of the treatment placed on the Heart, Liver and Spleen. Failure of Vital Energy of the Kidney at seven times seven years of age is a normal physiological phenomenon. To restore the Vital Energy of the Kidney to normal by medications would have been to work against the normal progression of human physiological functions. The major role traditional Chinese medicine played in the treatment was to regulate the imbalance of Yin and Yang and to restore the harmony between the Qi and Blood.

The excess of Fire in the Heart and Liver, though incidental, was pathological. During the course of treatment, one must distinguish the pathological from the physiological, the primary from the secondary and yield to the laws of nature. Such logic will ensure an appropriate therapeutic measure and recovery from the disease.

The principles of replenishing the Yin and dispelling pathogenic Heat are used to treat the Heart. Commonly employed herbs for this purpose are Rhizoma coptidis, Radix ophiopogonis, Fructus tritici levis, Radix glycyrrhizae, Herba lophatheri, Radix salviae and others. For dispelling pathogenic Heat from the Heart, Huanglian and Maidong are more effective. In the prescription, Rhizoma coptidis was used to dispel pathogenic Fire from the Heart and Radix ophiopogonis to nourish its Vital Energy. In TCM teaching, sweat is the fluid of the Heart. When Heart Fire subsides and excessive sweating stops, fidgetiness disappears and sound sleep returns.

For the treatment of the Liver, Radix paeoniae alba and Radix ampelopsis were used to nourish the Vital Essence and soothe the Liver, which in turn overcame the rigidity (to quench the Fire in the Liver). Also given in the prescription were Cortex moutan radicis and Fructus gardeniae which possess excellent effects in eliminating irritability and relieving depression. Os draconis was used to dispel pathogenic Heat and to subdue the hyperactivity of the Heart and Liver.

When Spleen deficiency is present with symptoms of tastelessness and gastric discomfort, Herba agastachi and Fructus amomi can be used. They are effective in resolving Dampness, invigorating the Spleen and regulating the Stomach function. In addition, Radix rehmanniae, Radix scrophulariae, Herba ecliptae, Fructus ligustri lucidi and the like can be added to the prescription to nourish the Liver and Kidney.

In short, herbs used to treat this condition are, more or less, cold in property.

In our case, because of correct analysis by symptom-complex differentiation and application of appropriate prescriptions, the patient recovered completely from the condition after only three visits.

11.2 SECONDARY AMENORRHEA (AMENORRHEA OF THE DEFICIENCY TYPE)

Wang Dazeng

Longhua Hospital, Shanghai College of Traditional Chinese Medicine, Shanghai

Zhang, 24, female, Han nationality, single, worker. Medical record number: 295. Date of first consultation: September 7, 1982.
CHIEF COMPLAINT: Amenorrhea for more than three months.

HISTORY OF PRESENT ILLNESS: Menarche at age 17, menstruation cycle once in several months. LMO, May 30, 1982 (after injection of progesterone). PMP, February 8, 1982. Menstruation ceased for more than three months. The patient also complained of dizziness, fatigue, anorexia, backache and thin leukorrhea.

PAST HISTORY: Non-contributory.

PERTINENT PHYSICAL EXAMINATION & LABORATORY FINDINGS: Well-developed, lustreless skin complexion, body weight 47 kg and height 163 cm. Gynecological examination: both breasts well developed with several coarse and long hairs on the areola. External genitalia well developed, pubic hair in adult distribution. Vaginal orifice mucosa slightly hyperemic. Rectal examination: uterus smaller than normal, in midposterior position and movable. Both lateral fornices were negative. Routine blood examination: hemoglobin, 11.3 gm%; RBC, 4.5 M/mm^3; WBC, 7,000/mm^3; polymorphs, 62%; lymphocytes, 33%; eosinophils, 5%. Vaginal smear: mainly midlayer cells. Pneumoperitoneograph: both ovaries were larger than 1/3 size of the uterus, suggesting polycystic ovaries.

INSPECTION OF TONGUE: Tip red with thin fur.

PULSE CONDITION: Thready and fast.

MODERN MEDICINE DIAGNOSIS: Secondary Amenorrhea (PCO).

TRADITIONAL CHINESE MEDICINE DIAGNOSIS: Amenorrhea (Insufficiency of Qi and Blood, Deficiency of the Liver and Kidney).

THERAPEUTIC PRINCIPLES: Reinforce the Vital Energy and Blood, regulate and tonify the Liver and Kidney.

PRESCRIPTION: Gui-Qi Menstruation Regulating Decoction (A-A Decoction). Radix angelicae, 30 gm; Radix astragali, 30 gm; Herba epimedii, 15 gm; Semen cuscutae, 30 gm; Rhizoma zingiberis recens, 3 slices; and Fructus ziziphi jujubae, 10 pieces. Once a day in two divided doses, morning and evening.

FOLLOW-UP/COURSE OF TREATMENT:

Third consultation on October 12, 1982: After two weeks of medication, amount of leukorrhea had increased and was transparent in appearance. BBT elevated. Menstruation returned on September 27, lasting for five days, moderate in amount, dark in colour with some clots. Menstrual period was accompanied by slight distention in the lower abdomen. No other discomfort reported. Manifestations of the tongue and pulse were normal. Continued the previous prescription.

Sixth consultation on November 27, 1982: The patient had taken a total of 70 doses of A-A Decoction since the first visit. Menstruation returned for the second time on November 10 and lasted for five days. Amount of menstrual discharge moderate with blood clots markedly decreased. Abdominal distention minimized. BBT biphasic. Vitality improved. Tongue thinly coated and pulse soft. Continued the same prescription.

Eighth consultation on January 15, 1983: Menstruation returned for the third time on January 9, 1983. Amount and colour of discharge normal. No accompanying abdominal distention. BTT biphasic. Preparation changed to Gui-Qi Medicinal Granules (composed of Radix angelica, 30 gm, Radix astragali, 30 gm, Rhizoma zingiberis, 3 slices, Fructus ziziphi, 10 pieces) to tonify the Vital Energy and Blood. One dose twice daily after the granules were dissolved in boiling water. Another medicine, Congrong (Cistanche) Tablet (each tablet containing 0.5 gm of Herba cistanchis) was prescribed at the dosage of 5 tablets t.i.d. to tonify the Liver and Kidney.

Eleventh consultation on February 5, 1983: The patient's general condition and vitality further improved after several months of medication. Appetite increased. Menstrual cycle shortened to one and a half to two months. BTT biphasic. Tongue and pulse conditions normal. The patient was asked to discontinue the medication and to have regular follow-up.

Twelfth consultation on May 14, 1983: Medication had been discontinued for three months. During this period, menstruation occurred twice, on March 10 and April 17. Amount and colour of discharge normal. General condition good.

DISCUSSION: The main component of menstruation is Blood. Its formation, storage and circulation are initiated and regulated by the Vital Energy. The Vital Energy in turn is nourished by Blood. Once deficiency in Vital Energy and Blood occurs, deficiency in the Chong (Vital) and Ren (Front Midline) Channels and inadequacy of the Blood reservoir will result, often leading to amenorrhea. Furthermore, Vital Essence of the Kidney governs the growth pattern as well as the developmental and reproductive functions. Vital Essence and Blood can transform mutually. These facts demonstrate the importance of Vital Energy, Blood and the Kidney in the pathophysiology of menstruation.

Based on these teachings, A-A Decoction was formulated accordingly. Through clinical observation in 31 cases, this prescription has proven to be of good therapeutic effect in treating deficiency-type amenorrhea. The prescription, with Radix angelicae and Radix astragali as the main ingredients for tonifying the Vital Energy and Blood, was supplemented by Herba epimedii and Semen cuscutae to tonify the Liver and Kidney. Rhizoma zingiberis and Fructus ziziphi, pungent and sweet in nature, respectively, were also used to mediate the nutrients and Blood.

By TCM symptom-complex differentiation, this case was classified as deficiency of both the Vital Energy and Blood as well as deficiencies of both the Liver and Kidney. Menstruation became normal after five months of medication and stayed normal over the next three months, after which the medication was discontinued. The therapeutic effect in this case was stable.

Vital Energy and Blood in traditional Chinese medicine have wide implications. Xu (insufficiency) means inadequacy, both functionally and materially. Data gathered from 19 cases have shown that A-A Decoction does have an effect in elevating the hemoglobin level and number of RBC's. This blood-enriching effect of A-A Decoction may be attributed to vitamin B_{12}, folic acid, vitamin B_2, vitamin C and iron contained in Radix angelicae, Radix astragali and Fructus ziziphi, since these elements are all essential for normal hemopoiesis. Examinations of desquamated vaginal epithelium before and after treatment in 23 cases revealed higher eosinophil index and pyknotic nuclei index in the post-treatment specimens. The vaginal epithelium undergoes periodic changes under the influence of ovarian hormones. Nuclear pyknosis and eosinophilic reaction of desquamated vaginal epithelial cells can reflect the estrogen level in the body. These findings suggest that A-A Decoction can raise the estrogen level of the body.

It is our experience that most of the amenorrheic patients are of the deficiency type, and the deficiency is mainly of the Vital Energy and Blood. So long as the case does not manifest symptoms and signs of the excess symptom-complex clinically, reinforcement measures should be included in the treatment.

11.3 COMPENSATORY MENSTRUATION (VICARIOUS MENSTRUATION, MENOXENIA)

Wang Minghui

Hunan Academy of Traditional Chinese Medicine and Materia Medica, Changsha

Liu Zinian, 29, female, Han nationality, teacher. Medical record number: 78159. Date of first consultation: May 10, 1961.

CHIEF COMPLAINT: Menstruation disorders with lumbago and epistaxis during menstruation for about three years.

HISTORY OF PRESENT ILLNESS: Since 1958, menstruation had been irregular, lasting around 15 days, with each phase 8 to 10 days. This year, bilateral sole pain was experienced occasionally, it being worse in winter. The patient consulted more than once the Department of Medicine of our hospital where she was treated as a case of erythromelalgia and peripheral neuritis. She also consulted the TCM clinic, where she was given more than 20 doses of Xiaoyao Powder, Decoction of Four Drugs and Modified Decoction for Warming. These medications were able to afford temporary relief, but symptoms never really remitted. A few days prior to this consultation, the patient experienced lumbago, low abdominal pain, tinnitus, headache and dizziness, irritability, palpitation, constipation and yellowish, short-stream urine, though her appetite and sleep were good. The amount of menstruation discharge was noted to have increased markedly, occasionally accompanied by bleeding from the nose or mouth and distending feeling over the right hypochondrium.

PAST HISTORY: Menarche at age 16. Menstruation regular. Married for seven years. Both husband and child healthy.

PERTINENT PHYSICAL EXAMINATION & LABORATORY FINDINGS: Conscious, cooperative during physical examination; developmental and nutritional status good, cheeks flushed. Voice smooth and respiration regular. Complete physical examination revealed no abnormalities.

INSPECTION OF TONGUE: Red tongue substance with white to yellowish fur.

PULSE CONDITION: Wiry, slow and powerful.

MODERN MEDICINE DIAGNOSIS: Compensatory Menstruation; Menstruation Disorder.

TRADITIONAL CHINESE MEDICINE DIAGNOSIS: Flaring of Fire in the Liver and Gallbladder; Menoxenia.

THERAPEUTIC PRINCIPLES: Purge the Liver-Fire, nourish the Yin and suppress the Sthenic Yang.

PRESCRIPTION: Modified Decoction of Radix Gentiane for Purging Liver-Fire. Semen plantaginis, 15 gm; Rhizoma alismatis, 10 gm; Radix bupleuri, 10 gm; Radix scutellariae, 10 gm; Radix rehmanniae, 15 gm; Radix angelicae sinensis, 10 gm; Caulis akebiae, 15 gm; Fructus gardeniae, 15 gm; Concha ostreae, 15 gm; Radix gentianae, 15 gm; Carapax trionycis, 15 gm; and Radix glycyrrhizae, 3 gm.

After three doses of this prescription, the patient recovered completely from the condition and the symptoms did not recur during the next three years of follow-up.

DISCUSSION: The patient in this case suffered from Blood stasis in the menstrual cycle, irritability, distending sensation over the hypochondrium, lumbago, sensation of heat on the centres of the soles of the feet, flushed face, lips and tongue, tinnitus, palpitation, wiry and powerful pulse and vicarious menstruation from the mouth and nose. These signs and symptoms indicated presence of evils in the Liver and Gallbladder classified as sthenic Fire-syndrome. The strategy of the treatment called for purging of the sthenic Fire in the Liver and Gallbladder and nourishing the Yin and suppressing the sthenic Yang.

In the prescription given, Radix bupleuri has effective in purging the sthenic Fire of the Liver and Gallbladder; Radix scutellariae and Fructus gardeniae removed Heat from the Three Burners; while Caulis akebiae and Semen plantaginis removed Wetness from the small intestine and the bladder. In addition, Rhizoma alismatis was used to dissipate Kidney Wetness, Radix angelicae sinensis and Radix rehmanniae to nourish the Blood and invigorate the Liver and Radix glycyrrhisae to protect the Kidney from all these purging and expelling agents which are bitter and cold in nature. Carapax trionycis nourished the Yin and suppressed the sthenic Yang, while Concha ostreae was used to clear away the Heat.

Ordinarily, this is an important prescription used chiefly for clearing away Heat and eliminating Wetness from the Lower Burner and as an analgesia. Currently, it is often used to treat symptoms of inflammation, congestion and pain in the lower abdomen involving organs of the pelvis. It is particularly effective for cases of inflammation of the urogenital tract and sexual hormone glands.

From past experience and pharmacological studies, it has been shown that Radix angelicae sinensis is a Blood-nourishing herb, containing mainly volatile oil, vitamin B_{12}, folic acid and nicotinic acid. It elevates the circulatory estrogen level and is effective in correcting anemia. Radix rehmanniae is a Blood-cooling herb; its main components are secondary glycosides of catalpol, mannitol, etc. It is effective in lowering the blood sugar level in circulation and is also used as a diuretic. Caulis akebiae is a Heat-clearing herb and a diuretic, composed mainly of aristolochic acid, etc., and it is effective in inhibiting bacteria and cancer cells. Radix scutellariae is also a Heat-clearing herb made up mainly of baicalin, caicalein and wogonoside, wogomin, etc., and has sedative, anti-bacterial and diuretic effects. Semen plantaginis, with its chief components of plantain acid, glycosides of plantain seed, succinic acid, adenine and choline, is a diuretic which also inhibits the actions of the secretory glands. As can be seen here, this modified prescription based on a correct symptom-complex differentiation has excellent therapeutic effects in treating the condition of vicarious menstruation.

Ye Tianshi of the Qing Dynasty once indicated that menstruation, which does not present itself in its proper lower location but comes from the mouth and nose, is called retromenstruation. Compensatory menstruation, as one of the menstruation disorders, is frequently accompanied with epistaxis before or during the menstrual period, and some occurrences of this condition may even be complicated with hemorrhage of the retina or the gastrointestinal tract. Traditional Chinese medicine considers dispelling the Heat, cooling the Blood and inducing the menstruation to go down as the principles of treatment for cases where menstruation is found in the upper locations secondary to Heat in the Blood. Herbs recommended for this purpose are fresh Rehmanniae glutinosa, Achyranthis bidentata Bl Charcoal, Burnt Gardeniae jasminodes ellis, Schizonepetae tenuifolia sprig charcoal, Paronia suffruticoca and Rcharcoal, Pteria margaritifera, Scutellariae baicalensis, Glycyrrhizae, Uralensis, etc. If the case is due to deficiency of Yin resulting in hyperactivity of Fire and impairment of the Chong and Ren Channels, the therapeutic principles should be those of nourishing the Yin, suppressing the Yang, clearing and cooling the Blood and leading the Blood to the lower locations. When deficiency of Yin is evident, the priority should be to invigorate the Yin. But when the condition is accompanied by presence of Heat, measures to clear away the Heat should be added. Likewise, measures to cool the Blood and activate the circulation should be instituted once overt Heat is present.

Our case suffered from Fire in the liver and Gallbladder. It was not a case due to asthenic Cold of the uterus or asthenia of Yin Blood, and it was not a case of compensatory menstruation caused by emotional disorder. As such, Modified Decoction of Radix Gentianae for Purging Liver Fire used in this treatment achieved the desired effect rapidly.

Generally, there are five conditions which can induce epistaxis. The first is the one seen in our case with the presence of irritation, thirst, flushing, hypochondriac pain and wiry and powerful pulse attributed to hyperaction of Liver-Fire and should be treated by Decoction of Radix Gentianae for Purging Liver-Fire. The next is due to invasion of Cold and Wind, where the Taiyang Channel is troubled by exogenous evils. The condition is reflected in epistaxis secondary to Shanghan Superficial Sthenic Syndrome. Treatment of choice is to expel superficial evils by diaphoresis using Herba Ephedrae Decoction administered at a time when there is no active bleeding. The third situation is epistaxis due to retention of Heat in the Lung and raising up of the Lung's air. Common symptoms are dry nose, severe thirst and cough. This condition is usually treated with herbs acrid in taste and cool in nature to open up the Lung, such as modified Decoction of Folium Mori and Flos Chrysanthemi. The fourth condition is epistaxis resulting from Lung Heat and Wind and internal retention of Heat. Symptoms are thirst, dryness and obstruction of the nose, cough, fever and headache, sweating with aversion to wind and floating pulse. Medication of choice is also Decoction of Folium Mori and Flos Chrysanthemi with the addition of Radix moutan radicis and Rhizoma imperatae, which are also acrid in taste and cool in nature, to dispel the Heat and cool the Blood. The last condition is epistaxis due to hyperactivity of Heat-Evil in the Yangming Channel with Wetness and Heat retention in the Stomach as evidenced by symptoms of thirst, malodorous breath, dryness of the nose, constipation and yellow tongue fur. Treatment of choice is to administer the modified Jade Maid Decoction for dispelling the Heat and cooling the Blood. In short, epistaxis can be managed satisfactorily with appropriate therapeutic principles once the symptom-complex differentiation is correctly established.

11.4 MENORRHAGIA
(UTERINE BLEEDING)

Sun Lihua

Xiyuan Hospital, China Academy of Traditional Chinese Medicine,
Beijing

Yang Shulan, 48, female, Han nationality, married, shop assistant. Medical record number: 29884. Date of first consultation: May 17, 1986.
CHIEF COMPLAINT: Menorrhagia for two years; slight vaginal bleeding for more than 10 days.

HISTORY OF PRESENT ILLNESS: For the past two years, the patient had menorrhagia described as profuse in amount, dark in colour and with clots. This was accompanied by lower abdominal pain. IMP, May 8, 1986, with condition characterized by excessive uterine bleeding and mild but persistent vaginal discharge, lassitude, palpitation, tinnitus, anorexia and nausea. Laboratory findings showed hemoglobin level to be 7.9 gm%; bleeding time, 5 minutes; clotting time, 2 minutes.

PAST HISTORY: History of chronic inflammatory pathology of the pelvis. Menarche at age 16 with interval between episodes being 29 days (16 28/5). Dysmenorrhagic. The patient got married at the age of 19. Two full-term, healthy children parturition and three miscarriages.

PERTINENT PHYSICAL EXAMINATION & LABORATORY FINDINGS: Gynecological examination: Cervix, uterus and adnexa were all within normal limits. No signs of pelvic infection.

INSPECTION OF TONGUE: Tongue with thin, white to yellow coating.

PULSE CONDITION: Deep.

MODERN MEDICINE DIAGNOSIS: Uterine Bleeding.

TRADITIONAL CHINESE MEDICINE DIAGNOSIS: Menorrhagia.

Symptom-complex differentiation: Deficiency of both Qi and Blood; weakness of the Chong and Ren Channels.

THERAPEUTIC PRINCIPLES: Tonify both the Qi and Blood, control the profuse uterine bleeding.

PRESCRIPTION: Modified Gui Pi Tang. Rhizoma atractylodis macrocephalae, 10 gm; Radix astragali, 10 gm; Radix codonopsis, 10 gm; Colla corii asini, 15 gm; Semen ziziphi spinosae, 10 gm; Radix glycyrrhizae, 6 gm; Radix paeoniae alba, 10 gm;

Pericarpium citri reticulatae, 10 gm; Radix ophiopogonis, 10 gm; Fructus schisandrae, 10 gm; Radix sanguisorbae, 10 gm; and Os sepiellae seu sepiae, 20 gm.

In this particular prescription, Radix codonopsis, Rhizoma atractylodis macrocephalae, Radix astragali and Radix glycyrrhizae were used to reinforce Vital Energy and invigorate the Spleen; Colla corii asini to stop bleeding by tonifying the Blood; Semen ziziphi spinosae to reinforce the functional activities of the Heart and Spleen; Radix ophiopogonis and Fructus schisandrae to replenish the Vital Essence; Pericarpium citri reticulatae to regulate the flow of the Vital Energy and revitalize the Spleen; Radix sanguisorbae to halt the bleeding by dispelling pathogenic Heat from the Blood; and Radix paeoniae alba to tonify the Blood. Os sepiellae seu sepiae was used to stop bleeding by removing Blood stasis.

On May 22, 1986, bleeding had stopped, though symptoms of lassitude, palpitation, pale appearance, pale tongue with white fur, and sinking pulse remained. Continued to tonify both the Vital Energy and Blood by using Radix astragali, 10 gm; Radix codonopsis, 10 gm; Radix paeoniae alba, 10 gm; Rhizoma atractylodis macrocephalae, 10 gm; Radix glycyrrhizae, 6 gm; Pericarpium citri reticulatae, 10 gm; Radix ophiopogonis, 10 gm; Colla corii asini, 15 gm; Fructus schisandrae, 10 gm; Rhizoma dioscoreae, 10 gm; and Radix rehmanniae praeparatae, 10 gm.

11.5 DYSFUNCTIONAL UTERINE BLEEDING (UTERINE BLEEDING)

Sun Lihua

Xiyuan Hospital, China Academy of Traditional Chinese Medicine, Beijing

Zhao Xiuzhen, 26, female, Han nationality, single, worker. Medical record number: 258113. Date of first consultation: June 11, 1986.

CHIEF COMPLAINT: Menstrual bleeding for 36 days.

HISTORY OF PRESENT ILLNESS: The patient's last menstruation was on May 5, 1986, and she had been bleeding for more than a month. She also experienced increased frequency of urination and bowel movement, weakness in the loins and legs, vertigo, thirst, feverish sensation, shortness of breath, dry stool, oliguria and anorexia.

PAST HISTORY: Non-contributory.

MENSTRUAL HISTORY: Menarche at age 16. The interval between the onset of successive menstruation was 25 days. (16 25/6).

PERTINENT PHYSICAL EXAMINATION & LABORATORY FINDINGS: Shallow face, no malodorous breath. Rectal examination showed normal uterus, ovaries and tubes. Slight vaginal bleeding.

INSPECTION OF TONGUE: Pale tongue substance with tooth prints at the borders, thin and yellow fur.

PULSE CONDITION: Soft and deep.

MODERN MEDICINE DIAGNOSIS: Dysfunctional Uterine Bleeding.

TRADITIONAL CHINESE MEDICINE DIAGNOSIS: Uterine Bleeding.

Symptom-complex differentiation: Deficiency of Yin of the Liver and Kidney, dysfunction of the Spleen and Stomach, damage of the Chong and Ren Channels. The kidney is the foundation of the original constitution and stores the essence of life. Liver stores the Blood, while the Spleen provides the material basis of the acquired constitution. The patient in this case suffered from deficiency of Blood and of the Liver and Kidney, and the foundation of the Chong and Ren Channels was not sustained. Hence the manifestation of persistent bloody vaginal discharge.

THERAPEUTIC PRINCIPLES: Nourish the Yin of the Liver and Kidney, invigorate the function of the Spleen, regulate the Stomach function and stop the profuse uterine bleeding.

PRESCRIPTION: Modified Liuwei Dihuang Decoction (adopted from *Key to the Therapeutics of Diseases of the Children* by Qian Yi) composed mainly of Radix rehmanniae praeparatae, Fructus corni, Rhizoma dioscoreae, Poria, Rhizoma alismatis, Cortex moutan radicis, Rhizoma alismatis and Fructus corni with the addition of Fructus ligustri lucidi, Herba ecliptae, Radix codonopsis, Colla corii asini, Radix paeoniae alba, Radix rehmanniae and Concha ostreae.

Radix rehmanniae was used to dispel pathogenic Heat by replenishing the Yin; Rhizoma dioscoreae and Radix codonopsis warmed the Kidney to activate the function of the Spleen; Radix paeoniae alba to nourish and soothe the Liver by tonifying the Blood; Poria to tonify the Heart and Spleen; Cortex moutan radicis to remove evil Heat to stop bleeding; Herba ecliptae and Nuzhenzi to nourish Yin to remove evil Heat; Colla corii asini to nourish the Vital Essence; and Poria to nourish the Vital Essence to subdue the exuberant Yang.

Therapeutic principles were to treat the cardinal syndrome due to exuberance of Yang secondary to deficiency of Yin by nourishing the Vital Essence in order to subdue the exuberant Yang, dispel pathogenic Heat from the Blood, regulate the exuberant Yang to stop the bleeding and stop the profuse uterine bleeding.

Radix codonopsis, 10 gm; Radix astragali, 10 gm; Poria, 10 gm; Rhizoma atractylodis macrocephalae, 10 gm; Herba ecliptae, 10 gm; Pericarpium citri reticulatae, 10 gm; Fructus ligustri lucidi, 10 gm; Pollen typhae, 10 gm; Radix rubiae, 10 gm; and Concha ostreae, 20 gm.

July 16, 1986: The patient had menstruation which lasted for six days. There was no excessive uterine bleeding. Tongue substance normal with white fur. Pulse deep and soft. Reinforced the Vital Energy and nourish the Blood to regulate the menstruation.

Radix codonopsis, 10 gm; Radix astragali, 10 gm; Poria, 10 gm; Radix rehmanniae, 10 gm; Radix rehmanniae praeparatae, 10 gm; Radix paeoniae alba, 10 gm; Herba ecliptae, 10 gm; Colla corii asini, 10 gm (taken after pouring water on it); Radix ophiopogonis, 10 gm; Pericarpium citri reticulatae, 10 gm; and Radix polygoni multiflori, 10 gm.

11.6 HABITUAL ABORTION
(HABITUAL ABORTION, HUA TAI)

Li Mingzhen

Institute for the Integration of Traditional and Western Medicine, Tongji
Medical University, Wuhan

*Guo Zhiyuan, 38, female, Han nationality, married, worker. Medical record
number: 91235. Date of admission: December 24, 1964.*

CHIEF COMPLAINT: Abortion nine times, menolipsis for 47 days with soreness
of the waist and tenesmus.

HISTORY OF PRESENT ILLNESS: Menstrual cycle of the patient had been
normal. She had nine abortions to date, and her last menstrual period was on
November 7, 1964, with menolipsis for 47 days. Recently, the patient experienced
dizziness, fullness in the stomach, nausea and occasional soreness of the waist and
tenesmus as well as frequent urination.

PAST HISTORY: The patient had natural labour in 1959, but the baby died at the
age of three months. Since then the patient had nine abortions. During her last two
pregnancies, she was hospitalized and restricted to complete bed rest with injection of
progesterone and administration of Chinese herbal medicines, but abortion still occurred
at gestation age of three to four months. The patient denied any systemic disease.

PERTINENT PHYSICAL EXAMINATION & LABORATORY FINDINGS:
Gynecological examination showed an egg-sized uterus. Urinary pregnancy test positive.

INSPECTION OF TONGUE: Tender and red tongue with thin and white fur.

MODERN MEDICINE DIAGNOSIS: Early Pregnancy; Habitual Abortion.

TRADITIONAL CHINESE MEDICINE DIAGNOSIS: Hua Tai (Habitual Abortion), Sunken Qi of the Middle Burner.

THERAPEUTIC PRINCIPLES: Invigorate the Spleen function and regulate the
vital function of the Stomach, supplement the Qi and elevate the sunken Qi of the
Middle Burner.

PRESCRIPTION: Modified Decoction for Reinforcing the Middle Burner and
Replenishing Qi. Radix codonopsis pilosulae, 9 gm; Radix astragali, 12 gm; Rhizoma
atractylodis macrocephalae, 12 gm; Radix glycyrrhizae praeparatae, 6 gm; Radix
angelicae, 9 gm; Rhizoma cimicifugae, 3 gm; Pericarpium citri reticulatae, 9 gm; and
Caulis bambusae in taeniam, 9 gm. Decoct in water and divide into two equal parts for
oral ingestion. Absolute and complete bed rest.

FOLLOW-UP/COURSE OF TREATMENT:

November 29, 1964: Symptoms such as soreness of the waist and tenesmus were
not alleviated. Dizziness, insomnia, frequency of nocturia, condition of the tongue and
pulse remained the same as before. Accordingly, Ramulus loranthi, 15 gm, and Cortex
eucommiae, 9 gm, were added to the original prescription in agreement with Suo Yi
Zai Pill to strengthen the Spleen and tonify the Kidney and to reinforce the Chong
Channel to ensure a successful pregnancy.

February 5, 1965: Having been treated with modified Suo Yi Zai Pill for more than one month, soreness of the waist and tenesmus was significantly alleviated, but frequent urination was still apparent. Semen cuscutae, 12 gm, was added to strengthen the Kidney and reinforce the Chong and Ren Channels.

March 10, 1965: Treated with the above modified decoction, all symptoms had disappeared. The patient was discharged from hospital to recuperate at home and was directed to take the prescriptions intermittently to consolidate the therapeutic effects.

August 17, 1965: A healthy, full-term baby girl was born.

Follow-up in 1984: The baby born in 1965 had grown up healthy. The patient was pregnant again in 1967 which resulted eventually in abortion and since then the couple has not conceived.

DISCUSSION:

1) Etiology of habitual abortion is quite varied, the most common one being disorder of the endocrine system. In view of this, routine treatment of the condition has been administration of progesterone. However, regulation of the female endocrine system is complicated, and the effect of complementary progesterone therapy is often unsatisfactory. This was a typical case.

2) In traditional Chinese medicine, habitual abortion is known as Hua Tai, and its pathogeneses are insufficiency of the Spleen, Kidney deficiency and Heat in the Blood. The Spleen serves as the source for the generation and transformation of Qi and Blood. Insufficiency of the Spleen causes depletion at the source of Qi and Blood, weakness and undernourishment of uterine collaterals which eventually results in habitual abortion. The Kidney is in charge of the original, or inborn, constitution of the body. Connected with the uterine collaterals, it reinforces the primordial Qi of the fetus. Debility of the Chong and Ren Channels due to insufficiency of the Kidney may lead to habitual abortion. In addition, Heat secondary to stagnation of Liver Qi, excess Yang or infiltration of exogenous Heat into the body can disturb the Chong and Ren Channels. As a result, Blood will be forced to flow unchecked, damaging the original Qi of the fetus and ultimately leading to habitual abortion. Among these pathogenic factors, Kidney and Spleen insufficiencies are the most common, but in clinical practice, many other factors may coexist with these insufficiencies.

3) Suo Yi Zai Pill was first prescribed by Chen Xiuyuan, who noted that "Rhizoma atractylodis macrocephalae is the main ingredient to strengthen the Earth, which is the origin and foundation of a multitude of other elements." The name of the prescription depicts this idea. In this prescription, Rhizoma atractylodis macrocephalae is the dominant ingredient with Ginseng, poria and Fructus ziziphi jujubae used to strengthen the Spleen and replenish the Qi and Cortex eucommiae and Ramulus loranthi to tonify the kidney and reinforce the Chong and Ren Channels. This prescription as a whole replenishes both the Spleen and Kidney. Strengthening and fortifying the Chong and Ren Channels will lead to a safe and sound baby. In pregnant women, tenesmus and frequent urination are signs of Spleen deficiency and sunken Qi of the Middle Burner. Soreness at the waist, dizziness and threatened abortion are symptoms caused by kidney deficiency and debility of the Chong and Ren Channels. Since the loins are the seat of the Kidney which is in charge of the bones and the generation of marrow,

the reservoir of which is the brain, symptoms of soreness at the waist and dizziness naturally result if there is Kidney deficiency. Furthermore, frequent urination, which may be a result of deficiency of the Spleen and sunken Qi of the Middle Burner, is closely related to Kidney deficiency. Kidney also controls the discharge and retention of both the urine and stool, so the symptoms of urinary frequency could be due to Kidney deficiency. By TCM symptom-complex differentiation, it is clear that this case belonged to deficiency of both the Spleen and Kidney, not the Spleen alone. On the first visit, Decoction for Reinforcing the Middle Burner and Replenishing Qi, which only strengthened the Spleen, was prescribed but to no obvious benefit. Following the formulation of Suo Yi Zai Pill, Cortex eucommiae and Ramulus loranthi were added to reinforce both the Spleen and Kidney. Symptoms began to be relieved gradually after administration of this prescription. This effect was further enhanced by addition of seed of Chinese dodder and red raspberry to strengthen the Kidney, invigorate the loins and reduce urinary frequency. The effect of these herbs were to focus on the Kidney more than the Spleen. Symptoms were subsequently relieved and primordial Qi of the fetus strengthened.

4) In the treatment of habitual abortion, the formulation of Suo Yi Zai Pill is usually modified according to clinical manifestations. If the condition is complicated by colporrhagia, Decoction of Four Ingredients and Ass-hide glue and Tolium artemisiae should be added to nourish the Blood and relieve metrostaxis. Rhizoma ligustici chuanxiong is often omitted lest bleeding be induced because of its pungent and fragrant nature. Fructus psoraleae, Radix pisaci, Herba cistanchis and Semen cuscutae which strengthen the Kidney, waist and knees and the Chong and Ren Channels, may be chosen for drastic relief of waist soreness.

Decoction for Reinforcing the middle Burner and Replenishing Qi should be added for tenesmus. In this prescription, Radix astragali and Rhizoma cimicifugae are used, the former in heavy dosage of at least 15 gm, to reinforce the Qi and elevate the sinking Qi of the Middle Burner. Shaoyao Gancao Decoction may be used to treat abdominal pain in which at least 15 gm of Radix paeoniae alba should be used to relieve spasms and pain. Two to three grams of Fructus amomi may also be used to regulate Qi to relieve pain and prevent abortion; Radix scutellariae and Radix rehmanniae, which dispel the interior Heat, may be appropriately administered for dry mouth and yellow fur of the tongue and signs of fetal heat. The prescription should be administered as soon as pregnancy is diagnosed. After the third month of gestation, dosage of the prescription should be reduced but should not be discontinued until the month at which habitual abortion usually takes place. During this period of time, the patient must pay particular attention to rest.

Numerous cases have been treated in our clinic following the spirit of the therapy just described. Some of these cases were treated with Anti-Abortion Pills fashioned after Suo Yi Zai Pill, and most of the fetuses of women suffering from habitual abortion reached full-term and were delivered safe and sound.

(The author acknowledges the cooperation and assistance of Shu Huying, Professor of Traditional Chinese Medicine of Tongji Medical University Teaching Hospital, in the treatment of this case.)

11.7 HABITUAL ABORTION
(HABITUAL ABORTION)

Sun Lihua

Xiyuan Hospital, China Academy of Traditional Chinese Medicine, Beijing

Fang Jinxiang, 27, female, Han nationality, married, worker. Medical record number: 28191. Date of first consultation: June 13, 1985.

CHIEF COMPLAINT: Cessation of menstruation for 45 days with discomfort in the lower abdomen.

HISTORY OF PRESENT ILLNESS: The patient had her last menstruation on April 28, 1985. On June 12, 1985, her urinary pregnancy test result was positive, and she had slight vaginal bleeding and soreness of the lower abdomen for the past eight days.

PAST HISTORY: History of habitual abortion.

MENSTRUAL AND OBSTETRICAL HISTORY: Menarche at age 14. Interval between menstruations was 30 days, each menstrual period lasting for four days. Amount of discharge moderate. No dysmenorrhea. Married at age 23. The patient had three miscarriages, two in 1982 and one in 1983, all occurring at 40 to 60 days after confirmation of pregnancy.

PERTINENT PHYSICAL EXAMINATION & LABORATORY FINDINGS: Slight yellowish discolouration of the skin. Aside from slight vaginal discharge, all other physical findings were negative.

INSPECTION OF TONGUE: Tongue substance pale with white and slimy coating.

PULSE CONDITION: Slippery and fine.

MODERN MEDICINE DIAGNOSIS: Habitual Abortion.

TRADITIONAL CHINESE MEDICINE DIAGNOSIS: Habitual Abortion.

Symptom-complex differentiation: Deficiency of the Kidney and lack of consolidation of the fetus.

THERAPEUTIC PRINCIPLES: Replenish the Vital Energy of the Kidney to stop the bleeding and consolidate the conception.

PRESCRIPTION: Modified Shou Tai Wan. Semen cuscutae, 15 gm; Radix dipsaci, 10 gm; Colla corii asini, 10 gm; Ramulus loranthi, 15 gm; Fructus lycii, 15 gm; Radix paeoniae alba, 25 gm; Pericarpium citri reticulatae, 10 gm; and Zhumagen, 30 gm.

In this prescription, Semen cuscutae, Radix dipsaci and Ramulus loranthis were used to replenish the Vital Energy of the Kidney and to prevent miscarriage; Colla Corii asini to nourish the Vital Essence; Radix paeoniae alba and Fructus lycii to nourish Yin and tonify the Kidney; Zhumagen to remove evil Heat in order to stop the bleeding; and Pericarpium citri reticulatae to regulate the flow of the Vital Energy and revitalize the Spleen.

FOLLOW-UP/COURSE OF TREATMENT:

June 28, 1985: Bleeding had stopped. There was no soreness of the lower abdomen and no nausea. Tongue substance pale with white coating; pulse slippery. Therapeutic principles applied were to resolve Phlegm to stop vomiting, replenish the Vital Energy of the Kidney and consolidate the fetus. Prescription made up of Rhizoma pinelliae, 10 gm; Poria, 10 gm; Radix dipsaci, 10 gm; Pericarpium citri reticulatae, 10 gm; Ramulus loranthi, 10 gm; Semen cuscutae, 10 gm; Radix paeoniae alba, 15 gm; Rhizoma atractylodis macrocephalae, 10 gm; Radix ophiopogonis, 10 gm; Radix scutellariae, 10 gm; and Fructus amomi, 6 gm.

August 12, 1985: The patient had been amenorrheic for three months. Complained of arthralgia. There was no bleeding. Dark colour and soft tongue with white coating, pulse slippery. These were signs of Kidney deficiency and unconsolidation of the fetus. Condition was treated by principles of activating the Blood circulation to stop pain. Prescription: Radix codonopsis, 10 gm; Radix angelicae, 6 gm; Cortex eucommiae, 10 gm; Radix glycyrrhizae praeparatae, 6 gm; Rhizoma atractylodis macrocephalae, 10 gm; Radix scutellariae, 10 gm; Ramulus loranthi, 15 gm; Semen cuscutae, 10 gm; Radix dipsaci, 15 gm; and Pericarpium citri reticulatae, 10 gm.

August 24, 1985: General condition of the patient good; there was no complaint of pain or bleeding. Pale tongue with white coating; pulse slippery. Prescription: Radix codonopsis, 10 gm; Radix paeoniae alba, 15 gm; Radix scutellariae, 6 gm; Rhizoma atractylodis macrocephalae, 10 gm; Ramulus loranthi, 15 gm; Semen cuscutae, 10 gm; Radix dipsaci, 15 gm; Cortex eucommiae, 10 gm; Colla corii asini, 10 gm; and Radix morindae officinalis, 10 gm.

October 26, 1985: Fetal movement and heart sound and strong. No specific complaint. Tongue substance pale with white coating; pulse slippery. Prescription: Radix codonopsis, 10 gm; Rhizoma atractylodis macrocephalae, 10 gm; Radix scutellariae, 6 gm; Pericarpium citri reticulatae, 10 gm; Radix paeoniae alba, 10 gm; Ramulus loranthi, 15 gm; Poria, 10 gm; Semen cuscutae, 10 gm; Radix dipsaci, 15 gm; Rhizoma pinelliae, 10 gm; and Rhizoma dioscoreae, 10 gm.

The patient was discharged from hospital on November 6, 1985, and gave birth to a full-term, healthy baby in February 1986.

11.8 HABITUAL ABORTION
(HABITUAL ABORTION)

Sun Lihua

Xiyuan Hospital, China Academy of Traditional Chinese Medicine, Beijing

Ma Suqin, 32, female, Han nationality, married, peasant. Medical record number: 24283. Date of consultation: May 29, 1985.

CHIEF COMPLAINT: Having had four miscarriages before and being pregnant at present, the patient sought protection from recurrence of miscarriage.

HISTORY OF PRESENT ILLNESS: Pregnancy test positive. Menstruation had ceased for 54 days. Last menstrual period began on April 5, 1986. The patient complained of pain in the lower abdomen, lassitude, soreness of the loin and tenesmus.

PAST HISTORY: Non-contributory.

MENSTRUAL AND OBSTETRICAL HISTORY: Menarche at age 14. Interval between onsets of successive menstruations was 25 days, each onset lasting for four days. The patient got married at age 24. She had four miscarriages, all between the second and fifth month of gestation. The miscarriages might have been due to physical overstrain.

INSPECTION OF TONGUE: Pale tongue substance with tooth prints at the borders; tongue fur white.

PULSE CONDITION: Fine and smooth.

MODERN MEDICINE DIAGNOSIS: Habitual Abortion.

TRADITIONAL CHINESE MEDICINE DIAGNOSIS: Habitual Abortion; Unconsolidation of the Fetus.

Symptom-complex differentiation: Deficiency of the Kidney in this case was caused by the previous four miscarriages. The Kidney is the foundation of the original constitution. Its deficiency results in weakness of the Chong and Ren Channels and is also responsible for symptoms such as lower abdominal pain and excessive movement of the fetus. Lassitude is a result of insufficiency of the Middle Burner. The patient's tongue condition, i.e., pale substance with tooth prints on the borders, was attributed to sthenia-syndrome of the Spleen. Smooth pulse was a characteristic manifestation of pregnancy, while the fine aspect of the pulse was due to deficiency of the Kidney and Spleen.

THERAPEUTIC PRINCIPLES: Replenish the Vital Energy of the Kidney to prevent miscarriage.

PRESCRIPTION: Modified Tai Shan Pian Shi San adopted from the 64-volume *Jing-Yue's Complete Works* written by Zhang Jiebin in 1624. Original recipe contained Radix ginseng, Radix angelicae, Radix rehmanniae praeparatae, Radix paeoniae alba, Rhizoma atractylodis macrocephalae, Fructus amomi, Radix glycyrrhizae praeparatae, Rhizoma ligustici, Radix dipsaci and Radix scutellariae.

Modification was effected by removing Radix ginseng, Fructus amomi and Rhizoma ligustici and adding Radix codonopsis, Radix astragali and Semen cuscutae. In this prescription, Radix codonopsis, Rhizoma atractylodis macrocephalae and Radix astragali reinforced the functions of the Spleen; Semen cuscutae and Radix dipsaci replenished the Vital Energy of the Kidney and prevented miscarriage; and Radix rehmanniae praeparatae and Radix angelicae nourished the Blood and prevented miscarriage. Radix astragali also prevents occurrence of miscarriage by its effect in removing evil Heat from the body, while Radix glycyrrhizae was used to invigorate the vital function.

During the course of treatment, the patient was strictly confined to bed.

FOLLOW-UP/COURSE OF TREATMENT:

June 6, 1985: The patient reported no loin pain or tenesmus. She felt well. Tongue substance pale with white coat. Smooth pulse. Principles applied at this stage were to warm and tonify the Kidney, invigorate Spleen functions and consolidate the fetus. Prescription: Shou Tai Wan and Sijunzi Tang. Radix codonopsis, 10 gm; Poria, 10 gm; Rhizoma atractylodis macrocephalae, 10 gm; Radix glycyrrhizae, 6 gm; Radix astragali, 10 gm; Radix dipsaci, 10 gm; Ramulus loranthi, 15 gm; Semen cuscutae, 10 gm;

and Colla corii asini, 15 gm.

In this prescription, Radix codonopsis, Poria, Radix astragali and Rhizoma atractylodis macrocephalae reinforced the functional activities of the Spleen; Semen cuscutae, Ramulus loranthi and Radix dipsaci replenished the Vital Energy of the Kidney; Poria and Radix glycyrrhizae invigorated the Spleen and the Stomach; and Colla corii asini tonified the Blood.

The patient was discharged on October 6, 1985, her fetal heart rate at the time being 150/min.

A full-term, healthy baby was born to the patient on her return visit.

11.9 ENDOMETRIOSIS
(DYSMENORRHEA, STAGNATION OF QI AND STASIS OF BLOOD)

Wang Dazeng
Longhua Hospital, Shanghai College of Traditional Chinese Medicine, Shanghai

Xie, 38, female, Han nationality, married, worker. Medical record number: 75868. Date of admission: September 12, 1986.

CHIEF COMPLAINT: Dysmenorrhea with progressive exacerbation for seven years.

HISTORY OF PRESENT ILLNESS: Dysmenorrhea with progressive exacerbation after induced abortion seven years ago, accompanied by nausea, vomiting, cold sweating, coldness of the extremities, dragging-down sensation in the lower abdomen together with sensation of defecation. Analgesic drugs were necessary for relief of the pain. The patient had been treated with Megestrum tablet in another hospital, but the results were not satisfactory. Menstruation was moderate in amount, deep red in colour, with presence of blood clots. Married at 27 years of age, she had one full-term delivery and two induced abortions. Menstruation returned the day before admission and was accompanied by abdominal pain, soreness in the loins and nausea.

PAST HISTORY: History of pyelonephritis, duodenal ulcer and antrum gastritis.

PERTINENT PHYSICAL EXAMINATION & LABORATORY FINDINGS: Well-developed, slightly lustreless complexion. Abdomen soft, external genitalia marital, cervix smooth, uterus normal size, in retroflexed position and not very movable. Left fornix thickened, right fornix negative. Posterior fornix presence of several bean-sized nodules with marked tenderness. Routine blood examination: Hemoglobin, 10.5 gm%; RBC, 2.44 M/mm^3; WBC, 6,900/mm^3; platelet, 135,000/mm^3; bleeding time, 2 minutes; coagulation time, 2 minutes; ESR, 16 mm/hr.

INSPECTION OF TONGUE: Plump, deep in colour, thinly coated with engorged veins at the undersurface of the tongue.

PULSE CONDITION: Thready and taut.

MODERN MEDICINE DIAGNOSIS: Endometriosis.

TRADITIONAL CHINESE MEDICINE DIAGNOSIS: Dysmenorrhea (Stagnation of Vital Energy and Stasis of Blood).

THERAPEUTIC PRINCIPLES: Activate the blood circulation by removing blood stasis, regulate the flow of Qi (Vital Energy) and relieve pain (during menstruation).

PRESCRIPTION: Modified Shaofu Zhuyu Tang (Decoction for Removing Blood Stasis from the Lower Abdomen). Radix angelicae sinensis, 9 gm; Rhizoma ligustici, 9 gm; Radix paeoniae rubra, 9 gm; Radix salviae, 9 gm; Corydalis tuber, 9 gm; Cortex cinnamomi, 3 gm; Shi Xiao Powder, 9 gm; Rhizoma cyperi, 9 gm; Resina ommiphorae myrrhae, 4.5 gm; and Resina boswelliae carterii, 4.5 gm. Decocted in water and administered orally twice a day. Continued taking the prescription till the end of menstruation. IV drip of Danshen (Salviae) once a day (eight ampules of Injection Danshen containing a total of 16 mg of Danshen diluted with 500 ml of 5% GS).

FOLLOW-UP/COURSE OF TREATMENT:

During the period between menstruations, herbs effective in reinforcing the Vital Energy, nourishing the Blood, eliminating Blood stasis and resolving the mass were given together with intravenous Danshen. Radix astragalis, 15 gm; Radix angelicae, 9 gm; Rhizoma ligustici, 9 gm; Radix paeoniae alba, 9 gm; Rhizoma cyperi, 9 gm; Fructus foeniculi, 3 gm; Shi Xiao Powder, 9 gm; Flos carthami, 6 gm; Resina draconis, 9 gm; Cortex cinnamomi, 3 gm; and Radix codonopsis pilosulae, 9 gm. Method of preparation and administration of the decoction same as above.

Intravenous infusion of Danshen, once a day, was started at the middle of the menstrual cycle and continued until the end of the next menstruation.

Menstruation returned on November 2 but was delayed. BBT biphasic and abdominal pain markedly alleviated. Nausea and vexation were relieved. Vaginal examination findings were same as before. Continued the same therapeutic measures.

On November 30, menstruation returned and was normal in amount. The patient complained of abdominal pain on the first day but it was milder than before and subsided the next day. No analgesic was used. Pulse was thin and taut. Herbs for regulating the flow of Qi and activating Blood circulation, eliminating Blood stasis and relieving the pain were prescribed as before. She was discharged on December 11, 1986, and instructed to have follow-ups in the outpatient department.

DISCUSSION: Endometriosis is a commonly encountered disease in gynecology. In recent years, the morbidity of this disease has tended to increase because of the improvement in diagnostic techniques and the increase in the number of induced abortions. The chief manifestations of endometriosis are menstrual irregularity, dysmenorrhea and sterility. It can also manifest itself in the form of pelvic mass (such as adenomyosis, chocolate cyst or ovary, pelvic adhesion and posterior fornix nodules). According to TCM symptom-complex differentiation, this was a case of Blood stasis and Blood mass. The principles of treatment were mainly those of activating Blood circulation to eliminate Blood stasis, regulating the flow of Qi, relieving the pain and softening and disintegrating the mass. Abdominal pain is the chief symptom of endometriosis. It can occur before or during menstruation as well as be a constant complaint during the time between menstrual cycles. However, some patients may have no abdominal pain. The pain is usually in the lower abdomen and fixed in location. As has been mentioned, it is due to Blood stasis. Herbs effective in activating Blood circulation and eliminating Blood stasis, such as Semen persicae, Flos carthami, Faeces trogopterorum, Resina commiphorae and Boswelliae, are generally indicated as well as medicinal materials originating from insects and worms, such as Hirudo tabanus. Abdominal pain is often accompanied by abdominal distention (due to pelvic congestion and adhesion resulting from endometriosis). Corydalis tuber, Fructus meliae, Radix and Fructus aurantii and other herbs of the same nature were indicated in this case to promote the flow of Qi and to invigorate Blood circulation. In general, herbs with warm and hot properties are more suitable for the treatment of this disease because they result in effective remission of the pain. Warmth and heat are beneficial for the circulation of Qi and Blood and can also enhance the function of these herbs in eliminating Blood stasis. Commonly used herbs with warm and hot properties include Cinnamomi and Fructus foeniculi, Cinnamomi oil contains Rougui which dilates blood vessels leading to improvement of blood circulation. To soften the hardness and dissolve the mass, Rhizoma sparganii, Rhizoma zedoariae, Sargassum, Thallus laminariae and Concha ostreae were used. The commonly used prescriptions were Guizhi Fuling Pills, adopted from Zhang Zhongjing by Wang Qingren, and Shaofu Zhuyu Tang (Decoction for Removing Blood Stasis from the Lower Abdomen). The main ingredient of these prescriptions, Radix salviae, which is effective in activating Blood circulation, can be administered by intravenous infusion to achieve a more direct and rapid outcome.

In this case, satisfactory therapeutic effects were achieved by administration of a combination of herbs effective in activating Blood circulation and removing Blood stasis. Intravenous administration of Danshen was used to treat Vital Energy disorder and to achieve an analgesic effect.

During her stay in the hospital, the patient's menstruation returned twice, abdominal pain was markedly alleviated and analgesics were not needed. The patient had an induced abortion on January 20, 1987. She continued to take the prescriptions after that. A follow-up visit in January 1988 showed her in good health with regular menstruation. Abdominal discomfort was minimal.

11.10 METRORRHAGIA AND METROSTAXIS (DYSFUNCTIONAL UTERINE BLEEDING)

Chen Kezhong and Zhang Jidong
Shandong Medical University Hospital, Jinan

Fang Wenshu, 45, female, Han nationality, married, worker. Medical record number: 177877. Date of first consultation: August 1, 1972.
CHIEF COMPLAINT: Irregular, lingering vaginal bleeding for more than four months.

HISTORY OF PRESENT ILLNESS: Four months prior to admission, the patient started to experience irregular vaginal bleeding lasting about 10 to 20 days each time. The amount of discharge was large and light in colour. Accompanying symptoms were lumbago, palpitation, shortness of breath, dizziness, insomnia, fatigue and poor appetite.

PAST HISTORY: Non-contributory.

PERTINENT PHYSICAL EXAMINATION & LABORATORY FINDINGS: Pallor evident; systolic murmur appreciated at the apex of the heart. Hemoglobin, 7.8 gm%; RBC, 2.5 M/mm^3.

INSPECTION OF TONGUE: Pale tongue proper thickly coated with greasy and white fur.

PULSE CONDITION: Fine and weak.

MODERN MEDICINE DIAGNOSIS: Dysfunctional Uterine Bleeding.

TRADITIONAL CHINESE MEDICINE DIAGNOSIS: Metrorrhagia and Metrostaxis.

THERAPEUTIC PRINCIPLES: Invigorate the Spleen and replenish the Vital Energy; stop the bleeding and enrich the Blood.

PRESCRIPTION: Guipi Tang Jiajian (Modified Decoction for Invigorating the Spleen and Nourishing the Heart). Radix astragali, 15 gm; Radix codonopsis, 15 gm; Rhizoma dioscoreae, 15 gm; Poria, 15 gm; Radix angelicae, 15 gm; Radix paeoniae alba, 15 gm; Rhizoma atractylodis macrocephalae, 18 gm; Colla corii asini, 12 gm; Charcoal Radix rubiae, 9 gm; Rhizoma polygonati, 30 gm; Radix dipsaci, 15 gm; Radix glycyrrhizae, 6 gm; Semen ziziphi, 14 gm; Cacumen biotae, 9 gm; and Jiaosanxian (malt, fruit of hawthorn and medicated leaven stir-baked to brown), 9 gm. To be decocted in water for oral dose. One dose per day.

FOLLOW-UP/COURSE OF TREATMENT:

Second consultation on January 12, 1973: Vaginal bleeding had ceased. The patient still felt weak in her extremities and had cough as well as oppressed feeling in the chest. Tongue substance fresh, thinly coated with white fur. Pulse sinking and thready. Prescription: Radix astragali, 15 gm; Radix codonopsis, 15 gm; Rhizoma dioscoreae, 15 gm; Radix angelicae, 9 gm; Radix paeoniae alba, 15 gm; Colla corii asini, 9 gm; Rhizoma atractylodis macrocephalae, 15 gm; Rhizoma polygonati, 30 gm; Semen amomi cardamomi, 9 gm; Folium eriobotryae, 30 gm; Endothelium corneium gigeriae galli, 9 gm; and Jiaosanxian, 9 gm. Five doses.

Third consultation on January 17, 1973: Vaginal bleeding had not recurred. Tongue substance pale with thin and white fur, pulse sinking and fine. Modified the prescription by removing Folium eriobotryae and adding Radix dipsaci. Five doses.

Fourth consultation on January 21, 1973. Having taken the medicine, the patient felt at ease and calm. Condition of the tongue and pulse remained the same. Five more doses of the same prescription.

Fifth consultation on January 27, 1973: Menstruation began with the normal amount of discharge. The patient still had lumbago and lower abdominal pain. Tongue substance pale with thin, yellow fur. Pulse sinking and fine. Continued the same prescription. Five doses.

Sixth consultation on January 31, 1973: Flow of menstrual discharge reduced. Abdominal and lumbar pain relieved. Tongue red with thin and white coating, pulse sinking and fine. Removed Semen amomi and added Rhizoma cyperi, 9 gm, to the prescription. Four doses.

Seventh consultation on February 5, 1973: Menstruation period lasted for seven days and discharge ceased. The patient's general condition was fairly good. She had moist and lustrous complexion. The tongue was pink with thin and white fur; pulse taut and thin. Routine blood examination showed hemoglobin, 10 gm% and RBC, 2.5 M/mm^3. Continued the same prescription. Five doses.

Eighth consultation on February 10, 1973: The patient's menstruation regular and normal in the amount of discharge. Appetite normal. She was discharged from hospital with six doses of the prescription as take-home medication.

DISCUSSION: Dysfunctional uterine bleeding belongs to the category of metrorrhagia and metrostaxis in traditional Chinese medicine. Its etiology and mechanism are largely due to unstableness of the Ren and Chong Channels caused by deficiencies of the Liver and Kidney as well as disturbance of the Blood and Vital Energy. In cases with heavy bleeding, the priority is to replenish the Vital Energy in order to stop the chronic hemorrhage. Once the bleeding is under control, focus of treatment should be placed on replenishing the Spleen and tonifying the Kidney to promote normal ovulation and menstruation. Empirical clinical experience demands that hemostasis be instituted in cases of heavy bleeding. In order to prevent the harmful effect of stasis, one should not institute hemostasis across the board in order to avoid abusing carbon-containing agents. On processing these agents, their medical properties must be kept in mind lest the formation of dry carbon results in the waste of drugs and a delay in the therapeutic effects. When prescribing medication, one or two of these agents, not more, may be chosen deliberately. It is useless to use more. Recent studies show that carbonated Caucumen biotae is effective in shortening both the bleeding and clotting time. It is more effective when applied raw than in carbonated form. Accordingly, raw Caucumen biotae was used in this prescription. Experimental studies also show that Radix rubiae possesses a mild hemostatic effect, and infusion of its root extract in warm water can shorten the time of bleeding and clotting in rabbits. When parched, the drug's effect is more obvious. This indicates the importance of keeping the medical property in parching. In cases of metrorrhagia and metrostaxis secondary to Blood stasis, the same effect can be obtained by applying the principles of removing stasis and regulating the circulation of Blood.

The patient in our case often worked long hours of hard manual labour and did not eat a regular diet. These factors can contribute to deficiency of the Vital Energy of the Spleen, disturbances in Blood regulation and generation as well as weakness of the Chong and Ren Channels. This condition is conducive to the occurrence of metrorrhagia and metrostaxis. Modified Decoction for Invigorating the Spleen and Nourishing the Heart was given in this case to invigorate the Spleen and produce Blood. As we know, the Spleen is the source of nutrients for growth and development. Invigoration of Spleen Vital Energy provides a rich source for production of Blood, and thus, anemia could be corrected naturally.

11.11 ENDOMETRIOSIS
(VICARIOUS HEMOPTYSIS)

Yu Jin

Gynecological Hospital, Shanghai Medical University, Shanghai

Yang Aihua, 31, female, Han nationality, married, worker. Medical record number: 83-53661. Date of first consultation: January 3, 1983.

CHIEF COMPLAINT: Hemoptysis with menorrhagia for one year.

HISTORY OF PRESENT ILLNESS: The patient had a normal delivery three years ago. A year later, she noted her menses was very profuse. One year prior to consultation, during one of her heavy menses, she experienced itchiness of the throat and subsequently coughed up a large amount of blood. Chest X-ray and routine blood examinations at the time were both normal. She also complained of dizziness, backache and irritability. Treatment received had been mainly hemostatic agents, but there was no evident effect.

PAST HISTORY: Non-contributory.

PERTINENT PHYSICAL EXAMINATION & LABORATORY FINDINGS: Pale in appearance; blood pressure, 110/90 mmHg. General physical examination findings normal. Pelvic examination: uterine cervix, mild erosion; uterus, anteposed and normal in size; left adnexa tender with cystic mass 3 cm in diameter, right adnexa negative. Routine blood examination findings negative.

INSPECTION OF TONGUE: Reddened tongue proper with purple dots on the tip.

PULSE CONDITION: Fine, string-like, tight and rapid.

MODERN MEDICINE DIAGNOSIS: Endometriosis.

TRADITIONAL CHINESE MEDICINE DIAGNOSIS: Vicarious Hemoptysis.

THERAPEUTIC PRINCIPLES: Replenish Yin of the Kidney and Lung, remove pathogenic Fire from the Lung.

PRESCRIPTION: Halstrum testudinis, 15 gm; Carapax trionycis, 12 gm; Concha ostreae, 30 gm; Rhizoma rehmanniae, 12 gm; Rhizoma anemarrhenae, 6 gm; Rhizoma coptidis, 3 gm; Radix ophiopogonis, 6 gm; Rhizoma polygonati odorati, 12 gm; Mulberry bark, 6 gm; and Cortex mori radicis, 6 gm. One dose per day for seven days.

FOLLOW-UP/COURSE OF TREATMENT:

Second consultation on January 10, 1983: Symptoms significantly relieved, but tongue and pulse conditions remained the same. Modified the previous prescription by adding herbs effective in removing Blood stasis in order to prevent heavy menses. Pollen typhae, 12 gm, and Flos sophorae, 12 gm. One dose per day for seven days.

Third consultation on January 17, 1983: LMP January 11, 1983. Amount of menstrual discharge significantly reduced or normal. No blood or sputum was coughed up during the menstruation period. The patient felt all right except for a mild headache. Tongue proper not as red and pulse fine and with regular rate and rhythm. She was instructed to continue using the prescription of the first consultation in the same dosage.

Fourth consultation on February 10, 1983: The patient's menstruation was due four days ago on February 6, 1983. Amount of discharge normal. There was no hemoptysis. During the menstruation period, blood-streaked sputum was coughed up once. She was satisfied with the progress of her recovery and asked to continue traditional medicine treatment at home.

In 1986, through the mail, the patient informed us that her condition was stable, and she had not coughed up any blood since the last visit.

DISCUSSION: Hemoptysis is a symptom of endometriosis, though it is seldom encountered. Transplantation of blood vessels secondary to endometriosis is thought to be the cause. Hemostatic agents, progestin and others are usually used in treatment. In *Yi Zong Jin Jian (The Golden Mirror of Medicine)*, vicarious hemoptysis and menorrhagia are defined as symptoms due to deficiency of Yin accompanied by flaring up of evil Fire. This evil Fire injures the Yang Collateral (pulmonary vascular system) and the Yin Collateral (uterine vascular system). An important teaching in TCM therapeutics is "treat a disease by looking into both its root cause and its symptoms or complications." In our case, the manifestations were hemoptysis and menorrhagia, and the fundamental cause of these symptoms was deficiency of Yin. Herbs effective in replenishing Yin of the Kidney and Lung and in removing evil Fire from the Lung, not hemostatics, were used. After a relatively short period of administration of this prescription, we were able to achieve a satisfactory therapeutic effect. Another case in our hospital (medical record number: 84-17740) with cyclic nasal bleeding was also cured with this method. This patient suffered from nasal bleeding and menorrhagia for 13 years with 100-200 ml of blood lost during each menstruation. Chest film and nasal examination did not show any positive findings, and endometriosis was diagnosed after pelvic examination. Medications such as adrenaline and antibiotics were given but to no avail. By TCM symptom-complex differentiation, her case was classified as deficiency of Yin accompanied by presence of evil Fire. After one month of traditional medicine treatment (using a prescription similar to the one above), all symptoms were relieved and the patient recovered fully. She was followed up for three years during which she had taken traditional medicines intermittently, and there had not been any abnormal menstruation or nasal bleeding.

11.12 INFECTION OF UTERINE CAVITY (HEAT JUE)

Kang Ziqi

Department of Medicine, Peking Union Medical College Hospital, Beijing

Wu, 36, female, married, peasant. Date of first consultation: May 17, 1985.

CHIEF COMPLAINT: Gestation 13 weeks, high fever for two days after failure of induced labour.

HISTORY OF PRESENT ILLNESS: The patient had been pregnant for 13 weeks and requested termination of the pregnancy. Eleven hours after induction of labour with water sac in a local hospital, she had cold and shivers accompanied by lower abdominal pain. Body temperature, 39.3°C; blood pressure, 90/70 mmHg; and white blood cell count 13,000/mm³ with 96% neutrophils. She received a large dose of antibiotics for 10 days, but symptoms became worse, body temperature ranging between 39-40°C persistently. She experienced dryness of the mouth and craved for cold drinks. She had not had any bowel movement for 10 days. Urine was scanty and red, abdomen swollen, painful and tender. Uterus could not be clearly palpated. She had a sick facies and yellowish complexion.

PAST HISTORY: Weak physique with multiple pregnancies.

INSPECTION OF TONGUE: Dark tongue proper with dry and yellowish fur.

PULSE CONDITION: Slippery and rapid.

MODERN MEDICINE DIAGNOSIS: Infection of Uterine Cavity.

TRADITIONAL CHINESE MEDICINE DIAGNOSIS: Heat Jue.

Symptom-complex differentiation: The patient had been weak in the past with multiple labours. There was disturbance of the relationship between Qi and Blood. Damp-Heat and toxic pathogens invaded the uterus. She had cold extremities secondary to excessive pathogenic Heat impairing the tissue fluid and interfering with the circulation of Yang to the extremities.

THERAPEUTIC PRINCIPLES: Dissipate the heat and detoxify, cool the Blood, eliminate the stagnation and activate the Blood.

PRESCRIPTION: Radix scutellariae, 10 gm; Radix rehmanniae, 12 gm; Poria, 15 gm; Radix scrophulariae buergeruanae, 15 gm; Radix ophiopogonis, 13 gm; Radix glycyrrhizae, 12 gm; Herba schizonepetae, 10 gm; Fructus aurantii, 10 gm; Radix et rhizoma rhei, 13 gm; Semen persicae, 10 gm; and Natrii sulfas, 10 gm. Decocted for oral ingestion. Discontinued administration of antibiotics.

FOLLOW-UP/COURSE OF TREATMENT:

The patient had diarrhea once the night after taking the prescription. By 23:00 p.m., vaginal bleeding appeared and fetus was discharged later. At this stage, she had heavy sweating and body temperature rose to 40.3°C accompanied by shivering, cold extremities and a blood pressure reading of 96/60 mmHg. After three days of continuous infusion and three more doses of the TCM prescription, body temperature returned to normal and the abdomen was soft and non-tender. WBC count was 6,500/mm³. Vaginal secretion culture positive for B. coli.

DISCUSSION:

The characteristics of this case were:

1) Excessive Fire. The patient had persistent high fever of 40°C accompanied by thirst and a craving for cold water. Urine was scanty and red, and she also suffered from constipation and profuse sweating. Feet and hands were cold and purplish in colour. Sensation of chills and shivering as well as drop in blood pressure were also evident. These symptoms point to accumulation of Heat inside the body. It is known as "true Heat and false Cold."

2) Distention and fullness of the abdomen with pain and tenderness. Firmness and fullness in the hypochondrium.

3) Blood stasis. The patient had dark tongue proper, cyanosis of the lips and

extremities. Lower abdominal pain was also present. These were signs of invasion of Chamber (uterus) by Heat resulting in stagnation of Blood. Death of the fetus in the uterus was treated by eliminating the stasis of Heat and Blood from the large intestine.

Semen persicae, which is bitter in nature, was the main ingredient in the recipe for the treatment of this case. It has the function of breaking the Blood stasis and eliminating the stagnation. Its application in this case was to relieve Blood stagnation, constipation and invasion of the Heat to the Blood Chamber. Radix et rhizoma rhei, a bitter and cold herb, cleared the stagnant Qi of the Stomach and Intestine, dissipated the evil Heat from the Blood, eliminated stagnation and activated the Blood. Fructus aurantii, a pungent and bitter herb, was effective in eliminating the Phlegm and dissolving the mass, relieving the distention and breaking the stagnant Qi to treat pain and distention of the hypochondrium and abdomen. Fructus aurantii induced contraction of the smooth muscle of the uterus, important in promoting the delivery of the fetus.

Remarks about Rhubarb:

1) Rhubarb (Radix et rhizoma rhei) contains alkali of rhubarb. It stimulates the large intestine to facilitate peristalsis and promote bowel movement.

2) Rhubarb has a strong antiseptic effect on Staphylococci aurei, Escherichia coli, dysentery and tuberculous bacillus.

3) Rhubarb, when used together with Semen persicae, can penetrate the Blood. Rhubarb cools the Blood and removes the stasis, while Semen persicae eliminates the stagnation and activates the Blood. The dosage of Rhubarb was small in this case because of the patient's weak constitution.

11.13 INFLAMMATORY PELVIC MASS (ZHENG-JI)

Zhang Yuxuan

Department of Traditional Chinese Medicine, Peking Union Medical College Hospital, Beijing

Shen, 22, female, Han nationality, single, worker. Medical record number: G231365. Date of admission: December 15, 1981.

CHIEF COMPLAINT: High fever accompanied by abdominal pain for 18 days.

HISTORY OF PRESENT ILLNESS: On November 17, 1981, the patient suddenly developed chills and fever (39°C) accompanied by dull lower abdominal pain. Her stool became loose and increased in frequency, but this condition subsided later after taking gentamycin and erythromycin. On December 5, 1981, she was hospitalized in Beijing's Jishuitan Hospital because of persistent high fever and abdominal pain. She was treated as a case of tuberculous peritonitis and was given rimifon and kanamycin. Ten days later, her condition did not improve and her body temperature was still 39°C. She was subsequently transferred to our hospital. On admission, the patient had hyperpyrexia associated with distending pain in the lower abdomen. Her appetite was poor and she complained of thirst but was not willing to drink.

PERTINENT PHYSICAL EXAMINATION & LABORATORY FINDINGS: Acute sickness facies with flushed appearance; temperature, 39°C; and pulse rate, 96/min. Heart and lungs findings negative. Lower abdomen appeared slightly bulging with an uneven bordered mass palpable; no pain or tenderness. Hemoglobin, 10.3 gm%; WBC, 6,100/mm^3; neutrophils, 75%; lymphocytes, 25%; and ESR, 105 mm/hr. Routine urinalysis and stool examination normal. Chest film negative. Ultrasound examination showed a cystic and substantial mass, 7.2 × 4.1 × 3.1 cm in size situated near the left upper border of the uterus; borders of the mass were not distinct, suggesting a mass inflammatory and adhesive in nature.

INSPECTION OF TONGUE: Tongue proper pale with a thick layer of white fur.

PULSE CONDITION: Deep and thready.

MODERN MEDICINE DIAGNOSIS: Pelvic Inflammatory and Adhesive Mass.

TRADITIONAL CHINESE MEDICINE DIAGNOSIS: Internal Accumulation of Dampness and Heat; Blood Stasis and Mass Formation.

THERAPEUTIC PRINCIPLES: Clear off the Heat and Dampness.

PRESCRIPTION: San Ren Tang. Semen armeniacae amarum, 10 gm; Semen coicis, 15 gm; Semen amomi cardamomi, 5 gm; Cortex magnoliae officinalis, 10 gm; Rhizoma pinelliae, 10 gm; Herba lophatheri, 10 gm; Rhizoma atractylodis, 10 gm; Herba agastachis, 10 gm; Herba eupatoii, 10 gm; Rhizoma acori graminei, 10 gm; and Liu Yi San (mixture of powder of talcum and Radix glycyrrhizae), 10 gm. Decocted and served one dose per day in two equally divided portions.

FOLLOW-UP/COURSE OF TREATMENT:

Second consultation on December 21, 1981: After taking six doses of the prescription, temperature had returned to normal, though conditions of the tongue and pulse remained the same. Gynecological examination revealed a cystic mass as big as a fetal head attached to the left anterior area of the uterus, high in tension, non-movable and non-tender, suggesting a twisted ovarian cyst. The patient was transferred to the gynecology ward and herbal medicine discontinued.

Third consultation on January 7, 1982: Peritoneoscopy established the diagnosis as inflammatory mass of the pelvic appendages, and this was proven by biopsy. During this period the patient again had fever for several days which was brought down after IM injection of penicillin and gentamycin for 11 days. Examination revealed no apparent change in the mass. She was then transferred back to our ward. She complained of impaired appetite, slight distention of the abdomen and heaviness of the lower extremities. Bowel movement and urination had been normal; tongue substance pale and greasy-looking; pulse deep and thready. Principles of treatment were to clear off the Heat and Dampness and activate Blood circulation to remove Blood clots.

Prescription: Semen armeniacae amarum, 10 gm; Semen coicis, 20 gm; Semen amomi cardamomi, 10 gm; Cortex magnoliae officinalis, 10 gm; Poria, 15 gm; Rhizoma pinelliae, 10 gm; Rhizoma alismatis, 12 gm; Rhizoma atractylodis macrocephalae, 15 gm; Radix angelicae sinensis, 10 gm; Radix paeoniae rubra, 15 gm; Rhizoma ligustici chuanxiong, 10 gm; Radix salviae miltiorrhizae, 20 gm; Rhizoma zedoariae,

10 gm; and Rhizoma corydalis, 10 gm. Method of preparation and administration same as above.

Fourth consultation on January 11, 1982: The patient had taken the last prescription for four days and felt fine. Tongue proper was light bluish in colour covered with a layer of white and thick fur. Pulse was still deep and thready. ESR had come down to 62 mm/hr. Principles of treatment modified to those of activating Blood circulation, softening the mass, clearing off the Heat and removing the toxins.

Prescription: Radix angelicae sinensis, 10 gm; Rhizoma ligustici chuanxiong, 10 gm; Radix paeoniae rubra, 10 gm; Radix paeoniae alba, 10 gm; Rhizoma zedoariae, 10 gm; Radix scrophulariae, 10 gm; Pulvis concha ostreae, 30 gm; Spica prunellae, 30 gm; Herba taraxaci, 30 gm; Herba patriniae, 30 gm; Herba violae, 30 gm; Poria, 30 gm; and Radix glycyrrhizae, 5 gm. Same preparation and administration methods.

In addition, the patient was given Radix salviae miltiorrhizae Co., 4 ml, IM, q.d.

Fifth consultation on February 3, 1982: After taking this prescription for 18 days, the patient felt well. ESR had come down to 22 mm/hr and hemoglobin level was 13 gm%. Ultrasound examination still showed no apparent reduction in the size of the mass. Tongue and pulse conditions remained the same. Discontinued the prescription and adopted Tao Ren Si Wu Tang with Gui Zhi Fu Ling Wan.

Prescription: Radix angelicae sinensis, 10 gm; Rhizoma ligustici chuanxiong, 10 gm; Radix paeoniae rubra, 10 gm; Radix paeoniae alba, 10 gm; Semen persicae, 10 gm; Flos carthami, 10 gm; Cortex moutan radicis, 10 gm; Ramulus cinnamomi, 10 gm; Poria, 12 gm; Rhizoma zedoariae, 15 gm; Radix linderae, 10 gm; Spica prunellae, 30 gm; Herba patriniae, 30 gm; Radix astragali, 15 gm; and Radix glycyrrhizae, 5 gm. Same preparation and administration methods.

In addition, Da Huang Zhe Chong Wan, half pill, b.i.d., in the morning and at night.

Sixth consultation on February 17, 1982: The last prescription had been administered for six days. The patient had no specific complaints. Tongue was pale with thin, yellow fur; pulse thready. On ultrasound examination of the abdomen, no definite mass could be seen. Continued the same prescription without Da Huang Zhe Chong Wan.

The patient was discharged on February 20, 1982. When last seen on July 19, 1982, she was well and had no complaints.

DISCUSSION: Traditional Chinese medicine considers presence of a definite mass of hard consistency to be Zheng and Ji which are located in the Xue (Blood) system, while masses of variable consistency and presence are considered Xia and Ju and are usually found in the Qi (Vital Energy) system.

In modern medicine, the etiology of masses is variable, and clinical manifestations and treatment are accordingly different. Occasionally, surgical procedures are indicated. As such, a simple diagnosis of Zheng and Ji is not sufficient. Modern medicine diagnostic procedures should be applied to further diagnose these Zheng and Ji. This is necessary not only to provide a sound basis of choosing the appropriate therapeutic measures but also as a basis for evaluating the therapeutic effects of traditional Chinese medicine.

Treatment of this case was divided into three stages:

The first stage involved differentiating the syndromes on the basis of high fever and the appearance of the tongue. Application of San Ren Tang to clear off the Heat and Dampness brought a satisfactory result. One must be reminded that prior to this, the patient had been treated with antibiotics for 10 days without satisfactory effects. With application of herbal medicine for only three days, fever was brought down to normal.

The second stage lasted from January 7 to February 3, 1982. The patient's general condition had improved significantly after applying the therapeutic principles of clearing off the Heat and Dampness and invigorating the Blood circulation to remove stasis. ESR had returned to normal, but there was no obvious reduction in the size of the mass. This could be attributed to under application of Blood-invigorating herbs.

The aim of the third age was to remove the mass. Therapeutic principles applied to achieve this goal were those of invigorating Blood circulation to remove stasis, softening the hardness and dissolving the mass. Clinical outcome was satisfactory with the mass disappearing after two weeks of herbal medicine administration. The herbs used in the prescription were adopted from the recipes of Tao Ren Si Wu Tang and Gui Zhi Fu Ling Wan. Also important was the administration of Da Huang Zhe Chong Wan. The successful outcome of this case was not unexpected since all the prescriptions applied contained herbs highly potent in invigorating Blood circulation and removing stasis, and they are commonly effective in treating Zheng and Ji, Pi Kuai and internal Gan Xue Zhen (conditions referring to presence of an abdominal mass).

11.14 POLYCYSTIC OVARY SYNDROME (STAGNATION AND FIRE IN THE LIVER)

Wang Dazeng

Longhua Hospital, Shanghai College of Traditional Chinese Medicine, Shanghai

Li, 24, female, Han nationality, married, worker. Medical record number: 423. Date of first consultation: February 3, 1987.

CHIEF COMPLAINT: Cessation of menstruation for two months.

HISTORY OF PRESENT ILLNESS: Having had her menarche at age 14, the patient usually had menstruations with different intervals. The amount of blood flow also varied greatly. LMP, November 18, 1986, and PMP on October 16, 1986 (after injection of progesterone). Pneumoperitoneograph in another hospital in January 1986 showed sizes of ovaries to be two-thirds and three-fifths of the uterine size. Polycystic ovary syndrome (PCO) was diagnosed. She was treated with clomiphene and HCG for three months. BBT was biphasic during treatment, but she was amenorrheic again shortly after the discontinuance of the hormonal treatment. The patient got upset and irritated easily.

PAST HISTORY: Non-contributory.

PERTINENT PHYSICAL EXAMINATION & LABORATORY FINDINGS: Well-developed and well-nourished. Height, 1.67 m, and body weight, 56 kg. Heavy eyebrows and acne on face. Gynecological examination: breasts well-developed; abdomen soft; external genitalia normal, unmarried in type with heavy pubic hairs of female distribution. Rectal examination: uterus normal in size, midpositioned and movable; left ovary palpable; right fornix negative.

Serum sex hormone determination (RIA):

Thirteenth day of menstruation period: FSH, 12 IU/ml; LH, 46 IU/ml; E_2, 132 pg/ml; T, 100 ng/dl; and P, 12.6 ng/ml. Twenty-third day of menstruation period: FSH, 10 IU/ml; LH, 76 IU/ml; E_2, 123 pg/ml; T, 132 ng/dl; and P, 15.5 ng/ml.

INSPECTION OF TONGUE: Tongue substance red and thinly coated.

PULSE CONDITION: Thready and taut.

MODERN MEDICINE DIAGNOSIS: Polycystic Ovary Syndrome.

TRADITIONAL CHINESE MEDICINE DIAGNOSIS: Stagnation and Fire in the Liver.

THERAPEUTIC PRINCIPLES: Quench the Fire in the Liver.

PRESCRIPTION: Long Dan Xie Gan Tang (LDXGT, Decoction of Gentianae to Purge the Liver). Radix gentianae, 6-9 gm; Radix scutellariae, 9 gm; Fructus gardeniae, 9 gm; Rhizoma alismatis, 9 gm; Caulis akebiae, 3 gm; Semen plantaginis, 9 gm; Radix angelicae, 9 gm; Radix rehmanniae, 6-12 gm; Radix bupleuri, 6 gm; and Radix glycyrrhizae, 1.5-3 gm. Decocted and served twice a day.

FOLLOW-UP/COURSE OF TREATMENT:

Course of treatment commenced on April 28, 1987: The patient took the prescription one dose a day and was followed up in the outpatient department once every two weeks. The last visit was on April 19, 1988. BBT was taken throughout the course.

Menstruation was normal after treatment, regular (once a month) and moderate in amount. BBT was biphasic (indicating ovulatory menstruation cycle). Her appetite was normal and irritability and emotional upset minimized. There was no other discomfort felt. Tongue condition normal, and pulse thready and taut.

Blood sample taken in August 1987 (six months after medication) showed the following results: Thirteenth day of menstruation period: FSH, 2 IU/ml; LH, 50 IU/ml; E_2, 66 pg/ml; and T, 171 ng/dl. Twenty-third day of menstruation period: FSH, 10 IU/ml; LH, 59 IU/ml; E_2, 99 pg/ml; and T, 38 ng/dl.

DISCUSSION: Polycystic ovary syndrome (PCO) is most prevalent in adolescent girls and young women. The main clinical manifestations are menstrual irregularity, amenorrhea, dysfunctional uterine bleeding, infertility, obesity and hirsutism. The cause of PCO is considered to be dysfunction of the hypothalamus-pituitary-ovary axis and abnormality in the synthesis of ovarian steroid hormones.

There are many reports of PCO treated by traditional Chinese medicine. By symptom-complex differentiation, some PCO cases are treated as accumulation of Phlegm-Dampness because of bilaterally enlarged ovaries with thickened outer layer, ovulation disturbance and obesity. Herbs used to resolve the Phlegm-Dampness, soften the hard masses and open up the Channels are Sargassum, Thallus laminariae, Squama manitis, Spina gleditsiae and others. Some cases are treated with the principle of tonifying the Kidney because of menstruation irregularity, ovulation disturbance and infertility. Others are treated by adding herbs to invigorate Blood circulation and eliminate Blood stasis during the period of ovulation to improve microcirculation and promoting ovulation.

The patient in our case was diagnosed as a case of PCO based on clinical manifestation, pneumoperitoneographic findings (both ovaries are larger than one quarter the size of the uterus) and blood sex hormone examination findings.

By TCM symptom-complex differentiation, signs and symptoms manifested in this case, i.e. strong and firm figure, hirsutism, rough skin with acne on the face, irritability, emotional upset, thready and taut pulse and red tongue proper, were indications of a syndrome of excessive Fire in the Liver Channel. LDXGT was prescribed accordingly to quench the Liver Fire.

In this prescription, Radix rehmanniae and Radix angelicae were used to nourish the Yin (Vital Essence) of the Liver; Radix bulpleuri to soothe the Liver and restore the normal functions of a depressed Liver; Radix gentianae, Radix scutellariae, and Fructus gardeniae to dispel the stagnant Fire from the Liver and Gallbladder and subdue the hyperfunction of Liver Yang; and Rhizoma alismatis, Semen plantaginis, and Caulis akebiae to dispel Dampness and Heat from the Liver and Gallbladder which in turn activated the function of the Spleen and Stomach with the result of removing the accumulated Phlegm and Dampness.

As a whole, this prescription had the effect of dispelling the stagnant Fire of the Liver and Gallbladder.

After more than one year's treatment, the patient's menstruation was essentially normal.

11.15 INFERTILITY
(INFERTILITY)

Wang Dazeng
Longhua Hospital, Shanghai College of Traditional Chinese Medicine, Shanghai

Wang, 30, female, Han nationality, married, office worker. Medical record number: 119860. Date of first consultation: November 14, 1985.

CHIEF COMPLAINT: Infertile after one and a half years of marriage.

HISTORY OF PRESENT ILLNESS: Married in April 1984, the patient was not able to get pregnant. She had history of evacuation of bilateral ovarian chocolate cysts on April 27, 1975. Hysterosalpingogram in September 1985 showed that both Fallopian tubes were not thoroughly patent. She received a short course of physiotherapy afterwards. Menstruation cycles were regular, profuse in amount and fresh in colour. Last menstruation period October 23-30, 1985. Basal body temperature was biphasic. Examination showed her husband's semen to be normal. The patient complained of fatigue, weakness, sensation of heat in the afternoon, constipation and diminished libido.

PAST HISTORY: Non-contributory.

PERTINENT PHYSICAL EXAMINATION & LABORATORY FINDINGS: Well-developed and well-nourished, slightly obese with dull complexion. Breasts well-developed, no mass and no tenderness. Abdomen soft. A surgical scar with keloid formation was seen at the midline of the abdomen below the umbilicus. External genitalia well developed with married-type vaginal orifice. Cervix smooth, uterus normal in size, in mid-position and movable. No palpable mass, no tenderness in both lateral and posterior fornixes.

INSPECTION OF TONGUE: Plump and thinly coated.

PULSE CONDITION: Deep and thready.

MODERN MEDICINE DIAGNOSIS: Infertility.

TRADITIONAL CHINESE MEDICINE DIAGNOSIS: Infertility.

THERAPEUTIC PRINCIPLES: Reinforce the Vital Energy and replenish the Vital Essence; activate Blood circulation and eliminate the stagnation in the Channels; nourish the Liver and Kidney.

PRESCRIPTION: Radix astragali, 15 gm; Radix pseudostellariae, 12 gm; Radix angelicae, 9 gm; Radix paeoniae alba, 9 gm; Radix rehmanniae and praeparatae, 15 gm; Radix cynanche atrali, 9 gm; Herba cistanchis, 9 gm; Herba epimedii, 15 gm; Radix salviae, 9 gm; and Fluoritum, 12 gm. One dose per day in two equally divided portions.

FOLLOW-UP/COURSE OF TREATMENT:

Second consultation on December 12, 1985: Menstruation on November 20, 1985. Symptoms alleviated after medication. BBT elevated. Tongue plump and thinly coated, pulse weak. Continued the same prescription. Cortex cinnamomi, 3 gm, was added to reinforce the vital function. During menstruation, another prescription of an "activating circulation and regulating menstruation' nature was prescribed instead in order to promote circulation and regulate and accelerate the elimination of the stagnation in the Channels. Prescription: Radix angelicae, 9 gm; Rhizoma ligustici, 9 gm; Herba lycope, 9 gm; Flos carthami, 9 gm; Radix achyranthis, 9 gm; Rhizoma cyperi, 9 gm; Herba leonuri, 15 gm; and Flos lonicerae, 3 gm.

Fourth consultation on December 26, 1985: In menstruation since December 22, 1985. Flow with ease and without abdominal discomfort, moderate in amount, fresh in colour and without clot. The patient felt well, manifestation of tongue and pulse normal. Ten doses of the prescription.

Fifth consultation on January 30, 1986: LMP December 22, 1985. BBT elevated for 24 days. The patient complained of belching of gas and sleepiness and preferred to take sour and salty food. Pulse soft and rapid, and tongue thinly coated. She was treated using the principle of nourishing the Liver and Kidney, regulating the function of the Stomach and depressing the upward-reverse flow of gas and food. Prescription: Herba epimedii, 15 gm; Fructus lycii, 9 gm; Herba cistanchis, 9 gm; Radix angelicae, 9 gm; Radix paeoniae alba, 9 gm; Herba agastachis, 9 gm; Radix rehmanniae, 15 gm; and Fructus amomi, 3 gm. Seven doses. Decocted and taken as before. Blood HCG examination ordered.

Eighth consultation on February 20, 1986: Menstruation had ceased for two-months. Complained of occasional nausea. Appetite normal. Tongue picture normal, and pulse soft and slippery. Vaginal examination: cervix soft and hyperemic, uterus two-month pregnancy size and soft in consistency, antepositioned and movable. Serum HCG (RIA) level, 101 ng/ml. Early pregnancy was diagnosed. Medication discontinued.

A male baby was born by Ceasaerean section because of prolonged labour on October 13, 1986. Birth weight was 3.65 kg.

DISCUSSION: *Canon of Internal Medicine* records that "if the Ren Channel is unhindered and the Chong Channel full, menstruation will be regular and pregnancy will result." Traditional Chinese medicine holds that fertilization is related to the fullness of the Chong Channel and the absence of hindrances in the Ren Channel. Chong is the reservoir of Blood, while Ren is in charge of the uterus and conception. Both Ren and Chong originate from the uterus and are under the control of the Liver and Kidney.

This patient got married one and a half years ago and was not able to conceive. She complained of dizziness and tinnitus and other signs of insufficiency of the Liver and Kidney. she was treated by tonifying the Liver and Kidney and regulating the Ren and Chong Channels.

The patient had history of endometriosis and bilateral overian chocolate cysts which were removed by surgical operation. This past history inevitably lowered the chance of conception. Hysterosalpingogram showed partial obstruction of both Fallopian tubes. According to TCM symptom-complex differentiation, the patient had syndrome of Blood stasis resulting in obstruction of the Channels and Collaterals and infertility. Therefore, measures to invigorate the Blood circulation and remove the obstruction of the Channels were applied in order to remove Blood stasis, clear obstruction of the Channels and their Collaterals and to increase the chance of pregnancy. Symptoms of fatigue, weakness, sensation of heat in the afternoons, constipation, plumpness of the tongue and thready pulse pointed to deficiency of Qi and Yin, and accordingly, herbs effective in reinforcing the Vital Energy and replenishing the Vital Essence were added.

In the prescription, Cistanche, Epimedium and Amethyst were effective in nourishing the Liver and Kidney; Radix angelicae sinensis and red sage root in invigorating Blood circulation and removing the obstruction from the Channels; and Radix astragali, Radix pseudostellariae, Radix rehmanniae, Radix paeoniae alba and Radix cynanche in reinforcing the Vital Energy and replenishing the Vital Essence.

On the second visit, a small amount of Cortex cinnamomi was added. It contains cinnamomi oil which dilates the blood vessels, promotes body functions and plays an important role in warming up the vital function of the Kidney. The property of this herb is extremely pungent and hot, but it is warm and blossoming if applied in a small quantity.

This patient was pregnent after two menstrual cycles and eight visits using the above method of treatment.

12. PEDIATRIC DISEASES

12.1 SUMMER FEVER IN CHILDREN (SEPTICEMIA)

Zhan Wenliang

First Affiliated Hospital, Wenzhou Medical College, Wenzhou

Zhen Jingyan, female, Han nationality. Medical record number: 86109. Date of admission: August 31, 1979.

CHIEF COMPLAINT: Irregular fever of more than one month duration.

HISTORY OF PRESENT ILLNESS: The patient was noted to have fever, sneezing, rhinorrhea on August 13, 1979. She ran a temperature of 38.5°C and was thought to have a common cold. She was brought to a nearby hospital where she was treated with traditional medications. Chest X-ray revealed increased pulmonary markings and lymphopathy in the left hilum. Treatment was changed to streptomycin, Rimifon and vitamin B_6, but it was not effective. Fever persisted and the patient was admitted to our hospital as a case of fever and septicemia.

PAST HISTORY: Born by normal delivery, the patient was the fourth child in the family. Healthy in the past with no history of infectious disease.

PERTINENT PHYSICAL EXAMINATION & LABORATORY FINDINGS: Conscious, emaciated. High temperature could be felt on the forehead, chest, trunk, abdomen and extremities. Skin and sclera were normal. There was no subcutaneous hemorrhage. Neck supple. Chicken-breast chest. Bilateral breath sounds accentuated. Cardiac auscultation normal. Liver and spleen not palpable. Other physical examination findings normal. Findings of routine blood examination, urinalysis and stool examination were all within normal limits. Blood culture positive for staphylococcus aureus.

INSPECTION OF TONGUE: Red tongue with thin fur.

PULSE CONDITION: Fine and frequent.

MODERN MEDICINE DIAGNOSIS: Septicemia; Rickets.

TRADITIONAL CHINESE MEDICINE DIAGNOSIS: Summer Fever in Children; Deficiency of Both Vital Energy and Yin.

FOLLOW-UP/COURSE OF TREATMENT:

Initial treatment consisted of penicillin, 6,000,000 u, IM, b.i.d. Later on, kanamycin, 200 mg, IM, b.i.d. and chlormycetin syrup orally were instituted. The patient's temperature continued to spike to 38°C. On September 8, administration of erythromycin, 500 mg, dexamethasone, 5 mg, lincomycin and nystatin was started, but the patient continued to run a fever and became weaker. Her condition was getting apparently worse. On September 14, she was referred to our clinic for further diagnosis and treatment. She was thin, weak and sometimes agitated. She had poor appetite and her temperature was 38.9°C. Some erosive spots could be noted on the oral cavity and surface of the tongue. Tongue substance was red with scanty amount of body fluid. As it was summer, a diagnosis of summer fever in children was given with accompanying deficiency of Vital Energy and Yin. The aim of the treatment was to tonify the Qi and Yin and to dissipate and relieve the summer Heat.

Prescription: Zu Ye She Gao Tang. Herba lophatheri, 6 gm; Gypsum fibrosum, 20 gm; Radix panacis quinquefolii, 6 gm; Radix ophiopogonis, 6 gm; Herba dendrobii, 6 gm; Rhizoma imperatae, 8 gm; Rhizoma coptidis, 3 gm; Radix scutellariae, 5 gm; Flos lonicerae, 8 gm; Poria, 6 gm; Fructus sectariae germinatus, 8 gm; and Fructus hordei germinatus, 8 gm. One dose per day.

In addition, Zi Xue Shan was prescribed for oral ingestion, once a day.

Second consultation on September 17, 1979: The patient was apparently on the mend. She had an improved appetite and temperature had gone down to below 38°C. Because of oral erosions caused by administration of antibiotics, her family requested that antibiotics be discontinued and that she be treated only with traditional Chinese medicines. Her pulse was fine and frequent. Tongue picture was better with virtual disappearance of the white fur. Blood culture still showed positive growth of staphylococcus aureus. On this ground, the diagnosis of septicemia was definitely established. Modern medical treatment involved choosing appropriate antibiotic agents based on culture and sensitivity. However, having been treated with antibiotics many times, the child still did not take a turn for the better which eventually resulted in the deterioration of her condition because of imbalance of the bacteria and the complication of mouth infections. Modern medicine puts too much emphasis on planning the therapeutic strategy based on the disease and does not adequately consider an organic approach to the overall analysis of the illness and the patient's condition.

Since the prescription was effective, another three doses were prescribed. The patient was discharged on September 18, 1979, from the hospital.

Third consultation on September 18, 1979: The patient looked well, though her appetite had not improved fully and she still ran a low fever with an occasional cough. Urine and bowel movement normal. Tongue substance red with thin and white fur, and pulse fine. Prescription: Radix panacis quinquefolii, 5 gm; Radix ophiopogonis, 6 gm; Herba lophatheri, 6 gm; Flos lonicerae, 6 gm; Herba ephedrae, 2 gm; Semen armeniacae amarum, 4 gm; Radix stemonae, 5 gm; Pericarpium trichosanthis, 3 gm; Fructus hordei germinatus, 3 gm; Fructus crataegi, 8 gm; Massa fermentata medicinalis, 8 gm; and Radix glycyrrhizae, 2 gm.

Three doses were prescribed. Blood culture taken later on in the outpatient department was negative. The patient continued to be followed up in the outpatient department and she has been healthy.

DISCUSSION: This was a case of summer fever of Damp-Heat disease according to TCM symptom-complex differentiation. The treatment was planned based on the principles of Wei Qi Ying and Xue. The patient was very young and weak. Initially, she was influenced by the exogenous pathogenic factors. Because of deficiency of Vital Energy, the pathogens could not be driven away. She had been inflicted by pathogens and fever for a long time, resulting in exhaustion of Vital Energy and Yin. Eventually, deficiency of both Vital Energy and Yin appeared.

The organic understanding of disease is the outstanding feature of TCM therapy. The course of a disease is considered a contest between Vital Energy and exogenous pathogenic factors. Healthy energy in the body can successfully fend off invasion by the pathogenic factors, while these evil pathogens and the general debility of the body make it vulnerable to attack by evil pathogens.

TCM treatment takes a comprehensive approach in considering the overall analysis of diagnosis, the disease course and the patient's condition. Doctors should always consider the rival forces of the body's Vital Energy and the pathogens, individual patient differences and the time of the seasons.

To cure a disease is not only to drive out the pathogens but also to pay attention to Vital Energy. The rise and fall of Vital Energy and pathogens are relative. They can change each other. The fall of Vital Energy is corrected whenever it is detected in order to induce production of positive factors in the body to build up resistance to disease.

The prescription used in this case was based on the Gypsum and Henonis staptex Rendle recipe. It is used to treat late-season exogenous febrile diseases associated with deficiency of Vital Energy. It is also indicated in cases with deficiency of both Yin and Vital Energy, weakness and shortness of breath, dry mouth and red and uncoated tongue. All febrile diseases, such as measles, pneumonia, influenzal encephalitis, summer fever and sunstroke, with deficiency of both Yin and Vital Energy can be treated by this prescription.

In this prescription, the dosages of Pinelliae and Glycyrrhizae were reduced and Flos lonicerae, Radix coptidis, Radix scutellariae and Zi Xue Shan were added in order to enhance the effectiveness of the prescription in dissipating Heat and detoxifying. Herba dendrobii and Rhizoma imperatae were added to tonify the Yin and to produce body fluid. Poria, Hordeum vulgare L. and Oryza sativa L. were added to strengthen the Spleen and regulate the Stomach energy as well as to improve digestion and appetite.

By using this prescription, high fever and symptoms were relieved rather quickly. In this prescription, Radix panacis quinquefolii played an important role in tonifying the Yin and Vital Energy, and producing body fluid; Flos lonicerae, Radix coptidis, Radix scutellariae, Gypsum fibrosum, Henonis and Zi Xue Shan eliminated the evil factors, dissipated the Heat and detoxified. Many of these herbs, in addition to their function of dissipating Heat and detoxifying, are also effective in suppressing viruses and bacteria. Flos lonicerae has been shown to be effective in enhancing the function of white cells in engulfing S. aureus. The efficacy of this prescription in treating this case was instantaneous, indicating a correct choice of appropriate medicinal herbs as therapeutic agent.

12.2 ARRHYTHMIA, VIRAL MYOCARDITIS (DEFICIENCY OF BOTH CARDIAC VITAL ENERGY AND YIN, REGULAR AND IRREGULAR INTERMITTENT PULSE)

Tong Huanxiang, Yu Peilan and Zhang Baolin

Department of Pediatrics, First Affiliated Hospital, Hunan Medical University, Changsha

Liu, 9, male, Han nationality. Medical record number: 31306. Admitted on February 23, 1988.

CHIEF COMPLAINT: Palpitation of three years duration, exacerbated in the past six months.

HISTORY OF PRESENT ILLNESS: In early 1985, the patient developed palpitation without apparent cause. It became worse and was accompanied by a compressive sensation over the chest as time went on. Symptoms aggravated when he got up from bed; he sometimes had dizziness and fatigue as well as dyspnea on exertion. In December 1987, he had three episodes of syncope when he got up to pass urine at night. During each of these syncopic episodes, he was unconscious for one to five minutes. Symptoms became worse six months prior to admission; he could not go up stairs by himself ever since. He frequently had profuse sweating during the daytime. He got wet from sweat while eating, even in winter. His appetite, sleep and spirits remained fair. No fever was noted. Stool and urine were normal.

PAST HISTORY: No arthritis or sore throat in the past.

PERTINENT PHYSICAL EXAMINATION & LABORATORY FINDINGS: Temperature, 36.7°C; pulse rate, 90/min; respiratory rate, 28/min; blood pressure, 100/50 mmHg; and body weight, 27 kg. Well developed and fairly well nourished. Slightly pale. No engorgement of neck veins. Throat clear. No rales. No enlargement of the heart. Heart rate 90/min with 10 to 115 extrasystoles per minute. A soft grade II systolic murmur could be appreciated over the apical region, P2 › A2. Liver and spleen not palpable. Hemoglobin, 11.9 gm%; WBC, 3,700/mm³; neutrophils, 63% ; lymphocytes, 36%; eosionophils, 1%. Routine urinalysis and stool examination normal. ECG: multiple ventricular extrasystoles with couple rhythm or triple. LDH, 372 u; C-reactive protein negative; mucoprotein, 4.7 mg/dl. Ultrasonographic cardiogram: internal diameter of the right ventricle slightly increased. Chest X-ray showed normal size of heart shadow.

INSPECTION OF TONGUE: Tip of tongue red in colour, with thin, white to yellowish fur over the root of the tongue.

PULSE CONDITION: Thready and rapid with alternate regular and irregular rhythm.

MODERN MEDICINE DIAGNOSIS: Multiple Ventricular Extrasystoles; Viral Myocarditis.

TRADITIONAL CHINESE MEDICINE DIAGNOSIS: Deficiency of Heart Vital Energy and Yin; Regular and Irregular Intermittent Pulse.

THERAPEUTIC PRINCIPLES: Tonify the Qi and Yin, regulate the pulse.

PRESCRIPTION: Modified Zhi Gan Cao Decoction. Radix glycyrrhizae praeparatae, 12 gm; Radix codonopsis pilosulae, 10 gm; Radix rehmanniae, 10 gm; Rhizoma atractylodis, 10 gm; Radix salviae, 10 gm; Radix ligustici, 6 gm; Fructus cannabis, 10 gm; and Fructus hordei, 10 gm. Oral decoction, one dose per day.

Other management: Vitamin C, Vitamin B_1 and ATP, taken orally. CoEnzyme A, taken intravenously.

FOLLOW-UP/COURSE OF TREATMENT:

Second consultation: After admission the patient was instructed to maintain complete bed rest and was given modern medications for eight days. There was no response to this regimen. After taking seven doses of Zhi Gan Cao Decoction, he reported that dizziness had been significantly relieved and sweating was reduced. Heart rate 80 to 90/min with extrasystoles 7 to 8/min. Continued the same prescription.

Third consultation: After taking 15 doses, ultrasonographic cardiogram was normal; the patient was discharged in an improved condition and was followed up in the outpatient department.

DISCUSSION: Extrasystole is a common type of arrhythmia in children. Occasional asymptomatic extrasystole may occur in a normal child. As for this patient, he had frequent extrasystoles with couple or triple rhythm accompanied by severe palpitation and shortness of breath. He was not able to go up stairs, indicating impairment of the cardiac function. There were three episodes of fainting which might have been induced by poor blood supply to the brain. Ultrasonographic cardiogram showed slight dilatation of the right ventricle. All these findings suggested organic heart disease —viral myocarditis —which is the most common cause of arrhythmia in children.

After admission, there was no improvement in symptoms after rest and taking modern medications for eight days. But after taking seven doses of herbal medicine, the patient reported significant relief from the symptoms. Doctors noted a reduction of frequency of extrasystoles. After 15 doses, dilatation of the right ventricle disappeared, too. The prescription had been shown to be effective in treating this case.

Zhi Gan Cao Decoction is also known as the Prescription for Resumption of the Pulse. It tonifies the Yin and resumes the pulse and is the prescription of choice for treatment of palpitation, shortness of breath and irregular pulse. Our prescription was based on the original recipe. We modified it by removing Rhizoma zingiberis and adding Radix angelicae, Rhizoma salviae, Fructus hordei, Rhizoma ligustici, Radix astragali and Rhizoma atractylodis. Radix glycyrrhizae praeparatae, Radix codonopsis pilosulae and Fructus ziziphi jujubae in the prescription tonified the Spleen and Qi; Ramulus cinnamomi warmed up the Heart Yang and opened up the vessels; Radix rehmanniae, Colla corii asini and Radix ophiopogonis nourished the Yin and Blood, while Fructus cannabis moistened the stool.

Though this is an old prescription first reported by Zhang Zhongjing in the TCM classic *On Febrile Diseases*, it is still quite effective and is usually indicated in a modified form to treat arrythmia in children.

Digitalis is contraindicated in cases with myocarditis and/or cardiac failure. Instead of digitalis, we have treated similar cases by using this prescription for a comparatively longer period of time in the ward or in the outpatient department. Results have been fairly satisfactory, indicating that this prescription can supplement some of the insufficiencies of modern therapeutic regimens.

12.3 EPIDEMIC DIARRHEA OF NEWBORN INFANTS (HEAT DIARRHEA WITH INSUFFICIENCY OF MIDDLE WARMER ENERGY)

Yu Peilan, Li Yiding and Yu Li
Department of Pediatrics, First Affiliated Hospital,
Hunan Medical University
Hunan Children's Hospital

Cao, a four-day-old girl of Han nationality. Date of first consultation: June 28, 1988.

CHIEF COMPLAINT: Diarrhea and fever.

HISTORY OF PRESENT ILLNESS: The patient was born full-term by spontaneous delivery on June 24, 1988. She started to cry feebly 30 seconds after delivery. Birth weight was 2.5 kilos. Sucking power was good and she took 20 millilitres of 10% glucose solution two hours after birth and was fed alternately by breast feeding and artificial formula composed of water and cow's milk in a ratio of 2:1. During pregnancy, II degree calcification spots on the placenta were shown by ultrasound examination.

Four days after birth, the patient began to have diarrhea at a frequency of more than ten times a day. Stool was described as watery, yellow or greenish in colour, large in amount with foul smell and pieces of undigested milky substances. She developed a fever of 38.5°C. She was noted to be thirsty and liked to suck water. She frequently passed flatus and was restless and cried a lot at night. Urination was likewise quite frequent with large amounts of clear urine. There was an outbreak of epidemic diarrhea in the nursery with eight to 10 cases of diarrhea discovered.

PERTINENT PHYSICAL EXAMINATION & LABORATORY FINDINGS: Temperature, 38.5°C; small and thin, weak cries, cold extremities; deep-yellow discolouration of the skin of the entire body and sclera; normal turgor. Anterior fontanel 2.5 × 2.5 cm in size. Throat clear. Normal breath sound over the lungs. Heart rate 130-140/min, no murmur appreciated. Abdomen distended and soft. Umbilical cord stump dried. Liver palpable 1.5 cm below the right costal margin.

INSPECTION OF TONGUE: Red tongue with thick and yellowish fur.

PULSE CONDITION: Examination of the venules of the finger showed stagnant and light purple colour of the small superficial venules of the index finger reaching up to the Qi Guan.

MODERN MEDICINE DIAGNOSIS: Neonatal Epidemic Diarrhea; Small for Gestation Age.

TRADITIONAL CHINESE MEDICINE DIAGNOSIS: Heat Diarrhea and Insufficiency of Middle-Burner Energy.

THERAPEUTIC PRINCIPLES: Clear away Heat to stop diarrhea, invigorate both the Vital Energy and Yin.

PRESCRIPTION: Ge Gen Qin Lian Decoction. Radix puerariae, 9 gm; Radix scutellariae, 2 gm; Rhizoma coptidis, 15 gm; Radix codonopsis pilosulae, 4 gm; Medicated leaven, 3 gm; and Herba artemisiae scopariae, 8 gm.

Other management: Oral kanamycin, 10 mg/24hr in two equally divided doses and Cephalexinum, 60 mg/24hr in two equally divided doses were administered alternately.

FOLLOW-UP/COURSE OF TREATMENT:

Second consultation on June 30, 1988: On the sixth day of life, the patient had diarrhea as before, but fever started to subside and jaundice was relieved slightly. Tongue substance red with thin and yellowish fur, thick on the root of the tongue. The small superficial venules of the index finger were purple in colour, stagnant and reaching up to Qi Guan. Temperature, 37.5°C, cold extremities; numerous white, flaky plaques covering the oral cavity; mycotic-like rash on the skin of the buttocks. Distention of the abdomen. Umbilical cord had dropped. Routine examination of stool was normal.

Modern medicine diagnosis: Neonatal epidemic diarrhea; small for gestation age; and candidiasis of buccal mucosa and skin of the buttocks. TCM diagnosis: Insufficiency of Middle-Burner energy and accumulation of pathogenic Wetness-Heat. Principles of treatment were to invigorate the central Vital Energy and clear away the Wetness. Prescription: Modified Shen Qi Qin Lian Decoction. Radix codonopsis pilosulae, 5 gm; Radix astragali, 4 gm; Tuckahoe Poria, 6 gm; Rhizoma coptidis, 2 gm; and Fructus aurantii, 1.5 gm. Other management: Nystatinum and vitamin C, vitamin Bco, vitamin E and vitamin D.

Third consultation on July 4, 1988: On the tenth day of life and after taking four doses of the herbal prescription, the patient's general condition had improved significantly. She was able to drink more milk and her cries were louder. Diarrhea started to subside, stool was slightly foul in smell and small in amount, five to six times per day. She was fed a 2:1 ratio of cow's milk, 50-60 ml, every one to two hours. She was restless and still cried a lot at night. Tip of the tongue was red with thin and yellowish fur, thick on the root of the tongue. The small superficial venules of the index fingers were red and slightly stagnant, reaching the Qi Guan on the right and the Fu Guan on the left. Physical examination showed a slightly chubby face and loud cries. Jaundice had subsided completely and abdominal distention was significantly relieved. Extremities warm. Symptom-complex differentiation revealed diarrhea due to asthenia of the Spleen and dyspepsia. Therapeutic principles applied at this stage were to invigorate the Spleen and eliminate Wetness-Evil, promote digestion and relieve dyspepsia. Prescription: Shen Lin Bai Zhu Decoction. Radix codonopsis pilosulae, 5 gm; Poria, 5 gm; Rhizoma atractylodis macrocephalae, 1.5 gm; Radix glycyrrhizae, 2 gm; Pericarpium citri reticulatae, 1.5 gm; Rhizoma dioscoreae, 5 gm; Semen nelumbinis, 4 gm; Fructus crataegi, 2 gm; Herba euphorbiae humifusae, 5 gm; and Medicated leaven, 3 gm.

Fourth consultation on July 10, 1988: On the sixteenth day of life and after taking six doses of the last prescription, stool was soft and yellow but thin, sometimes watery, three to four times per day. Good appetite with a 1.5:1 ratio of cow's milk, 100 ml each feeding. Polyuria. Often crying and irritable at night. Body weight 2.51 kg. Slightly chubby face and extremities, crying loud, strong movements of the neck and extremities. In supine position, she could change body postures by herself.

Modern medicine diagnosis: Neonatal epidemic diarrhea (convalescent stage). TCM diagnosis: Diarrhea due to asthenia of the Spleen accompanied by Fire in the Heart. Treated by invigorating the Spleen, eliminating Wetness-Evil and tranquilizing the mind by nourishing the Heart. Prescription: Modified Shen Lin Bai Zhu Decoction. Added Semen ziziphi spinosae, Cortex albiziae and Ramulus uncariae cum uncis to the prescription of July 10, 1988.

Fifth consultation on July 15, 1988: On the twenty-first day of life and after taking four doses of the last prescription, the patient cried less and was peaceful most of the time. No diarrhea. She was well-developed and well-nourished and back to normal growth and development.

Sixth consultation on July 24, 1988: On the thirtieth day of life, her body weight was 3.7 kg. General condition was good, stool well formed and yellow in colour.

DISCUSSION: The diagnosis of neonatal epidemic diarrhea was confirmed in this case based on findings of abrupt onset of diarrhea on the fourth day of life accompanied by fever and the outbreak of epidemic diarrhea in the nursery. Common microorganisms responsible for epidemic diarrhea of the newborns are E. coli, salmonella, ECHO virus and adenovirus. This patient was treated with oral kanamycin and cephalexin during the first two days, but there was no relief of the symptoms, and she subsequently developed candida albicans infection of the mouth and buttocks.

Based on findings of low body weight, thin, delicate build and weak cries at birth as well as history of placental calcification during pregnancy, congenital deficiency of various bodily functions was considered. After birth, she suffered from acute infectious diarrhea with fever, coldness of the extremities and increasing weakness. These are all signs of asthenia syndrome. Watery diarrhea, fever, red tongue coated with thick and yellow fur, stagnant venules of the fingers, foul-smelling stool, thirst and deep-yellow, stained skin suggested internal stasis of Dampness and Heat. Therefore, initial treatment was to clear away the Heat and stop the diarrhea. Among the herbs added to the Ge Gen Qin Lian Decoction, Radix puerariae, Radix scutellariae and Rhizoma coptidis were used for their effects in clearing away the Heat and their bacteriostatic effects on E. coli and dysenteric bacilli; Radix codonopsis pilosulae and medicated leaven were used to invigorate the Spleen and promote digestion. Fever and jaundice were reduced after taking two doses of the prescription, but diarrhea persisted. Therapeutic regimen was changed to Shen Qi Ling Lian Decoction in order to invigorate the central Vital

Energy and to clear away the Wetness. After taking this prescription, the patient's general condition improved significantly. She drank more milk and her cries were getting stronger. This was followed by administration of Shen Ling Bai Zhu Decoction to invigorate the Spleen and central Vital Energy and to stop the diarrhea. On the thirtieth day of life, the patient had no more diarrhea and candidiasis was cleared completely. She had normal development and body weight had increased to 3.7 kg.

This case illustrates the effectiveness of traditional Chinese medicine in treating neonatal epidemic diarrhea in small newborns. In this case, the patient developed candidiasis of buccal mucosa and buttocks after antibiotics therapy. After discontinuation of antibiotics administration, nystatin, vitamin Bco, Vitamin C and herbal medicines were given to successfully control the candidiasis. Initially, the patient was very sick with diarrhea, weakness, cold extremities and fever, but she was able to recover completely with administration of traditional Chinese medications.

12.4 TOXIC DYSENTERY SECONDARY TO PROLONGED ENTERITIS (HEAT OF MUSCLES REMAINED AFTER HEAT EPIDEMIC TOXIC DYSENTERY AND PERSISTENT DYSENTERY)

Ye Xiaoli and Cao Yixiang
Fujian Provincial Hospital, Fuzhou

Wang Chongyu, 14 months old, male, Han nationality. Medical record number: 78813. Date of admission: October 10, 1970.

CHIEF COMPLAINT: Diarrhea and fever associated with convulsion for one day.

HISTORY OF PRESENT ILLNESS: The patient was noted to have high fever, pus-like stool, shortness of breath, restlessness, cyanosis, convulsion and loss of consciousness. On admission, he was given modern medicine for symptomatic treatment which was able to stop the convulsion and regain consciousness. Fever persisted at 38-39°C.

PAST HISTORY: Non-contributory.

PERTINENT PHYSICAL EXAMINATION & LABORATORY FINDINGS: Dehydrated-looking; temperature, 40.5°C. General physical examination findings negative. Stool examination: mucous, (+); pus cell, (++); RBC, few.

INSPECTION OF TONGUE: Tip of tongue deep red in colour.

PULSE CONDITION: Fine and rapid.

MODERN MEDICINE DIAGNOSIS: Dysentery; Chronic Enteritis.

TRADITIONAL CHINESE MEDICINE DIAGNOSIS: Heat Epidemic Toxic Dysentery; Heat of Muscles; Persistent Dysentery.

THERAPEUTIC PRINCIPLES: Dispel pathogenic factor from both the exterior and interior of the body.

PRESCRIPTION: Modified Ge Gen Qin Lian Tang. Radix puerariae, 6 gm; Radix scutellariae, 6 gm; Radix coptidis, 3 gm; Radix paeoniae, 6 gm; Radix scrophulariae, 3 gm; Fructus gardeniae, 9 gm; and Cortex magnoliae officinalis, 4.5 gm.

In this prescription, Radix puerariae was used to dispel pathogenic factors from the exterior and to clear up Heat from the interior of the body; Radix scutellariae was used to eliminate Heat in the stomach; Raw gardeniae and Radix scrophulariae helped Ge Gen Qin Lian Tang clear up the fever; Cortex magnoliae officinalis was used to promote the flow of Vital Energy. Persistent dysentery may result in Shangyin (impairment of Yin vital essence).

FOLLOW-UP/COURSE OF TREATMENT:

Second consultation on October 13, 1970: Fever had subsided after taking two doses of the prescription. Since the patient caught a cold and had a cough, Yanqiao Powder was given. Flos lonicerae, 9 gm; Fructus forsythiae, 9 gm; Fructus perillae, 4.5 gm; Radix scrophulariae, 9 gm; Radix ophiopogonis, 9 gm; Radix asparagi, 9 gm; Radix paeoniae alba, 4.5 gm; and Radix glycyrrhizae, 3 gm.

Third consultation on October 15, 1970: Cough was relieved. The patient had recovered fully and was discharged after two weeks of hospitalization.

Fourth consultation on October 21, 1970: Six days after discharge, due to improper feeding, diarrhea recurred and was not responsive to six days of modern medicine treatment. The patient was hospitalized again. Dehydration was evident. Frequency of bowel movement about ten times per day. Traditional Chinese medicine was used to treat the condition. Application of therapeutic principles of reinforcing the function of the Spleen, clearing up Heat and eliminating Dampness was achieved through administration of secretion-promoting herbs. Prescription: Secretion-promoting decoction plus modified Ge Gen Qin Lian Tang. Radix scrophulariae, 9 gm; Radix ophiopogonis, 9 gm; Radix asparagi, 9 gm; Radix puerariae, 6 gm; Radix scutellariae, 6 gm; Radix paeoniae alba, 6 gm; Radix glycyrrhizae, 4 gm; Semen dolichoris, 9 gm; Semen euryale, 9 gm; and Rhizoma dioscoreae, 6 gm.

Supplementary fluid therapy was also instituted.

Fifth consultation on November 6, 1970: Diarrhea was relieved but there was still undigested food seen in the stool. Herbs effective in promoting digestion and removing food stagnation were prescribed. Endothelium corneum gigeriae galli, 3 gm; Fructus crataegi, 9 gm; Poria, 9 gm; Radix glycyrrhizae, 3 gm; Euryale, 9 gm; and Germinated barley and millet, 9 gm each.

Diarrhea stopped after three doses of the last prescription. Examination of stool was normal on discharge.

DISCUSSION: This case was classified as Heat epidemic toxic dysentery. It had a sudden onset and the invading pathogenic factors were very toxic. Modern medical therapeutic regimen was instituted initially. This was followed by modified Ge Gen Qin Lian Tang to clear up the internal Heat. Persistent diarrhea resulted in insufficiency syndrome. This was treated by applying the principles of reinforcing the function of the Spleen, clearing up the Heat and eliminating Dampness by using secretion-promoting drugs. In this way, both the cause and the symptoms of the disease were treated, resulting in full recovery.

12.5 PROLONGED ENTERITIS (CHRONIC DYSENTERY, LOWERED YANG OF THE SPLEEN, PERSISTENT DIARRHEA)

Ye Xiaoli and Cao Yixiang

Fujian Provincial Hospital, Fuzhou

Wang Yu, one year old, male, Han nationality. Medical record number: 99717. Date of admission: June 14, 1972.

CHIEF COMPLAINT: Fever and diarrhea for four days.

HISTORY OF PRESENT ILLNESS: Four days prior to admission, the patient developed diarrhea and fever. Five days after admission his diarrhea became worse. The number of bowel movements was over 30 times per day. A one-week course of treatment using modern medications did not show any effect. Stool was watery and the patient had incontinence, anuria, irritability, thirst and severe dehydration.

PAST HISTORY: At seven months of age, the patient was admitted because of diarrhea of seven days duration with dehydration. He was cured after nine days of treatment. The month following this he was treated in the outpatient department for acute bronchitis.

PERTINENT PHYSICAL EXAMINATION & LABORATORY FINDINGS: Severely dehydrated, temperature, 39°C. Peripheral count showed WBC, 11,500/mm^3; polymorphs, 29%; lymphocytes, 68%; and eosinophils, 5%; monocytes, 1%. Few pus cells were seen on stool examination. Stool culture positive for salmonella growth.

INSPECTION OF TONGUE: Tongue substance coated with turbid fur.

PULSE CONDITION: Superficial veins of fingers red and barely visible, pulse soft.

MODERN MEDICINE DIAGNOSIS: Prolonged Enteritis; Severe Dehydration.

TRADITIONAL CHINESE MEDICINE DIAGNOSIS: Chronic Diarrhea; Lowered Yang of the Spleen.

THERAPEUTIC PRINCIPLES: Strengthen the Vital Function of the Spleen and arrest the discharge.

PRESCRIPTION: Modified Lizhong Decoction (Decoction to Regulate the Function of the Middle Burner, i.e. the Spleen and Stomach). Radix codonopsis pilosulae, 10 gm; Rhizoma atractylodis macrocephalae, 5 gm; Rhizoma zingiberis, 1.5 gm; Radix glycyrrhizae praeparatae, 3 gm; Umbellate Pore-fungus, 10 gm; Poria, 10 gm; Rhizoma alismatis, 10 gm; Halloysitum rubrum, 15 gm; and Semen plantaginis, 10 gm. In addition, fluid therapy was instituted.

In this prescription, Rhizoma zingiberis is the principal ingredient which provides therapeutic action. It was used to warm the Stomach and the Middle Burner and to disperse Cold from the interior. Radix codonopsis pilosulae is the adjuvant which helps to strengthen the principal action and also replenishes the Vital Energy of the Spleen, facilitates the circulation of nutrients and relieves the disturbance in upward and downward movement of functional activities. Rhizoma atractylodis and Radix glycyrrhizae praeparatae are the auxiliary ingredients which function as conduction vehicles in the prescription. Atractylodis promotes Spleen function and eliminates Dampness by drying, while glycyrrhizae reinforces the Vital Energy and regulates the Vital Function of the Spleen. Other herbs, Poria, Rhizoma alismatis and Semen plantaginis act as diuretics. Halloysitum rubrum causes contraction and arrests discharges and serves in this prescription as an antidiarrheal agent.

FOLLOW-UP/COURSE OF TREATMENT:

Second consultation on June 19, 1972: After the first prescription was given, diarrhea was alleviated markedly. Picture of superficial veins of the finger was getting better, pulse moderate. Tongue with turbid fur. Slight abdominal distention. Modified the previous prescription by eliminating Rhizoma zingiberis and adding Radix aucklandiae, 1.5 gm, and Semen dolichoris, 5 gm. Five doses.

Third consultation on June 21, 1972: Stool was normal. Conditions of the tongue and pulse normal and the patient regained his vigour. However, symptoms of weakness and anorexia remained. Prescribed herbs to regulate the Vital Function of the Stomach and reinforce the function of the Spleen. Poria, 10 gm; Rhizoma dioscoreae, 10 gm; Endothelium corneum gigeriae galli, 4.5 gm; Radix glycyrrhizae, 3 gm; Radix aucklandiae, 3 gm; Radix coptidis, 2 gm; Herba agastachis, 6 gm; Chung Sa, 2 gm; and Rhizoma atractylodis, 10 gm.

After taking three doses of the last prescription, the patient was cured and discharged after 13 days of hospitalization.

DISCUSSION: Prolonged enteritis is usually caused by insufficiency of Yang (Vital Function) of the Spleen. In our case, diarrhea was quite severe with a frequency of more than 30 times a day. TCM teaching holds that persistent diarrhea is secondary to insufficiency of Spleen Yang. Principles of treatment in this kind of case were to uplift the energy of the Spleen for treating chronic diarrhea, to induce contraction to halt the discharge and to warm the Spleen and Stomach in order to dispel the Cold. Deficiency syndrome should be treated by reinforcement or replenishment. Accordingly, Lizhong Decoction was used initially to reinforce the function and to enhance contraction. This was followed by administration of herbs effective in regulating Stomach Vital Function. Concurrently, measures were instituted to correct fluid and electrolyte imbalance of the patient. With this combined approach, the therapeutic effect was rapid and significant.

12.6 CIRRHOSIS OF THE LIVER, ASCITES, HYPERSPLENISM (BLOOD STASIS IN LIVER VESSELS, STAGNANT MASS AND ABDOMINAL TYMPANITIS)

Yu Peilan, Tong Huanxiang and Zhang Baolin

Department of Pediatrics, First Affiliated Hospital, Hunan Medical University, Changsha

Yu, 7, female, Han nationality. Medical record number: 19134. Admitted on November 3, 1975.

CHIEF COMPLAINT: Intermittent abdominal pain for 22 months, enlargement of abdomen for two months.

HISTORY OF PRESENT ILLNESS: The patient has had recurrent abdominal pain since January 1974. After treatment, she passed more than 10 ascarids and abdominal pain subsided. The liver was 1.5 cm below the costal margin, soft in consistency. In February 1975, the patient consulted our clinic again. The liver was now found to be 3 cm below the costal margin and rather hard in consistency. In September 1975, she developed paroxysmal abdominal pain and loss of appetite. Abdominal distention and enlargement were evident. The patient was in low spirits and complained of fatigue, irritability and had diarrhea intermittently. She was confined to bed. Urine deep-yellow in colour. The patient also reported burning sensation in the chest, palms and soles and had epistaxis occasionally.

PERTINENT PHYSICAL EXAMINATION & LABORATORY FINDINGS: Stretcher-born, chronic illness facies, emaciated and with dull complexion; temperature, 37.3°C; respiratory rate, 27/min; pulse rate, 120/min; blood pressure, 90/60 mmHg. Spider nevus noted over the dorsum of the left hand. Abdomen markedly distended with a circumference of 61 cm. Marked distention of superficial abdominal veins and pouting of umbilicus. Liver palpable 7 cm below right costal margin. Positive shifting dullness and fluid wave. Platelets, 63,000/mm^3. Stool examination: positive for presence of ascarid eggs, 0-1/hpf. SGOT, 193 u (normal range 0-35 u); CCFT, (+); A/GM ratio, 2.67/2.52; ß-ultrasound examination revealed hepatomegaly, splenomegaly and ascites. Chest film normal. Upper GI Series showed no esophageal varicosis.

INSPECTION OF TONGUE: Pale tongue substance with white greasy fur.

PULSE CONDITION: Weak, thready and rapid.

MODERN MEDICINE DIAGNOSIS: Cirrhosis of the Liver, late stage (Chronic Active Hepatitis); Ascites; Hypersplenism.

TRADITIONAL CHINESE MEDICINE DIAGNOSIS: Blood Stasis in Liver Vessels (Veins); Abdominal Tympanitis; Stagnant Mass; Deficiency of both Vital Energy and Blood.

THERAPEUTIC PRINCIPLES: Promote Blood circulation to remove Blood stasis, tonify the Qi and Blood.

PRESCRIPTION: Modified Xie Fu Zhu Yu Decoction. Radix bupleuri, 10 gm; Semen persicae, 10 gm; Flos carthami, 5 gm; Radix rehmanniae, 10 gm; Radix angelicae, 10 gm; Rhizoma ligustici, 10 gm; Radix paeoniae rubra, 10 gm; Radix achyranthis, 10 gm; Fructus aurantii, 6 gm; Herba artemisiae scopariae, 10 gm; Radix codonopsis pilosulae, 10 gm; and Fried Fructus crataegi, Massa fermentata and Fructus hordei vulgaris geminatus, 10 gm each. One dose per day.

Other management: Low-salt and high-protein diet; vitamins B, C and ATP, CoEnzyme A, inosine; traimterine for diuresis; penicillin and Herba ardrographitis for control of infection.

FOLLOW-UP/COURSE OF TREATMENT:

Second consultation: After taking five doses of the prescription, symptoms had improved markedly, and the patient's appetite had also improved. She could get up for bowel movement and urination by herself.

Third consultation: After taking 14 doses, abdominal distention significantly was reduced. Platelet count 65,000/mm^3.

Fourth consultation: After consuming a total of 21 doses of the same prescription, the patient felt well with abdominal distention markedly diminished. Umbilicus was flat. She had normal appetite and regained her vigour. Diarrhea had stopped and the patient passed formed stool once a day. However, she still complained of heat sensation in the chest, palms and soles, easy fatigability and deep-yellow discolouration of urine. Tongue substance pale with white and greasy fur; pulse weak, small and rapid. Several herbs were added to the prescription: Carapax trionycis, 10 gm; Radix salviae, 10 gm; Semen coicis, 10 gm; Poria, 10 gm; and Rhizoma atractylodis macrocephalae, 6 gm. One dose per day.

Fifth consultation: Symptoms continued to be alleviated after a total of 28 doses. Abdominal circumference reduced from 61 cm to 52.5 cm. The patient still complained of irritability and occasional pain over the right costal margin. Stool was dry and urine still deep-yellow in colour. Tongue substance red with thin yellow coating; pulse string-like and rapid. Liver 6 cm below costal margin with tenderness. Spleen palpable, 1 cm below the costal margin. No signs of ascites. TCM symptom-complex differentiation: Liver stasis and Spleen deficiency accompanied by Blood stasis. Condition treated by applying therapeutic principles of clearing the Liver, strengthening the Spleen and promoting Blood circulation to remove Blood stasis. Prescription: Xiaoyao San. Semen persicae, 10 gm; Flos carthami, 10 gm; Radix salviae, 10 gm; Radix bupleuri, 6 gm; Radix angelicae, 10 gm; Radix paeoniae alba, 6 gm; Poria, 10 gm; Rhizoma atractylodis macrocephalae, 6 gm; Carapax trionycis, 10 gm; Radix achyranthis bidentatae, 10 gm; and Rhizoma polygonati odorati, 10 gm. One dose daily. Twelve doses.

The patient had been under treatment in the ward for 54 days and had taken 40 doses of herbal prescriptions totally. No corticosteroid or intravenous fluid was given. She was discharged in fairly well condition. On discharge, she had normal appetite, good spirits and was playful. Stool and urine were normal. Liver and spleen palpable 5 cm and 1 cm, respectively, below the costal margin, rather hard in consistency. No ascites. Liver function tests and SGPT normal.

Outcome of the treatment course could be summarized as marked improvement of liver cirrhotic state, remission of ascites and status quo of hypersplenism. After discharge, the patient was followed up in the outpatient department for two months and took herbal medicine continuously during that time. Medications were discontinued thereafter. Two years after discharge, the patient suddenly lapsed into coma and died of hepatic coma in the emergency room of our hospital.

DISCUSSION:

1) Diagnosis: The diagnosis of late-stage liver cirrhosis was established definitely in this case based on clinical signs and symptoms of hepatomegaly and splenomegaly of hard consistency, elevation of SGPT, lowering of serum albumin, reduction of platelets, ultrasound findings of hepato-splenomegaly, splenomegaly and ascites.

2) Therapeutic effect: The patient showed rather quick and significant improvement after taking herbal medications. When she first came to our clinic, the patient was weak and stretcher-born, but after taking five doses of the herbal prescription, she was able to get up from bed and showed an improved appetite. At the end of the course of treatment, she was discharged in fair condition. This goes to show that careful planning of treatment course based on accurate symptom-complex differentiation can be beneficial in treating the late stage of liver cirrhosis in children.

3) Treatment based on symptom-complex differentiation: The patient was chronically ill for 22 months with dull complexion and depression. Liver and spleen were enlarged and hard in consistency with tenderness. Superficial abdominal veins were markedly distended and she had ascites, spider nevus and bruises on the tongue. All these signs and symptoms indicated serious Blood stasis in the Liver vessels. Liver was 7 cm below the costal margin and hard in consistency, suggesting stagnant mass resulting from Blood stasis. General therapeutic principle was to promote Blood circulation and to remove Blood stasis.

In traditional Chinese medicine, Vital Energy commands the Blood and its motion renders normal Blood circulation possible. In our case, the patient displayed both signs of Vital Energy stagnation (abdominal distention and pain below the costal margin) and Vital Energy deficiency (easy fatigability, anorexia, diarrhea, low-pitched voice, weak pulse and mental depression). Spleen insufficiency leads to impairment of the normal transport functions resulting in accumulation of Dampness and ascites. This combination of Blood stagnation and Dampness progressively aggravated the patient's condition. Accordingly, the patient was prescribed Radix achyranthis bidentatae, Semen persicae, Flos carthami, Rhizoma ligustici, Radix angelicae and Radix paeoniae alba to promote Blood circulation and to remove stasis; Radix rehmanniae to nourish the Yin; Radix bupleuri to disperse the stagnant Liver energy and to restore its normal function; Fructus aurantii to promote digestion and relieve dyspepsia; and Radix codonopsis pilosulae and Radix glycyrrhizae. After taking 21 doses of the original prescription, Carapax trionycis was added to soften the hard mass; Rhizoma atractylodis macrocephalae, Poria and Semen coicis to invigorate the Spleen and eliminate the Dampness (Wetness-Evil); and Radix salviae, Semen persicae and Flos carthami to promote regeneration of hepatic cells. After apparent relief of the symptoms and signs, the therapeutic principle was modified in such a way as to reinforce body resistance and to eliminate pathogens by administration of Xiaoyao San. Some of the herbs in this prescription are similar to those used in Xie Fu Zhu Yu Decoction. However, there are more herbs here to tonify the Blood (Radix angelicae and Radix paeoniae) and to nourish the Yin (Rhizoma polygonati odorati). In addition, this prescription is not as potent as the first prescription, which makes it suitable for prolonged administration during the convalescent stage.

There were two other patients with chronic active hapatitis with suspicious liver cirrhosis under our care at about the same time. One of them had four spider nevi, another seven, over their faces and forearms. The mode of treatment employed in these two cases was similar to this case. They took prescriptions (at first continuously and then intermittently) for eight to 10 years. SGPT in both cases returned to normal. They are more than 30 years old now, and there has not been any recurrence of the disease. We also used modified Xiaoyao San to treat 11 cases of chronic hepatitis of one to five years duration. Five of them were nearly cured and the rest experienced improved conditions. The courses of treatment for these cases were longer than one year.

Our clinical experience indicates that these prescriptions are quite effective in treating liver cirrhosis and chronic hepatitis in children.

4) Pharmacological effects and course of treatment: In cirrhosis, connective tissue spreads all over the liver. In 1986, an analysis was made of 146 cases of cirrhosis of the liver, of which, 63 belonged to the Blood stagnation group; the majority of them were accompanied by Blood stagnation or Qi deficiency, and all of them had high viscosity of the blood. Medications which are effective in promoting Blood circulation and removing stasis have also proven to be effective in inhibiting over-synthesis and growth of connective tissues, thus controlling degradation and absorption of connective tissues. In addition, they are effective in reducing blood viscosity, and they possess antimicrobial and immunology-regulating effects. All these effects are beneficial for the recovery of cirrhosis. However, these effects, especially those of connective tissue absorption and liver cell regeneration, require a period of two to two and a half years to become evident. Thus, the course of treatment should be longer than two years.

5) Application of Xie Fu Zhu Yu Decoction and Xiaoyao San should be successive. A long treatment course for chronic active hepatitis or liver cirrhosis in children usually has a better outcome because children possess less connective tissue than adults and because their tissue has greater ability for regeneration. The effect of the prescriptions used in the treatment course is rheologic rather than hasty. In our particular case, the symptoms started to be alleviated after a few days of treatment. But as for the absorption of connective tissue and liver cell regeneration, which require quite a long time to achieve, these did not materialize in this case because this patient did not pay attention to rest, nutrition and continuation of herbal medicine treatment. The patient eventually succumbed to hepatic coma.

12.7 ACUTE NEPHRITIS ASSOCIATED WITH HYPERTENSIVE ENCEPHALOPATHY (EDEMA DUE TO AFFECTION BY WIND, FLARING UP OF LIVER HEAT)

Ye Xiaoli and Cao Yixiang
Fujian Provincial Hospital, Fuzhou

You Changying, 8, female, Han nationality. Medical record number: 96305. Admitted on September 28, 1971.

CHIEF COMPLAINT: Edema and oliguria for the past seven to eight days; vomiting and convulsion for 30 minutes.

HISTORY OF PRESENT ILLNESS: Before admission, the patient had tea-like urine for seven to eight days which was associated with vomiting and persistent convulsion.

PAST HISTORY: Non-contributory.

PERTINENT PHYSICAL EXAMINATION & LABORATORY FINDINGS: Blood pressure, 170/140 mmHg. Unconscious with persistent convulsion. Presence of peri-oral cyanosis. ECG: Right bundle branch block; tachycardia. Urinalysis showed protein (+++); RBC, (++) and WBC, (++).

INSPECTION OF TONGUE: Reddened tongue substance.

PULSE CONDITION: Rapid and taut.

MODERN MEDICINE DIAGNOSIS: Acute Nephritis; Hypertensive Encephalopathy; Myocarditis.

TRADITIONAL CHINESE MEDICINE DIAGNOSIS: Edema due to Affection by Wind, Flaring Up of Liver Heat.

THERAPEUTIC PRINCIPLES: Subdue Liver hyperactivity and endogenous Wind.

PRESCRIPTION: Decoction of Ephedra, Fructus Forsythiae and Phaseolus seeds plus Uncaria Stem with Hooks.

Rhizoma uncariae cumunics, 3 gm; Fructus gardeniae, 6 gm; Flos chrysanthemi, 3 gm; Radix gentianae, 6 gm; Cortex magnoliae officinalis, 4.5 gm; Herba ephedrae, 3 gm; Fructus forsythiae, 9 gm; Semen phaseoli, 24 gm; and Purple snowy powder, 0.6 gm.

In this prescription, Ephedrae was used to ventilate and smooth the troubled Lung and to facilitate diuresis; Fructus forsythiae and Semen phaseoli to remove toxic Heat; and Rhizoma uncariae and Flos chrysanthemi to subdue hyperfunction of the Liver and the endogenous Wind. Purple snowy powder was used to resuscitate.

FOLLOW-UP/COURSE OF TREATMENT:

Upon admission, conventional medications were used to control the convulsion and the elevated blood pressure. This was followed by application of traditional medications. TCM symptom-complex differentiation indicated the etiology was an affection by endogenous Wind and a flaring up of Liver Heat. These pathological processes were responsible for symptoms such as dizziness, headache, nausea, vomiting, convulsion and coma. The method of treatment was to subdue hyperactivity of the Liver and the endogenous Wind.

Second consultation: The patient was lucid. Blood pressure 100/70 mmHg. Prescription: Mahuang Lianqiao Chixiao Dou Tang and Longdan Xia Can Tang. Talcum, 18 gm; Radix scutellariae, 9 gm; Radix Gentianae, 9 gm; Fructus gardeniae, 6 gm; Herba ephedrae, 3 gm; Fructus forsythiae, 9 gm; Semen phaseoli, 24 gm; Radix bupleuri, 4.5 gm; and Radix paeoniae alba, 6 gm.

Third consultation: After three doses of the above prescription, administration of Mahuang Lianqiao Chixiao Dou Tang was initiated to consolidate the effect. During the course of treatment, there was persistent hematuria. After complete tonsillectomy, the amount of RBC in the urine was reduced. The patient was discharged after staying in hospital for 57 days.

Fourth consultation: Modified Ejiao Powder was given to treat the residual fever and presence of RBC in the urine. Colla corii asini, 9 gm; Pollen typhae, 3 gm; Succinum, 9 gm; Rhizoma rehmanniae, 9 gm; Herba selaginallee, 9 gm; Cortex moutan radicis, 4.5 gm; Imperatae cylindrica, 24 gm; Nodus nelumbinis, 18 gm; and Herba agrimoniae, 9 gm. Colla corii asini contained Blood in the Channels, and when combined with Succinum, Pollen typhae and others were effective in nourishing the Vital Essence and consolidating the Blood.

DISCUSSION: Hypertensive encephalopathy is a severe complication of nephritis that can cause death. In this case, we adopted the principle of diagnosis and treatment based on an overall analysis of symptoms combined with symptomatic treatment of Western medicine and achieved a satisfactory therapeutic effect. This case was due to edema and a flaring up of Liver Heat. Clinical findings such as vomiting, convulsion, dizziness, red tongue and taut pulse, were due to accumulation and brewing of Dampness as well as Heat in the body and endogenous Wind stirring in the Liver. Anti-hypertensive and anticonvulsive medications were administered initially for symptomatic treatment and were followed by traditional Chinese medications. Mahuang Lianqiao Chixiao Dou Tang, Radix paeoniae, Rhizoma uncariae and others were used to treat convulsion and to subdue endogenous Wind. They were also used to smooth the nerves, quench the Fire and revitalize the Liver. This took care of the critical stage of the disease. However, persistent hematuria is a serious complication in the course of treating nephritis. Traditional Chinese medicine believes that hematuria is due to Kidney deficiency and fever secondary to deficiency of Vital Energy or Blood. Presence of RBC in the urine was a sign of residual fever. Modified Ejiao Powder was then employed, resulting in a satisfactory clinical outcome. Ejiao Powder can nourish the Vital Essence and consolidate the Blood. From an immunological point of view, donkey-hide gelatin, amber and cattail pollen are all effective in nourishing the Vital Essence, dispelling pathogenic Heat from the Blood and removing stagnant Blood. All these facilitate the inhibition of immunological reactions and enhance microcirculation.

12.8 ACUTE ENCEPHALOPATHY ASSOCIATED WITH BLINDNESS AND APHASIA (CONVULSIVE PARALYSIS, TYPE OF STRONG EVIL FIRE, BLINDNESS AND APHASIA)

Ye Xiaoli and Cao Yixiang

Fujian Provincial Hospital, Fuzhou

Xue Songqing, 4, male. Medical record number: 97982. Date of admission: March 11, 1972.

CHIEF COMPLAINT: High fever, convulsion, blindness and aphasia for two weeks.

HISTORY OF PRESENT ILLNESS: Two weeks prior to admission, the patient developed headache with high fever followed by persistent convulsion, unconsciousness and foaming from the mouth. After treatment in a local hospital, the fever had subsided and convulsion ceased. However, other symptoms such as restlessness, anorexia, constipation, blindness, aphasia and paralysis of the right limbs were noted. Treatment in the same local hospital for the past two weeks proved to be of no avail. The patient was subsequently admitted to this hospital.

PAST HISTORY: Non-contributory.

INSPECTION OF TONGUE: Reddened and prickly tongue.

PULSE CONDITION: Rapid pulse.

MODERN MEDICINE DIAGNOSIS: Acute Encephalopathy; Blindness and Aphasia.

TRADITIONAL CHINESE MEDICINE DIAGNOSIS: Convulsive Paralysis: Type of Strong Evil Fire; Blindness and Aphasia.

THERAPEUTIC PRINCIPLES: Febrifuge and detoxication; eliminate pathogenic factors.

PRESCRIPTION: White Tiger Decoction plus Decoction of Gentianae to purge the Liver. Radix gentianae, 9 gm; Radix scutellariae, 6 gm; Fructus gardeniae, 9 gm; Radix bupleuri, 4.5 gm; Caulis akebiae, 3 gm; Plantaginis, 9 gm; Gypsum fibrosum, 20 gm; Rhizoma anemarrhenae, 9 gm; Herba inulae, 4.5 gm; and Semen astragali complanati, 9 gm.

In this prescription, Chinese Gentian is of extremely bitter and cold property, which acts to remove the Fire from the Liver and Gallbladder. The other febrifugal and diuretic herbs of the prescription are used to clear up Heat and eliminate Dampness.

FOLLOW-UP/COURSE OF TREATMENT:

Second consultation: Symptom of restlessness was relieved and the patient recovered most of his appetite. Eyes were noted to be reactive. Prescription: Semen astragali complanati, 9 gm; Flos puerariae, 9 gm; Radix gentianae, 9 gm; Gypsum fibrosum, 24 gm; Rhizoma anemarrhenae, 9 gm; Radix glycyrrhizae, 3 gm; Radix scutellariae, 6 gm;

Fructus gardeniae, 9 gm; Rhizoma corydalis, 4.5 gm; Radix asparagi and ophiopogonis, 9 gm each; and Flos inulae, 4.5 gm.

Third consultation: After two doses of the last prescription, the patient had recovered his vision. He wanted to be held. A prescription to clear up the heat and nourish the Vital Essence was given. Rhizoma corydalis, 24 gm; Radix asparagi and ophiopogonis, 9 gm each; Semen astragali complanati, 9 gm; Flos buddlejae, 9 gm; Rhizoma anemarrhenae, 9 gm; Talcum, 18 gm; Radix Glycyrrhizae, 3 gm; Flos inulae, 4.5 gm; Flos Chrysanthemi, 6 gm; Fructus lycii, 4.5 gm; and Radix scrophulariae, 6 gm.

Fourth consultation: Having taken three doses of the above prescription, the patient could say some simple words and stretch out his hand to take an apple. The paralysis of the lower limbs had also disappeared. A prescription to nourish the Yin of the Liver and Kidney was given: Modified Pill of Rehmanniae-Chrysanthemum-Wolfberry. Fructus lycii, 9 gm; Flos chrysanthemi, 6 gm; Rhizoma alismatis, 9 gm; Poria, 9 gm; Rhizoma dioscoreae, 9 gm; Cortex moutan radicis, 2 gm; Rhizoma rehmanniae, 9 gm; Fructus ligustri lucidi, 18 gm; and Herba ecliptae, 9 gm. Four doses were prescribed.

A combination of acupuncture and moxibustion was also applied as part of the course of treatment. For blindness: Ganshu, Shenshu, Jingming, Qiuhou, Taiyang, Fengchi and Guangming points; for aphasia; Shanglianquan, Yamen, Hegu, Zusanli and Yongquan points; for paralysis: Baqiao, Huantiao, Fengshi, Yanglingquan, Yinmen, Futu, Taichong and Sanyinjiao points.

The combined therapy of traditional Chinese and Western medicine was also used in this case.

The patient's vision recovered after 12 days of admission; clear speech after 24 days; and functions of all limbs returned to normal after 43 days. He was able to pick up a pin from the ground.

DISCUSSION: The principal clinical manifestations of this case were headache, high fever, persistent convulsion, coma, vomiting and foaming of the mouth. Emergency symptomatic treatment was able to hold the convulsion and fever at bay, though symptoms and signs of restlessness, aphasia, blindness, paralysis, rough tongue substance and rapid pulse persisted. Traditional Chinese medicine believes that the cause of such a clinical condition lies in the presence of excessive evil Heat, accumulation of toxic Dampness and Heat stasis. At the initial stage of treatment, White Tiger Decoction with Gentian was administered to purge the Liver in order to clear the interior of the Heat. As the patient's condition improved, secretion-promoting decoctions were given. During the convalescent stage, Pill of Rehmanniae-Chrysanthemum-Wolfberry was given in order to reinforce Yin of the Liver and Kidney. Administration of all these prescriptions in that sequence completed the patient's course of treatment.

12.9 NEPHRITIC TYPE OF NEPHROTIC SYNDROME (DEFICIENCY OF KIDNEY YIN)

Yu Peilan, Tong Huanxiang and Zhang Baolin

Department of Pediatrics, First Affiliated Hospital, Hunan Medical
University, Changsha

*Zou Xuejun, 11, male, Han nationality, student. Medical record number: 111204.
Date of admission: September 24, 1964.*

CHIEF COMPLAINT: Descending edema of one month duration, exacerbated in the past three days.

HISTORY OF PRESENT ILLNESS: Since August of 1964, the patient gradually developed puffiness of the face which was more marked in the morning. Edema became worse and was accompanied by oliguria three days prior to admission.

PERTINENT PHYSICAL EXAMINATION & LABORATORY FINDINGS: Temperature, 37°C; respiratory rate, 20/min; and blood pressure, 120/80 mmHg. Chronic illness facies with generalized pitting edema. Throat slightly congested. Lungs clear. Heart sound normal. Abdomen markedly distended with positive detection of fluid wave. Hemoglobin, 10.0 gm%; RBC, 2.74 M/mm^3; proteinuria, (+++) to (+); RBC 0 to 1/hpf; Sp, 3.94 gm/dl; cholesterol, 608 mg/dl; and NPN, 88 mg/dl.

INSPECTION OF TONGUE: Red with less coating than normal.

PULSE CONDITION: Deep, thready and weak.

MODERN MEDICINE DIAGNOSIS: Chronic Nephritis; Nephritis Type of Nephrotic Syndrome.

TRADITIONAL CHINESE MEDICINE DIAGNOSIS: Deficiency of Kidney Yin.

THERAPEUTIC PRINCIPLES: Tonify and nourish the Kidney.

PRESCRIPTION: Rhizoma rehmanniae praeparatae, 15 gm; Rhizoma Dioscoreae, 10 gm; Fructus corni, 10 gm; Poria, 15 gm; Cortex moutan radicis, 10 gm; and Rhizoma alismatis, 10 gm. The prescription was made into tablet form by the Hunan Pharmaceutical Factory; 15-20 gm b.i.d. taken with water. This mode of treatment was prescribed for three years.

Other management: Prednisone, chloroquine, diuretics and antibiotics were used during the first six months of treatment.

FOLLOW-UP/COURSE OF TREATMENT:

From September 1964 to February 1970, the patient had recurrent edema and was admitted to our hospital on 11 separate occasions. During his tenth admission, the patient had uremia (NPN, 88 mg/dl). In addition to prednisone, chloroquine and mustard treatments were used. Drainage of the ascitic fluid was performed five times; a total of 21,000 ml of fluid was withdrawn. The patient was discharged in an improved condition. Three months after discharge, edema recurred and was accompanied by redness of the face, sweating, irritability and weakness in the lumbar region and lower extremities. The patient was admitted for the eleventh time (first consultation).

Second consultation: September 1973 to May 1974. The patient was 20 years old at the time. General condition fair. Apparently asymptomatic. Appetite very good and he could carry a weight of 75 kg for some distance. Physical examination: blood pressure, 120/60 mmHg; many (100+) white striae were seen over the abdomen and lumbar regions, otherwise normal. Blood NPN, 51.3 mg/dl and cholesterol, 175 mg/dl. This complete remission lasted for two years and six months after the second consultation. The patient was employed as a worker in a factory, and he could tolerate his work fairly well.

Third consultation: On August 24, 1987, the patient was admitted for the twelfth time. He was a man of 34, and he had been taking the prescription, continuously or intermittently, for 16 years. His health had been fairly good, and he had worked in the factory continuously for 16 years. Since August 1986, he experienced dizziness and fatigue. Blood pressure was 180/110 mmHg, and BUN increased to 45 mg/dl, 47 mg/dl and 56.5 mg/dl, successively. PSP was only 5%, and creatinine, 7.9 mg/dl-10.2 mg/dl. After a combination of Western medicine and TCM treatment, he was discharged in an improved condition.

DISCUSSION: This was a case of a nephritis type of nephrotic syndrome. The patient had repeated exacerbation from 1964 to 1970 and was admitted to our hospital 11 times. After long-term treatment with our recipe for three years, he had nearly complete remission for two years and six months. As he continued to take this prescription, he had almost no symptoms and carried on his daily work in a factory for 16 years. This indicates that these herbs are effective in stabilizing and consolidating the effect of prednisone and other medications for a fairly long time.

In our hospital, we had two other cases of nephritic type of nephrotic syndrome that we treated by the therapeutic principle of tonifying and nourishing the Kidney (using the above herbal medicines or variations thereof based on individual diagnosis and clinical manifestations). Both patients attained complete remission for a fairly long time. One of them is a 70-year-old woman pathologist now living in America who returned once in 1985. She had complete remission from nephrotic syndrome for more than 45 years.

12.10 SEVERE SCLERODERMA NEONATORUM (DEFICIENCY OF SPLEEN AND KIDNEY YANG)

Zhang Baolin, Yu Peilan, Wang Baoqiong and Tong Huanxiang
First Affiliated Hospital, Hunan Medical University, Changsha

Zhou Maomao, 4 days old, female, Han nationality. Medical record number: 218246. Admitted on June 22, 1978.
CHIEF COMPLAINT: Cold and hardened skin for two days.
HISTORY OF PRESENT ILLNESS: The patient was delivered prematurely (30-week gestation) at 11 a.m., June 18, 1978. Birth weight was 1,250 gm. Complicated with asphyxia after birth, she was very weak with faint cry. Her temperature remained

subnormal (under 35°C) since birth. On June 20, she was noted to have developed hardening of the skin and subcutaneous tissue accompanied by edema and coldness over the hip, extremities and face. Lips were cyanotic. The patient was fed milk by gavage and given penicillin, 100,000 u intramuscularly twice daily. On June 21, hardening and edema of the skin spread to about 80% of the body surface. On June 22, rectal temperature remained under 35°C. Her condition continued to deteriorate.

PERTINENT PHYSICAL EXAMINATION & LABORATORY FINDINGS: The patient appeared weak with premature neonate facies. Cardiac rhythm regular with relative bradycardia (100-110/min). Heart sounds weak. Both lungs and abdomen negative. CBC showed WBC count to be 10,800/mm^3. Differential count: neutrophils, 64%; lymphocytes, 34%; and monocytes, 2%.

INSPECTION OF TONGUE: Red and uncoated.

PULSE CONDITION: Faint and weak.

MODERN MEDICINE DIAGNOSIS: Severe Scleroderma (Sclerema) Neonatorum.

TRADITIONAL CHINESE MEDICINE DIAGNOSIS: Deficiency of Spleen and Kidney Yang; Stagnation of Qi and Blood Stasis.

THERAPEUTIC PRINCIPLES: Warm the Kidney and strengthen the Spleen, promote Blood circulation and eliminate the stagnation.

PRESCRIPTION: Modified Zhen Wu Decoction. Radix aconiti praeparatae, 0.3 gm; Poria, 1.5 gm; Radix astragali, 1.5 gm; Radix Ginseng, 1.5 gm; Rhizoma ligustici chuanxiong, 0.3 gm; Flos carthami, 0.6 gm; and Herba euphorbiae, 3 gm. Two doses (June 22 and 23). One dose daily by gavage (lukewarm).

Other management: Routine nursing schedule for prematures; intramuscular testosterone propionate once weekly.

FOLLOW-UP/COURSE OF TREATMENT:

Second consultation (June 24): The patient cried louder. Rectal temperature rose to 35.6°C. Subcutaneous tissue of the face and hip became softer. Stool formed. The tongue was still red and uncoated. Modified the prescription by adding Radix ophiopogonis, 1.5 gm, and Rhizoma polygonati odorati, 0.6 gm, and by changing the dosage of Herba euphorbiae to 5 gm. Three doses (June 24 to June 26).

Third consultation (June 27): Rectal temperature progressively rose to 36-37°C. Hardening and edema of the skin and subcutaneous tissue markedly reduced. Chinese herbal medicine discontinued temporarily for observation. The patient was to be monitored closely.

Fourth consultation (July 2): After discontinuation of herbal medicine, hardening and edema of the skin continued to regress. The patient could tolerate bottle feedings. She was weak and anorexic. Tongue remained red and uncoated. Prescription to tonify the Qi and Yin and strengthen the Spleen was given. Radix ginseng, 1.5 gm; Radix astragali, 1.5 gm; Radix ophiopogonis, 1.5 gm; Radix angelicae, 1.5 gm; Poria, 3.0 gm; and Herba euphorbiae, 9 gm. Seven doses (July 2 to July 8).

Fifth consultation (July 9): The patient's condition remained stable. Hardening of the skin had disappeared almost completely. Tongue substance pink in colour with thin, white coating. Continued the prescription.

Sixth consultation (July 13): The patient's condition was fair. Discontinued Chinese herbal medicine. The patient was discharged on July 19 in good condition.

DISCUSSION: Scleroderma neonatorum is a common disorder in the central and northern regions of China. It is manifested by widespread hardening and edema of the subcutaneous tissue and skin. Its occurrence is confined almost exclusively to premature and debilitated newborn infants, wherein most of the cases have a poor prognosis for life.

Traditional Chinese medicine considers scleroderma neonatorum under the realms of "Cold Fainting," "Blood Stasis" and "The Five Hards." The cause of the disease is attributed to "pathogenic cold factor." The highest incidence is seen in northern China during the winter season. Since premature infants are most susceptible to scleroderma neonatorum, it appears that deficiency of congenital vitality and deficiency of Kidney-Yang are the two most important pathogenic factors. Deficiency of Spleen-Yang in premature infants causes inadequacy of the transportation and digestion functions of the Spleen, resulting in edema. Weakness and insufficiency of Kidney-Yang prevents the Yang-Qi from reaching the skin and muscles, leading to coldness of the body and clammy limbs.

Coldness of the body due to deficiency of Yang, accumulation of Cold and stagnation of Qi which leads to Blood stasis are manifested as hardening of the skin with purple discolouration and cyanosis of the lips and extremities. All these signs were evident in our case.

When hardening, edema and coldness of the skin are marked, the therapeutic goal is to warm the Kidney and strengthen the Spleen, thus promoting Blood circulation and eliminating the stagnation. Once scleroderma is relieved, it's logical and necessary to tonify the Qi and Yin, in addition to strengthening the Spleen. Following this therapeutic regimen, we were able to attain a most satisfactory clinical outcome.

13. OTHER DISEASES

13.1 ACONITUM INTOXICATION (DIZZINESS SECONDARY TO ACONITUM INTOXICATION)

Chen Keji

Xiyuan Hospital, China Academy of Traditional Chinese Medicine, Beijing

Chen Jiageng, 84, male, Han nationality, married, merchant. Date of first consultation: August 6, 1956.

CHIEF COMPLAINT: The patient's relative informed us that after taking Wutou (Aconitum) compound prescription, the patient complained of numbness of the lips and tongue and nausea followed by vomiting. Twenty minutes later he entered a state similar to that of heavy drunkenness.

HISTORY OF PRESENT ILLNESS: The patient has been hypertensive for more than 30 years with usual blood pressure reading at around 180/100 mmHg. He constantly complained of dizziness and headache. He claimed to have a chronic, intractable "headache' and took Reserpine as a treatment in the dosage of 0.25 mg t.i.d. After a course of one week, dizziness subsided and the blood pressure was lowered to about 160/80 mmHg, but he still complained of migraine-like headache; other symptoms experienced and described as "intolerable" were general malaise and body weakness. His concerned relatives subsequently advised him to take the Wutou compound prescription which was indicated in the *Book of Prescriptions* to be the remedy for the type of headache the patient claimed to have. This compound prescription contains 75 gm of Radix angelicae dahuricae and 30 gm each of Rhizoma ligustici chuanxiong, Radix glycyrrhizae, Rhizoma gastrodize and Radix aconiti, the last one being a mixture of both the preserved and raw forms of the herb. Two preparations of this prescription were purchased. This compound prescription, according to the book, should be taken in powder form at a dosage of 3 gm per ingestion. Unfortunately, both the patient and his relatives misunderstood that the prescription should be taken in liquid form, and thus they prepared it using the usual decoction method and even had the two preparations decocted at the same time. In so doing, each serving of the prescription contained up to 60 gm of Chuan Wutou which resulted in, sequentially, numbness of the lips, and tip and body of the tongue about 10 seconds after ingestion. Fifteen minutes later, numbness was also felt in the fingertips followed by both upper and lower extremities. The patient complained of nausea and vomited some clear liquid as well as a small amount of the decoction; 20 minutes after ingestion he complained of intolerable heaviness of the head followed by general retardation of mentality, resembling a state of heavy drunkenness. He also displayed a swaying motion of the body.

PERTINENT PHYSICAL EXAMINATION & LABORATORY FINDINGS: It was three hours after ingestion that the patient was examined. Though conscious, he displayed a dull facies and a dazed look. Both pupils were slightly dilated and pupillary reflex sluggish. Temperature 36.2°C, respiratory rate 20/min and blood pressure 120/60 mmHg. Neck supple, cardiac rhythm normal, no hepatomegaly or splenomegaly. Bilateral knee jerks reflex normal and no pathological reflexes elicited.

INSPECTION OF TONGUE: Slightly reddened tongue substance.

PULSE CONDITION: Clear.

MODERN MEDICINE DIAGNOSIS: Wutou Intoxication.

TRADITIONAL CHINESE MEDICINE DIAGNOSIS: Dizziness and Stupor Secondary to Wutou Intoxication.

THERAPEUTIC PRINCIPLES: Strengthening the body resistance to detoxicate the invading toxins.

PRESCRIPTION: Radix panacis quinquefolii, 10 gm; Poria cum radice pino, 12 gm; Radix cynanchi atrati, 10 gm; Raw glycyrrhizae, 10 gm; Herba lophatheri, 5 gm; Roasted Fructus gardeniae, 5 gm; and Fresh Herba dendrobii, 18 gm; decocted in water and taken orally together with 0.1 gm of ground rhinoceros horn. In addition, green beans in tea form were served regularly as long as the patient could tolerate it.

Second consultation: The next morning, the patient had full recovery of his mentality, did not feel dizzy and did not look dazed; numbness of the extremities had also disappeared, but he still complained of a spastic aching sensation about the area of the right otic arch. Pulse manifestation changed to taut and strong. Blood pressure: 160/100 mmHg. In view of the patient's advanced age and perturbation of Yin, which thus classified him under "Yin Deficient and Yang Unsteady" syndrome, additional herbs in the forms of fresh Radix rehmanniae, 15 gm, and Ootheca mantidis and Radix achyranthis bidentatae, 10 gm each, were added to the original prescription to further replenish the Liver and Kidney.

Third consultation: After two servings of the above prescription, the headache was gone.

DISCUSSION:

1) Aconitum falls under the Ranunculaceae family and traditional herbal medicine studies describe its pharmacological properties as "highly pungent, hot and poisonous." It thus requires delicate handling in clinical applications. In several Wutou-containing prescriptions mentioned in *Jin Kui Yao Lue (Synopsis of the Golden Chamber),* the dosage of Wutou is generally greater than that of Fuzi (Radix aconiti praeparatae), but it requires a different method of preparation, such as to decoct it with honey in order to retard its medicinal properties or to have it boiled first in water to remove the undesirable residues and then to boil it again with honey. Another method of preparing it is simply by "prolonged boiling" in water. In our case, the amount of Wutou used was too large in the first place, and in the second place, it was prepared only in the

ordinary way without any precautions, thus leading to intoxication.

2) The course of intoxication in this case ran for about 20 hours, and the patient completely recovered the next day. Such quick recovery can be attributed to the rapid absorption and excretion of Wutou and to the application of the traditional therapeutic principles of strengthening the body resistance (using American ginseng) and detoxication (using rhinoceros horn, green peas and glycyrrhizae) which played a significant role in limiting the course of intoxication.

中医药学临床验案范例

陈可冀　主编

*

ⓒ外文出版社
新世界出版社
（中国北京百万庄路 24 号）
邮政编码 100037
北京外文印刷厂印刷
中国国际图书贸易总公司发行
（中国北京车公庄西路 35 号）
北京邮政信箱第 399 号　邮政编码 100044
1994 年(16 开)第一版
（英）
ISBN 7 - 119 - 01661 - X /R·106（外）
08000
14 - E - 2843S